APPLYING RESEARCH EVIDENC

Applying Research Evidence in Social Work Practice

Edited by
Martin Webber

 macmillan education palgrave

First published 2015 by
PALGRAVE

Palgrave in the UK is an imprint of Macmillan Publishers Limited, registered in England, company number 785998, of 4 Crinan Street, London N1 9XW.

Palgrave Macmillan in the US is a division of St Martin's Press LLC, 175 Fifth Avenue, New York, NY 10010.

Palgrave is a global academic imprint of the above companies and has companies and is represented throughout the world.

Palgrave® and Macmillan® are registered trademarks in the United States, the United Kingdom, Europe and other countries

ISBN 978-1-137-27610-0

This book is printed on paper suitable for recycling and made from fully managed and sustained forest sources. Logging, pulping and manufacturing processes are expected to conform to the environmental regulations of the country of origin.

A catalogue record for this book is available from the British Library.

A catalog record for this book is available from the Library of Congress.

Printed in China

For Andrea, my inspiration

Contents

PART II   APPLYING RESEARCH EVIDENCE IN DIFFERENT SOCIAL WORK CONTEXTS

7   Safeguarding children   III

Karen Broadhurst and Andrew Pithouse

8   Working with looked-after children   127

Robin Sen

List of illustrative material

Boxes

Practice reflections

Case scenarios

Foreword

Perfect timing! This book arrives at an exciting moment in the historic relationship between practice and research in social work. To many students and
practitioners that might sound hard to believe. As someone who has taught the
required research courses that few students – if any – wanted to take, I suspect
'excitement' is hardly the word that comes to mind in opening this book. To
practitioners, who have been criticised and ridiculed by research academics in
the classroom, in their agencies or in continuing education workshops for not
being 'scientific' enough, returning to the primal scene of the educational
crime cannot be encouraging.

Nonetheless, it's true and let me tell you why. After years of painful and
painfully boring debate about the 'science' of research versus the 'art' of practice, over evidence-based practice versus practice-based research, over qualitative versus quantitative research, over randomised controlled trials versus
non-experimental designs, over original versus available data-collection,
agency versus academy, etc., etc., ad nauseum, academics in their wisdom
have agreed – not totally, because they're academics, but mostly – that they
all have a legitimate place in the integration of social work practice and
research. Whether justified through claims to methodological pluralism,
evidence-informed practice or other high sounding concepts, the important
point is that they all have a place and they all serve the purpose of providing
better service.

In fact, I am writing this Forward on the cusp of presiding over the Third
International Conference on Practice Research at which researchers who study
practice and practitioners who do research from 20 different countries will be
joining together in New York City to share the work they do and how they do
it. Rather than hurl ideological bricks at each other, the theme of the conference is 'Building bridges, not digging pipelines: Promoting two-way traffic
between practice and research'.

The editor of this book is an invited Plenary Speaker at that conference. A
seasoned practice researcher and research scholar, Martin Webber has seized
this historic moment and, together with numerous research colleagues,
produced a text that first defines, explains and applies the central concepts and
techniques that practitioners must have to intelligently consume research and
use it in their practice decision-making. The second portion of the book illustrates how research can be used in various practice and policy 'domains' of
social work – e.g., children at risk of various kinds, adults with substance
abuse problems, those with mental health issues, offenders, the disabled, the
elderly, etc.

Bringing together the various contributors to this book would make a conference in itself. They by no means agree on every point and their disagreements lend valuable complexity to this collection. But, as Webber points out in his forward moving concluding chapter, this is an especially opportune time for social work practitioners in the UK to embrace rather than reject research, and to use it in the interests of those whom they serve.

IRWIN EPSTEIN
Helen Rehr Professor of Applied Social Work Research
(Health & Mental Health)
Silberman School of Social Work at Hunter College
City University of New York

Preface

This book has two distinct, though related, parts. The first part provides a generic overview of the key debates and critical challenges in using research in social work practice. The second part builds on this knowledge by exploring how research is implemented in a wide variety of specialist practice domains. Reflecting the social work curriculum of a broad knowledge base applied to specific social work practice areas, you are encouraged to read all of Part I (Chapters 1 to 6) to gain a full understanding of how research evidence can be used to inform social work practice. Then, you can select the specific practice domains of interest to you from Chapters 7 to 14 in Part II to explore how research can be used when working with different service user groups. Coming back together at the end, Chapter 15 invites you to breach the research–practice divide and either undertake your own research, or share insights from this book with your colleagues about how evidence from research studies can inform your practice.

I chose to bring together people with considerable expertise in their fields to write this book, rather than do it all myself, to ensure you are provided with the best knowledge in each practice domain. This blend of methodological and subject expertise enriches the text as each chapter starts afresh with new insights and enthusiasm. Each chapter features practice reflection points to keep you thinking, and case scenarios or examples to help you apply some of the more conceptual aspects of the topic to real-life practice. The unique style of each author has been retained so you can benefit from their passion and interests, but I have carefully edited each chapter to provide consistency and continuity throughout the book.

This is not a social work research methods textbook. (If this is what you are interested in, please see the recommendations at the end of Chapter 1.) Instead, this book responds to a call from practitioners who feel distant from research, or who have not read a research paper since undertaking their university degree, to provide a critical, yet accessible, introduction to applying research findings in their practice. This book seeks to shed light on the research world, which can sometimes appear mystical or distant from practitioners. Further, as the process of applying research in practice is not always foremost in social work qualifying or post-qualifying programmes, this book will be useful for students and practitioners alike who are searching for suggestions about how they may draw on research to inform their practice.

I do not subscribe to a model of a one-way pipeline of research expertise from academic ivory towers feeding into social work practice. I see the role of research as critically interacting with practice environments, both shaping and being shaped by the realities of social work practice. Social work researchers have a responsibility to work alongside colleagues in practice to evaluate what works well and to share this so that service users' experiences and outcomes can be improved. Social work researchers also have a responsibility to ensure that the research agenda is shaped by the concerns of practitioners and service users to ensure it remains relevant to them. Finally, although there is not space to explore this in depth, practitioners should be provided with supported opportunities to undertake research themselves to answer their practice questions, develop their practice and contribute to social work knowledge.

This book plays a role in bringing research closer to practice so that it does not linger on dusty library shelves (or in the hidden recesses of bibliographic databases, or behind an internet paywall, as is the reality now). It adopts a practical and pragmatic approach to research evidence by arguing that, although individual studies may have their flaws and may not be immediately relevant to practice, insights gained from social work research have the potential to contribute to students' and practitioners' knowledge and expertise. Authors within these covers suggest how research findings can directly influence practice by illuminating particular approaches or interventions which may be more effective than others. However, we also suggest that knowledge of relevant research can be integrated with tacit knowledge and practitioner wisdom to enhance practice in subtle, yet real, ways.

Individual authors view the practice–research interface in different ways and I have not imposed an editorial uniformity of approach to research methodology, or the notion of evidence-based practice. Some authors are more critical than others about hierarchies of evidence, different research methodologies, or the role that research plays in social work practice. As you read through the chapters, I encourage you too to be critical. Think critically about what you read and, more importantly, how you can find, appraise and use research evidence to inform your practice.

Then, if you like, please contact me via my blog (www.martinwebber.net), twitter (@mgoat73), or at the University of York, with your thoughts about the practice–research interface and how social work researchers and practitioners can better work together to improve outcomes and experiences for users of social work services. I shall be happy to share good ideas and examples of good practice on my blog.

MARTIN WEBBER

Acknowledgements

I am indebted to the erudite contributions of the authors of chapters in this book. In order of appearance:

Sarah Carr, Paul Ross, Lisa Bostock, Mark Hardy, Tony Evans, Victoria Hart, Karen Broadhurst, Andrew Pithouse, Robin Sen, Steven Walker, Wulf Livingstone, Sarah Galvini, Nick Gould, Tom Lochhead, Hannah Morgan, David Smith and Jill Manthorpe.

I am very grateful that they made the time to contribute to this book, amidst very many competing demands. They have been responsive to my editorial changes and requests, and have carefully written to the brief provided to them. Above all, they have been patient while I have carved out time to undertake my editorial duties. Thank you.

I am also very grateful to the commissioning editors at Palgrave who have gently nudged this work to its conclusion. I wish to acknowledge the work of Lloyd Langman who approached me to put it together, advised on the shape and focus of the book, and moved it from proposal to reality. Latterly, Helen Caunce has patiently overseen the completion of the book. I can only apologise that it has taken so long – thank you for your patience.

My colleagues and students in the Department of Social Policy and Social Work at the University of York have intellectually nourished me throughout the gestation of this book. My ideas have been shaped through our interactions, for which I am most grateful.

Finally, it is my family – Andrea, Caitlin and Freya – who have sustained me throughout the process of pulling this book together. As usual when I am locked away in the study working towards deadlines you have reminded me that there is life beyond my work. From helping with homework to coaxing escaped hamsters out from underneath the sofa, your distractions have taken my mind off writing, helping me to return to it with renewed energy. I am sorry that I have been tired and grumpy. Thank you for putting up with me.

Andrea: You keep me grounded. Your creativity and vision astound me. Thank you for being my life partner.

Caitlin: Thank you for the cups of tea. I hope that this helping phase will endure.

Freya: Thank you for asking questions. Your inquisitiveness will take you a long way.

Martin Webber

The authors and publisher would like to thank the following individuals and organisations for permission to reproduce copyright material:

Colin Barnes and the University of Leeds for permission to reproduce 'Approaches to Welfare' from Oliver, M. (2004) 'The Social Model in Action: If I Had a Hammer', in Barnes, C. and Mercer, G. (eds), *Implementing the Social Model of Disability: Theory and Research* (Leeds: Disability Press) (this material is freely available to download at the Disability Archive UK: disability-studies.leeds.ac.uk<http://disability-studies.leeds.ac.uk). The book also contains public sector information licensed under the Open Government Licence v2.0.

Notes on Contributors

Lisa Bostock is an experienced social researcher specialising in integrated working between health, housing and social care who works for her own research and practice development consultancy Social Care Research Associates (SCRA).

Karen Broadhurst is Senior Lecturer in Socio-Legal Studies at the School of Nursing Midwifery and Social Work, University of Manchester.

Sarah Carr formerly worked at the Social Care Institute for Excellence but is now an independent social care and mental health knowledge consultant who holds honorary academic posts at the Universities of Birmingham and York.

Tony Evans is a registered social worker and Professor of Social Work at Royal Holloway, University of London whose research focuses on discretion, policy and moral economies of practice.

Sarah Galvani is a registered social worker and Assistant Director of the Tilda Goldberg Centre for Social Work and Social Care at the University of Bedfordshire.

Nick Gould is Emeritus Professor of Social Work at the University of Bath and combines ongoing academic and professional commitments with work as a member of the Mental Health Tribunal.

Mark Hardy is Lecturer in Social Work at the University of York, and author of *Evidence and Knowledge for Practice* (with Tony Evans, Polity Press, 2010) and *Governing Risk – Care and Control in Contemporary Social Work* (Palgrave Macmillan 2014).

Victoria Hart is a registered social worker with a background in mental health social work currently working in regulation of mental health services.

Wulf Livingston is Senior Lecturer in Social Work with specific research interests in alcohol, professional knowledge acquisition and service user involvement.

Tom Lochhead is Mental Health Professional Lead for Social Work in Bath & North East Somerset and served on the latest NICE Guideline Development Group for Schizophrenia and Psychosis

Jill Manthorpe is Professor of Social Work at King's College London and Director of the Social Care Workforce Research Unit, where she conducts a range of research covering adult social care and undertakes a variety of professional development activity with social workers.

Hannah Morgan is a Lecturer in Disability Studies in the Department of Sociology at Lancaster University where she teaches on the qualifying social work programmes.

Andrew Pithouse has practised in and written extensively about child and family services and currently combines a research post at Cardiff University's School of Social Sciences with a secondment to Welsh Government as policy adviser on social services.

Paul Ross is a Chartered Senior Information Specialist at the Social Care Institute of Excellence who describes himself as a social and cultural scientist (professionally) and a loveable nuisance (personally).

Robin Sen is a Lecturer in Social Work with research interests in child protection and out-of-home care.

David Smith was appointed in 1976 to a Lectureship in Lancaster University, after working as a probation officer, where he is now Emeritus Professor of Criminology.

Steven Walker has worked for 30 years in child protection, specialising in child and adolescent mental health services as a frontline worker and later as a Principal Lecturer (CAMHS), gaining his MPhil in 2009 as Programme Leader of a National Training Strategy Accolade (TOPSS) for most innovative multi-disciplinary training.

Martin Webber is a registered social worker and Reader in Social Work at the University of York, with research interests in the development and evaluation of social interventions for people with mental health problems.

List of Abbreviations and Acronyms

ACT	Assertive Community Treatment
ADHD	Attention-Deficit Hyperactivity Disorder
AMHS	Adult Mental Health Services
AOT	Assertive Outreach Team
ASSIA	Applied Social Sciences Index and Abstracts
AUDIT	Alcohol Use Disorders Identification Test
BCODP	British Council of Organisations of Disabled People
CAF	Common Assessment Framework
CAMHS	Child and Adolescent Mental Health Services
CBT	Cognitive Behavioural Therapy
CCN	County Councils Network
CMHT	Community Mental Health Team
CPA	Care Programme Approach
CPD	Continuing Professional Development
COS	Charity Organisation Society
CPA	Care Programme Approach
CPI	Connecting People Intervention
CQC	Care Quality Commission
CRD	Centre for Reviews and Dissemination
CREDOS	Collaboration of Researchers on the Effective Development of Supervision
CRP	Crime Reduction Programme
CST	Cognitive Stimulation Therapy
CTO	Community Treatment Order
EBP	Evidence-based practice
EHRC	Equality and Human Rights Commission
EPPI-Centre	Evidence for Policy and Practice Information and Co-ordinating Centre
ESRC	Economic and Social Research Council
FGC	Family Group Conference
GEO	Government Equalities Office
GMC	General Medical Council
GP	General Practitioner
HCPC	Health and Care Professions Council
HSCIC	Health and Social Care Information Centre
HV	Health visitor

IBA	Identification and Brief Advice
IBSS	International Bibliography of the Social Sciences
IPPR	Institute for Public Policy Research
IPS	Individual Placement and Support
IPT	Interpersonal Therapy
IRISS	Institute for Research and Innovation in Social Services
IT	Information Technology
JRF	Joseph Rowntree Foundation
LGA	Local Government Association
LGBT	Lesbian, gay, bisexual and transgendered
MeSH	Medical Subject Headings
MI	Motivational Interviewing
MST	Multi-Systemic Therapy
MST-CAN	Multi-Systemic Therapy for Child Abuse and Neglect
MTFC-P	Multi-Treatment Foster Care for Pre-schoolers
NALC	National Association of Local Councils
NAO	National Audit Office
NCIL	National Centre for Independent Living
NCVO	National Council for Voluntary Organisations
NEF	New Economics Foundation
NHS	National Health Service
NICE	National Institute for Health and Care Excellence
NIHR	National Institute for Health Research
NQSW	Newly Qualified Social Worker
ONS	Office of National Statistics
OPCS	Office of Population, Census and Survey
PCF	Professional Capabilities Framework
PICO(T)	Population/Intervention/Comparison/Outcome/(Time)
POET	Personal Outcomes Evaluation Tool
PTSD	Post-Traumatic Stress Disorder
PSSRU	Personal Social Services Research Unit
RCT	Randomised Controlled Trial
REC	Research Ethics Committee
RIP	Research in Practice
RIPFA	Research in Practice for Adults
RNR	Risk, need and responsivity
SAP	Single Assessment Processes
SBNT	Social Behaviour and Network Therapy
SCIE	Social Care Institute for Excellence
SCWRU	Social Care Workforce Research Unit
SCO	Social Care Online
SMART	Specific/Measurable/Achievable/Realistic
SPICE	Setting/Perspective/Intervention/Comparison/Evaluation
SPRU	Social Policy Research Unit
SSCI	Social Science Citation Index
SSRG	Social Services Research Group
SWA	Social Work Abstracts

TAPUPAS   Transparency/Accuracy/Purposivity/Utility/Propriety/
           Accessibility/ Specificity
TLAP   Think Local Act Personal
TSP   Thinking Skills Programme
UPIAS   Union of the Physically Impaired Against Segregation

Key Issues in Applying Research Evidence in Social Work Practice

Introduction to Part I

Part 1 introduces some of the key issues, debates and considerations related to applying research evidence in social work practice. You are encouraged to read through the chapters in sequence, though each can be read individually if you are interested in particular issues.

Chapter 1 blends expertise from the worlds of practice, research and lived experience to provide a critical introduction to the notion of 'evidence-based practice' and its adoption in social work. Martin Webber and Sarah Carr explore the hierarchy of evidence and the primacy of randomised controlled trials in determining 'what works', taking a critical approach to the apparent denigration of qualitative research. Finally, they explore different approaches to the use of research evidence in social work.

Chapter 2 is written by Paul Ross, an information specialist, who takes us through the steps of searching electronic databases to locate research evidence to answer a practice-based question. He discusses how to develop a potentially answerable question and translate this into concepts for database searching. He demystifies some of the technical approaches to searching databases and provides a number of handy hints to help you find appropriate sources.

Chapter 3 is co-authored by social care research analysts Sarah Carr and Lisa Bostock, who are both experienced in appraising social care research and presenting it in a digestible format to practitioners. They introduce critical appraisal techniques and discuss a method for systematically extracting data from papers to help determine their usefulness for practice.

Social work academic Mark Hardy explores the role of research in assessments in Chapter 4. He reviews debates about the art and science of social work assessments and, consequently, the role that research evidence might play. He argues that research evidence represents one of a variety of sources of knowledge that practitioners might draw on to inform their assessments, together with service user and practitioner knowledge, as well as organisational and policy frameworks.

This is followed in Chapter 5 by social work academic Tony Evans with an exploration of how research evidence informs decision-making. The decisions social workers make vary in their urgency, with some decisions offering more opportunities for practitioners to consult research evidence than others. However, this chapter explores the key roles of discretion – understood as freedom and as professional judgement – and intuition in the context of evidence-informed decision-making within contemporary public services.

Finally, a practitioner perspective is provided by Victoria Hart in Chapter 6 on the realities of using research in social work practice. She discusses the practical issues of balancing a busy caseload with being an evidence-based practitioner and working within organisational structures that do not always promote the use of evidence in practice. Importantly, though, she provides some suggestions and examples for students on placement and practitioners, particularly related to building learning into the culture of a team and into one's own practice.

CHAPTER 1

Applying Research Evidence in Social Work Practice: Seeing Beyond Paradigms

Martin Webber and Sarah Carr

Introduction

Social work knowledge is derived from multiple sources including social theory, social research and the experiential knowledge of individuals, families, communities and human service organisations. Additionally, social work is informed by many disciplines – psychology, sociology, anthropology or psychiatry to name just a few. The inherent complexity of social work means that practitioners are required to draw on many diverse sources of knowledge to inform their practice; rarely is one source of knowledge alone sufficient. Whether their knowledge is derived from legislation or policy, research, service users or carers, or their own experience, social work practitioners need to be equipped with the skills to engage with each type and source of knowledge. Furthermore, they need to know when, and how, to use different types of knowledge in their practice.

Knowledge derived from research plays an important, though frequently hidden, role in social work practice. Although practitioners may not routinely read research papers, the domains of research and practice are interwoven in social work. Many aspects of social work theory, social policy, legislation and practice guidance, for example, have been informed by research at some point in their development. By its very nature as an applied social science discipline, social work research is informed by practice, and vice versa. Arguably, the domains of research and practice in social work are inseparable and interdependent. However, there is a perceived gap: social work researchers are seen as distant from practice, and practitioners are criticised for not being aware of recent research findings or using them in their practice.

This book aims to bridge the gap – perceived or real – between the domains of practice and research in social work. It is primarily written for social work students and practitioners as an accessible, yet critical, introduction to engaging with and applying research in practice. It discusses how practitioners may critically engage with research and explores its relevance for their practice. However, it also brings researchers closer to practice by asking them to apply their research knowledge in different social work domains to specific case scenarios. Above all, it challenges the 'pipeline' assumption of a one-way transfer of social work research knowledge from the heights of the 'ivory towers' of academia to the 'real world' of social work practice, although this may be erroneously assumed by the title. If readers put the book down (after reading it!) understanding more about the inter-relationship of research and practice in social work, it will have achieved its aim.

The backdrop to this book is the desire to make practice more 'evidence-based' or 'evidence-informed'. This chapter provides a critical introduction to these concepts and their common use of the notion of 'evidence' in the context of social work practice. It engages briefly with the history of evidence-based practice and its adoption in social work. It then critically interrogates the notion of a hierarchy of evidence and the primacy of randomised controlled trials in determining 'what works', particularly the denigration of qualitative research. It explores the debate between protagonists of evidence-based and evidence-informed practice, while avoiding a discussion of semantics. First, though, it explores the professional requirements for social workers to use research in their practice with a little historical context.

Using research in social work practice

Social workers are required to draw on research in the course of their practice. In England, it is a requirement of registration with the Health and Care Professions Council (HCPC) that social workers meet standards of proficiency, which include the ability to use research evidence to inform practice (Health and Care Professions Council, 2012). The requirement to use research in practice is woven into the Professional Capabilities Framework (PCF) for social workers in England (College of Social Work, 2012) and the National Occupational Standards for Social Work (TOPPS UK Partnership, 2002) in Wales, Northern Ireland and Scotland. Some examples of requirements from these professional frameworks can be found in Box 1.1. Similar requirements can be found in the United States (Council on Social Work Education, 2008) and Australia (Australian Association of Social Workers, 2013), for example.

If you were to read through a whole professional framework, rather than just extracts such as those in Box 1.1, you would see that social workers are required to draw on many other sources of knowledge in addition to research. But the inclusion of the requirement to use research in practice raises some interesting questions. Is research so under-utilised in practice that practitioners have to be reminded in their professional frameworks to engage with it? Has the paradigm of evidence-based or evidence-informed practice been so influential that it has successfully permeated the fabric of the profession? Has research knowledge been identified as so important that it is essential for practitioners to utilise it to transform the lives of the clients with whom they work? While these questions may be rhetorical, it is clear that the profession views

BOX 1.1 USING RESEARCH IN PRACTICE: EXAMPLES FROM PROFESSIONAL FRAMEWORKS

Standards of Proficiency: Social workers in England

Registrant social workers must:

- be able to engage in evidence-informed practice, evaluate practice systematically and participate in audit procedures (12.3);
- be able to gather, analyse, critically evaluate and use information and knowledge to make recommendations or modify their practice (14.1);
- be aware of a range of research methodologies (14.5);
- recognise the value of research and analysis and be able to evaluate such evidence to inform their own practice (14.6).

Examples are drawn from across the 'Health and Care Professions Council Standards of Proficiency' (2012).

Professional Capabilities Framework

Social workers must be able to:

- demonstrate a comprehensive understanding and use of knowledge related to the area of their practice, including critical awareness of current issues and new evidence-based practice research;
- recognise the contribution, and begin to make use, of research to inform practice;
- demonstrate a critical understanding of research methods.

Examples are drawn from the knowledge domain of the social worker level of the Professional Capabilities Framework (College of Social Work, 2012).

National Occupational Standards for Social Work

Performance criteria:

- Use supervision and teamwork to identify different sources of knowledge that can inform best practice (18.2.a);
- Use procedures and practices, and prioritise time and commitments, to ensure that you have sufficient time to:
  - □ access and review literature;
  - □ access and review guidance on best practice;
  - □ review and evaluate the effectiveness of team practice (18.2.c);
- Continually evaluate and learn from current and emerging research (18.3.b).

Examples are drawn from Unit 18: Research, analyse, evaluate, and use current knowledge of best social work practice (TOPPS UK Partnership, 2002).

research as important. However, the connections between research and practice are not new. From the origins of the profession in the nineteenth century to the present day, social workers have used methods that some have likened to those used by qualitative researchers. Additionally, the influence of social research on the profession is quite apparent.

The Charity Organisation Society (COS) founded in 1869, to which the origins of contemporary social work in the UK can be traced, boasted of its use of 'scientific principles' to 'target relief where it was most needed' (Rees, 2001: 193). COS became known for its social casework, which involved thorough investigation of individual and family needs and the targeting of resources towards those most in need. COS aimed to address the 'human weakness of the social workers' (Young and Ashton, 1956: 93) who gave relief to anyone who appeared distressed, rather than according to their actual need. They trained their workers in the process of social investigation which, although over one hundred years old, has a surprisingly contemporary feel about it:

> Their spokesmen were determined to rid themselves of vague generalizations and opinions not based on evidence, and to substitute careful enquiry into the facts of the economic and social life of the family, its previous history, its friends and relations, and above all a clear understanding of the way the client himself thought he could be helped. (Extract of a description of the COS Annual Report in 1895, Young and Ashton, 1956: 103)

The process of social investigation in social work informed the early work of the Chicago School (of sociology) in the 1920s and 1930s. Researchers in this tradition used life histories of marginalised groups collected by social workers in the course of their work. The 'thick description' (Geertz, 1973) of human behaviour provided by these social work case notes, which also examined the social context of the individuals and families concerned, provided fertile material for these social researchers. The resultant insights into the role of social structures and physical environmental factors in human behaviour have been influential in the development of social work theory and practice throughout the twentieth century.

Social work methods of investigating complex social problems within their wider social, economic and cultural contexts are not dissimilar to ethnographic field methods used by social anthropologists and other social scientists. Ethnography provides an understanding of human behaviour and culture through a process of researchers immersing themselves within the groups or communities being studied. Although social workers are not ethnographers – and the relationship between the methodologies of qualitative research and social work practice is complex and contested (see Shaw and Gould, 2001, to explore some of these arguments) – there are undoubtedly some synergies between the practice of social work and the methods of undertaking research that inform it. After all, social work is an *applied* social science discipline that informs and draws on research from cognate disciplines to intervene in the lives of vulnerable people to safeguard them and enhance their well-being.

The relationship between research and practice in social work is complex and this book highlights the importance of a critical interrogation of research findings, rather than a simplistic acceptance and uncritical adoption of them in practice. From the origins of social work in COS in the UK to the present day, social work has taken a critical stance towards research. For example, the maps of the extent and location of poverty in London produced by Charles Booth (1889) or the studies of poverty in York by Seebohm Rowntree (e.g. Rowntree, 1901) contained a wealth of data about the living conditions of the poor with whom social workers were working. These studies revealed the extent of poverty and were influential in shaping government responses, but they were not universally embraced by the early social workers. COS was critical of Rowntree's (1901) study, which revealed that poverty was mainly caused by low wages, or by not having a household member in work. As his findings ran counter to the COS principles of self-help and beliefs that the poor were poor of their own accord, they rejected his report. It is clear that not accepting research findings that challenge preconceived ideas has a long heritage.

Using evidence in social work practice

The concept of 'evidence' is used repeatedly throughout this book, so it is worthwhile spending a few moments to consider what it means. Box 1.2 contains a few definitions.

Common to these definitions is the assertion that evidence is used to prove or disprove something, or to discover the truth. It is most frequently applied in court proceedings to help establish the facts in a case. In criminal proceedings, evidence is used to establish the guilt or innocence of a defendant. Evidence is tested under cross-examination in criminal courts to establish its reliability. Generally, evidence provided by professionals – for instance, forensic scientists – is seen as more reliable than that provided by witnesses of the crime or others personally involved in the case, for example. Key hallmarks of reliable evidence are that it is objective, scientific and independent. However, evidence is rarely 100 per cent reliable and there are notable cases where it has subsequently been found to be flawed.

In family courts, mental health tribunals or other civil proceedings involving social workers, evidence is used to support the argument of a practitioner to help them achieve the outcome they are seeking. The evidence that is presented to the court often relates to the history of the presenting problem and the social circumstances or behaviour of the people involved. Evidence is typically gathered about the case from the individual or family concerned, other professionals working with them or from previous case notes.

BOX 1.2 DEFINITIONS OF 'EVIDENCE'

The available facts, circumstances etc. supporting or otherwise a belief, proposition etc., or indicating whether or not a thing is true or valid (*Concise Oxford Dictionary*)

That which tends to prove or disprove something; ground for belief; proof (*dictionary.com*)

Evidence, broadly construed, is anything presented in support of an assertion. This support may be strong or weak. The strongest type of evidence is that which provides direct proof of the truth of an assertion (*Wikipedia*)

Occasionally, relevant research is introduced as evidence to inform the court's decision-making. Social workers' evidence is tested by those adjudicating the court case, so it needs to be as robust and reliable as possible to ensure it can withstand scrutiny.

This book is about the use of *research* evidence in routine social work practice. It is concerned with how the findings of research can inform social work assessments, decision-making and interventions. We must be aware, though, that the use of the word 'evidence' in this context implies there exists an objective truth that can be discerned through research. This view is derived from empiricism, a theory of knowledge that gives primacy to sensory experience and the role of experiments in deriving our knowledge about the world. Favoured by natural scientists, empiricism has been influential in the development of the notion of 'evidence-based practice'. As we shall discuss, this favours experimental evidence over experiential evidence. Empiricism has an important place in the canon of social work knowledge, but it must be appreciated that empirically derived data only becomes knowledge when it is referred to theory for understanding. (As this is not a textbook on the theories of social work knowledge or social work theory, we do not have the space here to explore this in full; however, we can point the reader to many good books that do – e.g. Lishman, 2007; Payne, 2014.) Suffice it to say that social work cannot live on empiricism alone.

Social work textbooks contain a plurality of theories as it is recognised that no one single theory can guide practice. Social work students often find that applying theory to practice during their placements is not a straightforward process, as the development of 'professional artistry' (Schon, 1987) in social work takes time and experience. It requires exposure to many complex situations characterised by uncertainty and uniqueness to develop the tacit knowledge that qualified practitioners come to rely on in their daily practice. Tacit knowledge lies just beneath the surface of professional practice and is often referred to as 'practice wisdom' in social work (Sheppard, 1995). Tacit knowledge is acquired through experience of practice, but it is not written down, is seldom made explicit and people are often unaware that they have it (Polanyi, 1958). It accounts for the automatic way in which decisions are made, frequently represented as intuition in social work practice (Carew, 1987). Practitioners place a high value on their tacit knowledge (Martinez-Brawley and Zorita, 2007), though one study has found that it does not lead to improved outcomes for users of services (Enguídanos and Jamison, 2006).

Practice learning in social work is aided by the process of reflection, which provides the practitioner with the opportunity to illuminate their practice with knowledge derived from theory and research to deepen their understanding of what they did and what intervention options they have going forward. As we have mentioned, there are many books on social work theory that support students and practitioners in applying knowledge derived from theory in their practice. This book seeks to do the same for research by helping social work students and practitioners to better understand how they can use research findings to inform, enrich and support their practice so that they become as familiar with using research as they are with using their intuition and tacit knowledge in making decisions.

Our use of the word 'evidence', therefore, is a reference to any research findings that can support the development of social work practice, rather than a narrow search for objective truth. 'Evidence' has entered the social work lexicon through the notion of 'evidence-based practice', to which we now turn our attention.

Origins of evidence-based practice

The notion of 'evidence-based practice' has its origins in medicine. It can be traced to a book published by the British epidemiologist Archie Cochrane about how decisions are made in the National Health Service (NHS) (Cochrane, 1972). He argued that his colleagues generally based their decisions on opinion and tradition, rather than evidence, and that this could lead to inequality, inefficiency and ineffectiveness. He proposed that:

> allocations of funds and facilities are nearly always based on the opinions of senior consultants, but more and more, requests for additional facilities will have to be based on detailed argument with 'hard evidence' as to the gain to be expected from the patients' angle and the cost. (Cochrane, 1972: 82)

However, Cochrane was also critical of research, particularly that which had little practical use:

> British science divided itself into pure and applied [research] … this has had a detrimental effect … I remember being advised by the most distinguished people that the best research should be utterly useless. (Cochrane, 1972: 9).

Finally, he argued that for 'applied research' the experimental randomised controlled trial (RCT) is the most reliable and robust study design for health services and interventions because the design minimised the impact of bias. However, he conceded that 'the assessment of the "quality of life" in such trials has proved very difficult' (Cochrane, 1972: 24), which potentially raises issues about its applicability in social work.

Cochrane's ideas were largely discredited during his lifetime and it was not until the 1990s that findings from RCTs were routinely appraised and synthesised to summarise the effectiveness of particular health interventions and inform medical practice. Exploring the process of applying research in medical practice, Sackett *et al.* (1996) articulated the principles and practice of evidence-based medicine which, they argued, had its origins in the mid-nineteenth century. As Cochrane, they were critical of practice based only on opinion, but they introduced the idea that professional experience could have a valuable role to play alongside research evidence in decision-making. They warned against a purely mechanistic, generalised or inflexible approach:

> Evidence-based medicine is not 'cookbook' medicine. Because it requires a bottom up approach that integrates the best external evidence with clinical expertise and patients' choice, it cannot result in slavish, cookbook approaches to individual patient care. (Sackett *et al.*, 1996: 72)

With the caveat that Sackett *et al.*'s argument does not account for the importance of service user or patient expertise (see Beresford, 2003), they maintain
that outcomes for the individual should remain of central importance:

> Without clinical expertise, practice risks becoming tyrannised by evidence, for even
> excellent external evidence may be inapplicable or inappropriate for an individual
> patient. (Sackett *et al.*, 1996: 72)

They were critical of Cochrane's approach in so far as they were sceptical
about the general application and use of RCTs, warning that such a research
design was not necessarily the 'gold standard' methodology for all circumstances:

> some questions about therapy do not require randomised controlled trials or cannot
> wait for the trial to be conducted. And if no randomised controlled trial has been
> carried out for our patient's predicament, we must follow the trail to the next best
> external evidence and work from there. (Sackett *et al.*, 1996: 72)

Sackett *et al.*'s definition of evidence-based medicine (again, noting the
absence of service user and carer expertise alongside practitioner expertise) has
been highly influential in the development of evidence-based social work in the
UK:

> Evidence-based medicine is the conscientious, explicit and judicious use of current
> best evidence in making decisions about the care of individual patients. The practice
> of evidence-based medicine means integrating clinical expertise with the best avail-
> able external clinical evidence from systematic research. (Sackett *et al.*, 1996: 71)

In defining evidence-based social care, Sheldon and Chilvers barely changed
Sackett *et al.*'s (1996) conceptualisation:

> Evidence-based social care is the conscientious, explicit and judicious use of current
> best evidence in making decisions *regarding the welfare of those in need of social
> services* (our emphasis). (Sheldon and Chilvers, 2000: 5)

They argued that evidence-based social work requires practitioners to seek out
the best quality research evidence relevant to the practice situation with which
they are faced and use that to inform their decision-making, assessments or
interventions. Their definition carried three injunctions for practitioners:
conscientiousness, transparency and judiciousness.

First, social workers are to be conscientious in their use of research in their
practice. As reinforced by the professional frameworks discussed earlier in this
chapter (see Box 1.1), practitioners are required to keep up to date with relevant research so that they can use the most effective approaches in their practice.

Second, the use of research to inform decision-making in practice helps care
and support planning to become transparent, open and accountable. If
research evidence is used to inform decision-making, it can be presented to

BOX 1.3 FIVE STEPS TO EVIDENCE-BASED PRACTICE

1. Transforming information about a client and proposed courses of action to specific empirically answerable questions;
2. Searching bibliographic databases to find the best available evidence to answer the question;
3. Evaluating the obtained literature for quality and usefulness;
4. Considering unique client needs and preferences and applying the results of the appraisal to policy or practice decisions;
5. Evaluating the outcome.

(Gibbs and Gambrill, 2002)

explain why particular decisions are made as required by courts, service users or other professionals, for example. It is not always possible to be explicit about particular courses of action but, if research can be appropriately cited, it can promote transparency and the building of professional and trusting relationships.

Third, practitioners are expected to exercise their judgement in the use of research findings in their practice. Judiciousness requires practitioners to assess the strengths and weaknesses of the research they have found to inform the particular problem they are addressing. They need to apply their tacit knowledge and practice wisdom to assess whether the research could be applied in each particular situation. This also includes being informed by what service users prefer and the availability of interventions or approaches indicated as potentially the most effective.

Gibbs and Gambrill (2002) suggested evidence-based practice involves taking five steps (Box 1.3). Although this is not a textbook of evidence-based practice, we discuss steps 1 and 2 in Chapter 2, step 3 in Chapter 3 and step 4 in Part II. Step 5 requires a whole book in its own right!

Hierarchy of evidence

Randomised controlled trials

Evidence-based practice assumes that research can be placed in a hierarchy according to its methodology. Sitting towards the top of this hierarchy are RCTs, which are considered 'gold standard' in evaluating what works best. They are used widely in the physical sciences to test the effectiveness of clinical interventions. For example, a trial of a new drug for clinical depression will involve:

- recruiting people with a diagnosis of clinical depression;
- assessing all research participants across a range of outcome measures;
- allocating them to either an intervention or control group by random selection, preferably by someone independent of the research and clinical teams;
- prescribing the new drug to members of the intervention group;

- prescribing the best treatment currently available, or a placebo if there is no best treatment in place, to members of the control group;
- assessing all the research participants against the outcome measures after a period of time has elapsed;
- ensuring where possible that the researchers collecting the data, the doctors prescribing the drugs and the research participants do not know in which group individual participants have been placed.

RCTs have strong internal validity as they minimise selection bias through the allocation of participants to groups at random. The blinding of participants and researchers to group allocation minimises bias in the data collection. Further, the interventions provided are standardised through the use of treatment manuals, which allow trials to be replicated elsewhere to evaluate the effectiveness of interventions in different contexts. The method favours interventions which can be more easily manualised and delivered consistently, such as medical or psychological therapies. As a result of this, evidence-based guidelines for working with people with mental health problems, for example, are lacking in social interventions (e.g. National Institute for Health and Care Excellence, 2014; National Institute for Health and Clinical Excellence, 2009).

RCTs are challenging to undertake in 'real-world' situations (Coulter, 2011), particularly with complex social interventions. Many social scientists view them with hostility – in part because of the ethics of randomisation, as one group is deprived of access to a potentially effective intervention. Trialists argue that it is ethically acceptable to randomise when there is genuine uncertainty about the effectiveness of the intervention and good pilot evidence that suggests that it may make a difference. Oakley *et al.* (2003) suggest that objections to the use of RCTs to evaluate social interventions 'ignore the history of the successful conduct of many thousands of such studies' (p. 179). Exploring recent examples, they argued that 'random allocation as a research technique for social intervention evaluation is sound on grounds of science, ethical acceptability, and feasibility' (p. 179). An example of a randomised controlled trial can be found in Box 1.4.

A further limitation with RCTs is that interventions evaluated under trial conditions may not be translatable into routine practice. Manualised interventions that require high levels of expertise and training, and produce positive outcomes when delivered by skilled practitioners in the context of a trial, may

BOX 1.4 A RANDOMISED CONTROLLED TRIAL

Brinkborg *et al.* (2011) evaluated the effectiveness of a brief stress management intervention on the stress and general mental health of social workers in Sweden. They stratified the sample of 106 social workers to high-level and low-level stress and randomised participants to an intervention group or a waiting-list control group. Of those with high levels of stress, the intervention significantly decreased levels of stress and burnout, and increased general mental health compared with the waiting-list control group.

BOX 1.5 A SYSTEMATIC REVIEW

Winokur et al. (2014) conducted a systematic review to evaluate the effect of kinship care compared with foster care on the safety, permanency and wellbeing of children removed from the home for maltreatment. They carefully searched for studies that met their inclusion criteria and included 102 quasi-experimental studies in their review. They found that children in kinship care experienced fewer behavioural problems, fewer mental health problems, better wellbeing and less placement disruption than those in foster care. However, the included studies had significant methodological weaknesses that raise concerns about the reliability of these findings.

be difficult to replicate in routine practice. However, by integrating practice wisdom and the tacit knowledge of practitioners into interventions when they are being designed, it is possible that they can be more readily applied in routine practice (Webber, 2014).

Systematic reviews

Evidence-based practice regards systematic reviews of RCTs as being at the pinnacle of the hierarchy of evidence. Named after the founding father of the paradigm, the Cochrane Collaboration publishes high-quality systematic reviews of RCTs of interventions for health problems: www.thecochranelibrary.com. Its sister organisation, the Campbell Collaboration: www.campbellcollaboration.org/lib, does the same for education, crime and justice, social welfare and international development. Either the Cochrane or Campbell Libraries should be the first place to look for evidence of the effectiveness of an intervention.

Systematic reviews use transparent procedures to find, evaluate and synthesise the results of relevant research. Studies included in a systematic review are screened for quality and the findings are combined to produce a single finding, or set of findings, about the effectiveness of an intervention, frequently in many different contexts. Systematic reviews do not have to include RCTs (see Box 1.5, for an example of a review of quasi-experimental studies) and could even be of qualitative research (Saini and Shlonsky, 2012). However, it is reviews of RCTs that are favoured by proponents of evidence-based practice.

Quasi-experimental studies

Studies that evaluate the effectiveness of interventions but where randomization is not possible are known as 'quasi-experimental' studies. They have many of the same features of RCTs, including a focus on a particular intervention or approach, a longitudinal design, and the use of standardised measurements to evaluate outcomes; they often involve comparison groups. They sit below RCTs and systematic reviews in the hierarchy of evidence because they are susceptible to selection bias, as participants are not allocated to intervention groups at random. When quasi-experimental studies do not include a

BOX 1.6 A QUASI-EXPERIMENTAL STUDY

Abel *et al.* (2013) evaluated the outcomes of an eight-week supportive-educational group programme to help children understand and cope more effectively with the stresses, changes and emotional challenges resulting from their parents' divorce or separation. They used a pre-post design and a waiting list control group involving a total of 91 children. They found parent-rated improvements on attending behaviours, social skills and distracting behaviours but no changes on the measures completed by teachers in comparison with the control group.

comparison or control group, it is difficult to ascertain whether any change was caused by the intervention or would have happened anyway, as is the case with the example provided in Box 1.6.

Pre-experimental/pilot studies

The next category of intervention studies are pre-experimental (or pilot) studies. These are usually single group pre-post test studies evaluating the outcome of an intervention, usually in a naturalistic setting. These studies are conducted prior to experimental studies to investigate whether an intervention is likely to produce positive outcomes, usually in a single group (see Box 1.7, for an example).

There are many aspects of social work practice that are not amenable to experimental studies (RCTs, quasi-experimental or pilot studies), notably statutory interventions. However, there are research designs that can produce reliable evidence to inform practice within statutory contexts. These are categorised as 'observation studies' in the hierarchy of evidence and include cross-sectional, cohort and case-control studies.

Cross-sectional surveys

Cross-sectional surveys are one of the most common types of quantitative research. They survey a defined group to explore the prevalence of particular attitudes, social problems or need amongst vulnerable groups, for example. They have multiple purposes, such as identifying where social work interven-

BOX 1.7 A PILOT STUDY

Sirey *et al.* (2012) piloted an intervention to increase the active participation of older adults with a diagnosis of depression in their treatment. ACTIVATE is a brief personalised psychosocial intervention to help people whose treatment for depression does not appear to alleviate their symptoms. It supports them to intensify their treatment by discussing augmenting their antidepressant medication or adding an extra service to their treatment. Two thirds of the 36 participants followed up after 12 weeks had taken a step to increase the intensity of their treatment and there was an overall decrease in depression severity in the sample.

BOX 1.8 A CROSS-SECTIONAL SURVEY

Stokes and Schmidt (2012) explored decision-making processes in child protection through a survey of 118 social workers. They used case vignettes to investigate how practitioners applied a risk assessment tool in their practice. They found no clear relationship between the decisions made and the source of knowledge on which those decisions rested, but knowledge derived from the case situation was more likely to be used when making decisions about risk level or service provision.

tion is required, or exploring the association between explanatory variables of a particular phenomenon. Large population surveys and small surveys specific to social work practitioners, services and service users are both valuable in informing social work practice. An example of a practitioner survey is given in Box 1.8.

Cohort studies

Cohort studies are longitudinal in nature and collect measurements from people over a period of time to identify change. They are particularly useful for exploring the association between risk factors and outcomes, as they can establish cause–effect relationships. Different types of cohort studies are used for different purposes, but each has relevance to social work practice.

'Classical' cohort studies study a single risk factor and follow a group of people over a period of time to measure whether a particular outcome occurs. For example, Warr and Jackson (1985) studied a large sample of unemployed men over a period of nine months to investigate the effect of unemployment on mental health. They found both the detrimental effect of unemployment and the positive impact of re-employment on psychological health. This seminal study has subsequently been influential in the development of supported employment schemes and other projects designed to support vulnerable people to find work.

Large population cohort studies investigate multiple risk factors and outcomes by asking a large cohort many questions over a long period of time. A good example of this is the Born in Bradford cohort of 13,500 children born between 2007 and 2010, who will be followed from pregnancy into adult life to investigate the many influences that shape our lives. Early findings from this cohort provide evidence to inform child protection proceedings, for example. Cooper *et al.* (2013) found an increased risk of babies being born small for their gestational age if their mothers were binge drinking during the second trimester of their pregnancy.

Finally, historical cohort studies use pre-existing data to look back in time at risk factors and outcomes. They permit investigation of social work practice questions, as illustrated by the practitioner research described in Box 1.9. However, they are limited by the quality of the data available in existing records, which were collected for different purposes.

BOX 1.9 A COHORT STUDY

Social work practitioner Richard Kingsford used an historical cohort study design to investigate whether social deprivation predicted the outcomes of a Crisis Resolution and Home Treatment (CRHT) team for adults with mental health problems (Kingsford and Webber, 2010). Exploring the outcomes of 260 people receiving a service from the CRHT, he found that increasing age and being referred from an enhanced Community Mental Health Team (CMHT) were associated with poorer outcomes. Those referred from the enhanced CMHT were more likely to live in socially deprived areas.

Qualitative studies

Of all the different types of research, social workers are likely to be most familiar with qualitative studies. As discussed earlier in this chapter, qualitative interviews have some synergies with social work interviews (although simplistic comparisons should be avoided). Qualitative studies require no understanding of statistics, which are rarely taught comprehensively on social work programmes, and are thus typically favoured by both social work academics and students. As qualitative research explores phenomena such as participants' experiences, values, attitudes and social work processes, for example, it is often viewed as directly relevant for practice. Qualitative research undertaken for social advocacy and activism is also preferred, particularly where it empowers users of social work services. However, it is controversially placed below quantitative research on the evidence-based practice hierarchy of evidence.

Debates between social work researchers specialising in qualitative or quantitative methods have been ongoing for many years. A recent editorial exchange by the leading qualitative social work researcher Ian Shaw (2012a) and his counterpart for quantitative social work research, Bruce Thyer (2012), discusses some of these arguments. Writing in each other's journal, they argued for the merits of the research approach with which they are least associated. As there is no space within this book to explore the debate in detail, I recommend reading their substantial textbooks to understand more about the full range of social work research methods (Shaw *et al.*, 2010b; Thyer, 2010).

PRACTICE REFLECTION 1.1

Research methods

Reflect on the research methods training you received, or are receiving, as part of your social work training. To what extent did this address the particular merits of qualitative and quantitative research methods? Reflect on the different methods used in social work research that you have come across so far and consider how these can be used to answer practice-based research questions.

BOX 1.10 A QUALITATIVE STUDY

Khoo and Skoog (2014) conducted in-depth interviews with eight foster carers to explore their experiences of placement breakdown. Their descriptions highlight that placement breakdown occurred as the consequence of a long series of events, rather than a single event. They also discussed a perceived lack of support from social workers, providing important messages for social work practice with looked-after children.

Qualitative studies in social work are diverse and have a wide-ranging impact on social work knowledge. Ethnography has been particularly influential. For example, from Rosenhan's (1973) classic study of psychiatric diagnosis, which used the observations of eight pseudo-patients to explore the consequences of labelling and depersonalisation in psychiatric hospitals, to Quirk *et al.*'s (2006) ethnographic study of life in contemporary psychiatric in-patient wards, observational methods have provided a wealth of valuable insights to inform mental health social work practice.

In-depth interviews, focus groups, discourse analysis and content analysis of narratives – amongst many more qualitative methods – are all useful for building theory, exploring the perspectives of practitioners and service users, or advocating for social change. Qualitative research can illuminate aspects of practice traditionally hidden from social workers' view, whether the focus is on social groups whose voice is seldom heard (e.g. Eriksson and Hummelvoll, 2012) or the in-depth experiences of carers with whom social workers work (see Box 1.10).

Preference is given to studies using quantitative methods in the hierarchy of evidence because of their potential to produce generalisable evidence. However, this is something of a misnomer, as the quality of each individual study is arguably just as important as the method used. A poorly-conducted experimental study (RCT or otherwise), where there was a low follow-up rate, or if inappropriate outcome measures were used, for example, is of less value than a robust, high-quality qualitative study investigating practitioner and service user experiences of an intervention. Each study needs to be appreciated for its particular strengths and unique contribution to social work knowledge, rather than relying on particular methodologies to provide us with all the answers. Thus, critical appraisal of research (considered in Chapter 3 and referred to throughout this book) is of paramount importance to ensure that high-quality research can be identified and more readily drawn on to inform practice.

Multiple methods studies

It is widely accepted that particular research methods are chosen to answer particular research questions. RCTs are not the answer to all practice questions. While good RCTs can provide useful evidence about the effectiveness of an intervention, qualitative studies can provide invaluable insights into the process of implementing the intervention in practice from the perspective of both practitioners and service users. In fact, social work researchers increasingly use

BOX 1.11 A MULTIPLE METHODS STUDY

Cattan et al. evaluated a national telephone befriending scheme for isolated or lonely older people using multiple methods (Cattan et al., 2010; Cattan et al., 2011). They used a pre-post telephone survey, health diaries, in-depth semi-structured interviews, focus groups and a Delphi survey. They found that telephone befriending helped participants to feel that life was worth living, provided assurance that there was a friend out there and reduced loneliness.

multiple methods in their studies to answer different research questions. For example, it is common to find both qualitative and quantitative methods used in evaluations, though they are often reported separately (see Box 1.11 and Scourfield et al., 2012, for examples of multi-method evaluations); or focus groups being used to explore themes emerging from quantitative data analysis (e.g. Furminger and Webber, 2009); or qualitative studies nested within RCTs to explore the feasibility and acceptability of interventions (e.g. Thomas et al., 2014). Additionally, qualitative methods are used to capture the practice wisdom of social workers to inform the design of interventions to be evaluated subsequently using experimental methods (Webber, 2014; Webber et al., in press). Qualitative and quantitative research methods both have a unique contribution to make to social work knowledge. Their respective locations in the notional hierarchy of evidence should not diminish or augment the respect to be accorded to either.

Evidence-based practice: a critique

Critics of evidence-based practice argue that practitioners' judgement is circumscribed, their expertise is not required and service users' values are ignored (Swinkels et al., 2002; Webb, 2001). In particular, Webb (2001) argues that evidence-based practice entraps practitioners within a mechanistic form of technical rationality. His argument suggests that practice could be constrained to using only a small range of interventions with proven effectiveness. As discussed above, RCTs are easier to conduct with interventions which can be clearly articulated and replicated, such as psychological or pharmacological interventions, or brief psychosocial interventions. Therefore, this critique envisages a practice landscape bereft of discretion or professional judgement with only limited proscribed intervention options available.

Webb's critique confuses evidence-based practice with a parallel development within the American Psychological Association in the early 1990s known as the Empirically Supported Treatments initiative. This reached consensus about how much evidence should be considered necessary to designate a therapy as 'empirically supported' and lists were compiled of those interventions. The idea that a certain level of evidence (such as that provided by two randomised controlled trials, for example) is sufficient to recommend a therapy, treatment or intervention is not dissimilar from the approach which the UK National Institute of Health and Care Excellence takes in its clinical guidelines. However, this is quite different from evidence-based practice and has had limited influence in UK social work. Rather than using lists of empirically-supported treatments (also known as 'empirically-validated' or 'research-supported' treatments), evidence-based practice requires practitioners to consult and appraise research evidence themselves and integrate this with service user preferences, ethical considerations, their own expertise and the availability of resources. If there is no research evidence available, then practice wisdom of experienced practitioners or credible theory is drawn on to decide if a particular approach or intervention is appropriate (Thyer and Pignotti, 2011).

A further critique is that evidence-based practice assumes that social workers are rational agents, ignoring the processes of deliberation and choice in their decision-making (Webb, 2001). However, literature about professional practice suggests the opposite (Gibbs and Gambrill, 2002). Practitioners do not routinely access new research findings and base their practice decisions on this in a way implied by rationalism. Evidence-based practice emphasises the uncertainty involved in decision-making and the importance of practitioners appraising options available to them. Chapter 5 explores this in more detail, particularly the role which research can play in informing decision-making.

Perhaps the most frequently cited limitation of evidence-based practice is simply not having enough evidence on which to base practice decisions (Magill, 2006). Social work research is rarely conclusive and is often of poor quality, which limits the ability of practitioners to be confident about its claims. This has important implications for social work researchers, who should focus their efforts on identifying under-researched practice domains and work with practitioners and service users to identify the relevant practice questions which require an answer. However, this should not prevent practitioners from appraising relevant research which is available and using it to inform decision-making.

Evidence-informed practice

Latterly, the notion of evidence-*informed* practice has been put forward as more appropriate for social work than evidence-*based* practice. This paradigm questions the hierarchy of evidence and the notion of what is 'best' evidence. It also questions practitioners' ability to appraise research and reach a judgement about it (which is, arguably, rather patronising) (Nevo and Slonim-Nevo, 2011). However, as Epstein suggests, evidence-informed practice:

> implies that practice knowledge and intervention decisions might be *enriched* by prior research but not *limited* to it. (Epstein, 2009: 224, emphasis in original)

Evidence is conceptualised as a more inclusive and non-hierarchical notion than proponents of evidence-based practice understand it. It equally values practice wisdom, tacit knowledge and all forms of knowing. It is thereby viewed as integrative, viewing practice and research less in opposition but more in support of one another. In particular, evidence-informed practice respects the role of practice research (Epstein, 2011), which is arguably the best way to integrate research and practice. This is a theme to which we will return in Chapter 15.

Pawson *et al.*'s (2003) typology of knowledge is not dissimilar to this perspective and has been very influential in the work of the Social Care Institute for Excellence (SCIE). It categorises knowledge by source, rather than in a strict hierarchy, and places equal value on organisational, practitioner, policy community, academic, and user and carer research. As Sarah Carr and Lisa Bostock discuss in Chapter 3, critical appraisal within this framework is based on notions of transparency, accuracy, purposivity, utility, propriety, accessibility and specificity. Each source of evidence is respected and appraised according to its own intrinsic merits.

In some regards, there are fundamental differences between evidence-based and evidence-informed practice, particularly in how they view 'evidence'; in others, there are synergies: both are interested in enhancing the role of research in social work practice. As you read this book, you will find both approaches represented. The notion of 'applying' research to practice, as suggested by the title of the book and this chapter, may suggest a leaning towards evidence-based practice. However, when you come to read the final chapter you may reach the opposite conclusion. We have not intentionally championed one notion over another and chapter authors have been given free rein to express their views on the matter. What we agree is important, though, is that research evidence is a valuable resource for social work practice and we should do what we can to ensure maximum value is gained from it.

PRACTICE REFLECTION 1.2

Relationship between research and practice

Having read this introduction to evidence-based practice and its critiques, what is your view on the relationship between research and practice? Has it changed? What do you think are the biggest challenges facing social workers in applying research evidence in their practice?

Conclusion

Research and practice in social work have a long and contested relationship. Many pages of academic journals are filled with debates about how one informs the other. Although this is taken up by some authors in this book, we have largely side-stepped it in favour of a pragmatic focus on what research is available and how this may assist practitioners in their work. Similarly, debates about evidence-based and evidence-informed practice help us to conceptualise the relationship between research and practice. However, as this book focuses on the practical realities and challenges of using research in practice, we have not explored these in depth. So, let us turn now to the important first stage in the process: searching for research evidence.

FURTHER READING

Newman, T., Moseley, A., Tierney, S. and Ellis, A. (2005) *Evidence-Based Social Work: A Guide for the Perplexed* (Lyme Regis: Russell House). A highly recommended introduction to evidence-based practice in social work: clear, concise and practical.

Thyer, B. A. (ed.) (2010) *The Handbook of Social Work Research Methods*, 2nd edn (Thousand Oaks: CA, Sage); Shaw, I., Briar-Lawson, K., Orme, J. and Ruckdeschel, R. (eds) (2010) *The SAGE Handbook of Social Work Research* (London: Sage). These multi-authored volumes are definitive guides to social work research methods and are 'must-reads' for those interested in finding out more about methodology.

Webber, M. (2011) *Evidence-Based Policy and Practice in Mental Health Social Work*, 2nd edn (Exeter: Learning Matters). Although the examples in this book are drawn from mental health social work, the chapters on critical appraisal of different research designs are generically applicable and accessible.

CHAPTER 2

Locating Evidence for Practice

Paul D. S. Ross

Introduction

The 'digital revolution' has provided us with access to a mind-boggling array of information and data, which was simply inconceivable before the creation of the World Wide Web. This direct access has become an implicit part of our lives and provides an immense source of knowledge for social work researchers, practitioners and clients alike. But for evidence-based practice to work as a process, we will need a methodical approach to the actions of searching, collecting and assessing relevant research for social work practice.

As discussed in Chapter 1, social workers are required to use the best available evidence to underpin and support professional knowledge, and to translate that evidence into their own practice in an ethical way. The skills for finding and using evidence are the same whether you are an undergraduate social work student or an experienced registered social worker. You can begin to use research evidence more effectively in routine practice by using your observational, critical and analytical skills in both your interactions with clients and with the evidence you seek. This is achieved by using the same systematic approach, but tailored to your source, and by recording this process by using a variety of tools and techniques which enable transparency and achieve professional quality standards.

This chapter will explain how to complete a systematic literature search focusing on social care information and discuss how to do this in an efficient, timely and cost-effective way. There are different approaches to searching for relevant research. The Cochrane Collaboration (2007), Social Care Institute for Excellence (Rutter *et al.*, 2010) and the EPPI-Centre (2010) all use different approaches, for example. However, no matter *where* or *how* you do your searching, you will want to do it in a way that not only provides the highest-quality evidence available, but also saves you time. Time is a significant factor for social workers, as their ability to keep their knowledge up-to-date is compromised by high caseloads and by a practice environment which questions the legitimacy of the task and sees both research and reflection on practice as a luxury in itself. Alongside this, there is urgency in the sector for cost-effectiveness at a time of severe public expenditure cuts and a need for ways of identifying high-quality evidence that improves both professional standards and reputation alongside others in the public sector (Nutley *et al.*, 2013).

We need to consider the similarities and differences in information across the disciplines of social care, health (including both public and mental health), housing, education, criminal justice and employment, as knowledge from these cognate disciplines may be useful in social work practice (Clapton, 2010). To do so, we will require a transparent systematic search process with a focused search strategy and a tested question to ensure that we can be confident in our approach methodologically.

Research evidence for social workers can be found in a variety of media and disciplines, which means that there is a diverse literature for practitioners to consider. The variety of terms used to describe social care and a lack of taxonomic standardization, such as the medical subject headings (MeSH) terms in health, can 'complicate the identification of useful information' (Grayson and Gomersall, 2003: 4) for social work practice. Standardization does exist in relation to Boolean search operators (see pp. 36–7) across the disciplines which are mainly for use within bibliographic databases. All provide similar search facilities varying from simple to advanced searching with nearly all having a thesaurus, or a taxonomy, which they use to classify and keyword their content. Standard classification across the databases can be a problem and 'experts warn against reliance on thesaurus-based searches and recommend combining them with free text searches' (Grayson and Gomersall, 2003: 8). As discussed in Chapter 1, systematic reviews are one way of focusing our literature search on a specific question, controlling the diversity of social care information and reporting transparently about what we find.

No matter what your enquiry is in relation to, by following simple rules you can systematically locate, appraise and apply research to your practice in a way that empowers you and the people with whom you work. We all have the ability to make computer enquiries at two basic levels; one as a consumer and one as a critic (Moore, 2002). However, each approach is vastly different in relation to evidence-based practice and this is generally to do with structure. By applying the following approach to both professional and personal enquiries, you will discover the ability to use a basic *structure* or *scaffold* to control and manage that information to assess its quality and value in relation to your question and subsequent practice. The critical framework this provides enables you to test the legitimacy of online sources of information alongside your own practice knowledge. My advice would be to assume you know nothing in an enquiry until you can qualify it, as Gordon *et al.*'s (2009) study highlighted there is a need for professionals to put their own current knowledge aside and to develop an open mind:

> I think if you've already decided on a conclusion before you've asked the question then you're not going to see other options. (Gordon *et al.*, 2009: 8)

> PRACTICE REFLECTION 2.1
>
> **Using research literature**
>
> *Research questions*
>
> Think about your work as a social worker. Are there any questions that arise from your practice that may be answered from the research literature? Are there topics you are curious to find out more about? These could be either general enquiries about a broad field of practice, or something very specific. Write down one or two; you can develop these as you read this chapter.

The critic

As a social worker, you will seek good-quality social care information from the internet and bibliographic databases in both study and practice, but this can be time-consuming and highly frustrating, especially if your approach is unstructured. You might not acknowledge it, but most of us are information-literate to a variety of levels, whether at home or at work, by ordering a pizza online, booking a holiday, writing an email, or even when researching and writing a report – we can all find information (CILIP Information Literacy Group, 2014).

So, what's special about searching for social care information? Can't I just Google it? Yes, you could just 'Google it' and some of the results may provide a good starting point to begin your search. However, for credibility purposes a quick search on Google might not be sufficient to locate research evidence that may impact on someone's life. I would suggest for those with the luxury of time, money and access that you use all the sources you have available, but if you have limited time and money, there are still ways to find a diversity of information from numerous free online sources.

The 'free gift' that Tim Berners Lee gave to the world has become an integral part of our lives, through the ways we interact, communicate, gain and share knowledge. However, this meld of human and machine can only be fully exploited if we understand that both have their limitations. In using the internet, we have to remember neither the human nor the machine is infallible, and this must be clear in our mind when searching the web or bibliographic databases and critically analysing content from them.

The major flaw in wanting to acquire credible information from the internet is, ironically, one of the web's strongest selling points: its operability, by anyone around the world, to say whatever they want (sometimes with little description of the methods used) and then publish this in a global public domain. Therefore, we have to always ask: 'What are the limitations of my source?'

Bias, inaccuracy and inequality of information exist within the web, which we need to be aware of as, unsurprisingly, the information online is not created or managed by one person. It is a collection of global knowledge that grows uncontrolled, unbounded and unaffected by many of the ethics of modern society. As users, we have to filter the information by being both critical and ethical at all times in both the actions of searching for information from the internet and the assessment of evidence from it. Being an evidence-based practitioner means you will need a systematic way to identify evidence relative to your field of enquiry, by searching and collecting information from a variety of sources and then critically assessing their relevance, using a variety of tools, to answer that enquiry.

Social care evidence could come from either the grey literature or peer-reviewed research. The first is likely to be informally published and not subject to set methodological conventions; the second is more likely to involve specific methods and has also been approved by their peers through the journal submission process. Box 2.1 outlines the types of evidence which may be found in each area.

BOX 2.1 TYPES AND SOURCES OF EVIDENCE

Types of evidence

Grey literature (generally free to access)

- Legislation, policy or guidance;
- Independent reports or reviews;
- National and local government reports;
- Thesis or conference proceedings;
- Legal reports or case law reports;
- News stories, blogs and websites.

Research literature (free to access but some full text is at a charge)

- Systematic or narrative literature reviews, meta-analysis;
- Qualitative or quantitative studies, or randomised controlled trials;
- Statistical data studies, or cost effectiveness studies.

Sources of evidence

- Online search engines and free or subscription databases;
- Peer reviewed journal sites and academia;
- Organisational websites and community third-sector groups;
- News sites and social media, including blogs, communities of practice and clearing houses.

Types of knowledge (Pawson et al., 2003)

Five sources:

- Organisations;
- Practitioners;
- The policy community; i.e. knowledge gained from the wider policy context;
- Research gathered systematically with a planned design;
- Service users and carers.

BOX 2.2 SAMPLE SEARCH RECORD TEMPLATE

Search record

Date	Terms	Question	Limits
15/03/14	Evidence-based practice, effectiveness, social work	How effective are social workers at implementing evidence-based knowledge into practice?	2004–2014

Sources

Databases

Date	Name	Search terms	Results	File saved
15/03/14	ASSIA	Evidence-based practice OR evidence-based treatments Limits 04–14	163 (32)	Assia1
15/03/14	Social Care Online	Evidence-based practice OR evidence-based treatments Limits 04–14	154 (98)	SCO1
15/03/14	PubMed	Evidence-based practice OR evidence-based treatments Limits 04–14	689 (689)	PUB1

Search Engines

Date	Name	Search terms	Results	Notes
15/03/14	Google	Evidence-based practice social work	42,400,000	Harvested
15/03/14	Bing	Evidence-based practice social work	101,000,000	To harvest

Organisations

Date	Name	Home page link	Notes	Notes
15/03/14	Economic and Social Research Council	http://www.esrc.ac.uk/	Key site	Research section
15/03/14	Social Care Institute For Excellence	http://www.scie.org.uk/	Key site	Publications section

Key documents

Date	Name	Link	Notes	Notes
15/03/14	'The Argument for Evidence-based Practice in Social Work'	http://www.communitycare.co.uk/2010/06/18/the-argument-for-evidence-based-practice-in-social-work/	Ref harvest	
15/03/14	'The Role of Relationships in Connecting Social Work Research and Evidence-Based Practice'	http://www.tandfonline.com/doi/full/10.1080/15433714.2013.845028#.UyTCvKtFDrc	Input RM	Good article about social researchers and practitioners

Journals

Date	Name	Search terms	Vol.	Notes
15/03/14	Evidence-based Mental Health	Social work	Vols 17–30	Hand-searched
15/03/14	Journal of Evidence-based Social Work	Implementation	Vols 1–11	To search

Tools of the trade

We must ensure that we search for evidence in a structured and systematic way, and we can do this by using a search record. This can help you to manage the process of searching and will provide you with the background to describe your methodological approach in the final stages of systematic report writing. It is also helpful for re-running searches and building search strategies across a variety of different sources. The best thing is to create a search template either in Excel or Word and to use a new template for each enquiry (Box 2.2). Why? You could use your favourites, online accounts, bookmarks and even save searches within the subscription databases. However, from experience, I would advise to keep it all in one place as it makes life much easier – especially when you come to report, or need to re-run an old search.

In searching a variety of literature, we will find large numbers of reports, journal papers, citations, references and abstracts that need to be managed and assessed at a later date. To do this efficiently, we need somewhere to house and manage them. There are a variety of reference management software packages available, such as Reference Manager, Endnote and Eppi Reviewer (available on the commercial market for a cost), along with a variety of free management systems such as Mendeley or Quippa. It will be very difficult to complete a systematic literature review without at least one of these. I would suggest you do a little research to investigate which is best for you and your operating system. If you are affiliated to a higher education institution, it should already have a licence for a reference management system, and I would advise you to test and explore its capabilities so that you are familiar with it before you start using it.

Many reference management systems work on the same basis, allowing you to input records from databases directly into them using a variety of selectable input types. Alternatively, some will require you to input your citation data manually and will allow you to remove duplicates. Each record contains details such as author, title, date of publication, journal citation, abstract and hyper-links – to name but a few sections. Reference management systems also help you to produce bibliographic outputs, which are especially useful when you need to generate a critical assessment of the collection of references at the later stages of the overall systematic process. Set up a new reference management library for each enquiry, as this will be your journal and document master reference database. Again, this saves time, provides structure to your decision-making process, and makes life that little bit easier.

Overall, these tools provide us, as critical evidence-based practitioners, with the ability to control the process of obtaining information in the pursuit of knowledge. They provide structure to the variety of sources available online and provide a framework in which to collect, record and conduct analysis. They can also help to structure your final report and can be used repeatedly, but the more organised and formulated your capture tools are, the quicker and easier the process becomes. You will be building your own personalised knowledge set by capturing references in this way, and you will use this to its full advantage when researching, writing and in practice.

Defining the question

As a student and as a practitioner, you will have many different enquiries in relation to your professional practice. In being an evidence-based practitioner, you will be expected to show that you are able to:

- produce a practice question;
- undertake a search of the evidence;
- critically appraise the research evidence;
- translate and implement into practice. (Webber, 2011)

There is some debate within social work about how to create an appropriate practice question which is answerable using desktop research. In health searches, the frameworks generally used are PICO (Patient or Population–Intervention–Comparison–Outcome), SPICE (Setting–Perspective–Intervention–Comparison–Evaluation) or CORE. In social science research, using these methods can be challenging. The main issue is that of the intervention and outcome parts; as in health, you could say that 'using drug x had the following outcomes on different types of people'. Interventions in social care, however, can be provided by a variety of professionals, over different periods of time, with many different outcomes, affecting different individuals, in a variety of unrelated ways, which are much harder to define, resulting in a greater complexity to social care research and intervention types. You could however use the SMART (Specific–Measurable–Achievable–Realistic–Timely) method to test whether your intended question is both relevant and credible.

The good news is – don't panic! Whatever question you formulated will be tested in the early stages of preliminary searching and you can refine it before you run the full systematic search. This is called an iterative process; it takes away the pressure to get it right first time and allows us to focus more on getting it right over a period of time by using our searching skills along with the evidence found at the early stages of preliminary searching.

At many times in your academic and professional career, you will need to make enquiries to find evidence on your desired topic, which will most frequently arise from your practice.

CASE SCENARIO 2.1

Jayne

On a regular visit to Jayne, a woman aged 72 with dementia, her family inform you that Jayne has been leaving the house more than usual and was recently found by the police confused and distressed in a neighbour's garden. The family discuss their concerns in relation to their mother's safety and ask if you can suggest anything that might help. They are clear, however, that they want their mother to stay with them.

Creating a search question

Taking Case scenario 2.1 as our example, we can create a search question to help us find relevant research evidence to inform practice decisions; for example:

> *How effective is assistive technology in keeping individuals with dementia safe and secure?*

The information you gather in the early stage of searching will enable you to assess whether the question is both relevant and feasible, given the variety of sources and information available. If it is not relevant and feasible, the information we possess from within the preliminary search will assist us to rewrite it. When you have constructed your question, you need to do one final thing before starting the preliminary search, which is to break the question down into different parts.

The science bit ...

The internet is a network of computers, which is nebulous in its collective formulation as a system. Searches on the internet can produce results via a variety of algorithms (ways of doing something). Many use keywords but, overall, they are different computer programs with different ways of collecting, constructing and arranging information, which exist as a global shareable source. The problem for a novice searcher is *how* they were constructed and *which* keywords to use to produce a tailored result.

Online bibliographic databases offer more structure than the World Wide Web, because they are constructed using a particular index which is used to arrange and classify the data. There are some exceptions but most indexing information, often referred to as a 'thesaurus', 'taxonomy', 'index' or 'directory', should be available within the database, online via its help section or in the main tool bar; copies can also be found in your academic or local library.

We need to break down our question to suit the sources we intend to use, by breaking it into keywords that are relevant to them. Again, this will be an iterative process and one we can refine after the preliminary search stage, as it is impossible to know all of the language and terminology used for social work and social care, both in the UK and abroad. First, because the language and terminology is vast and always changing but, second, because you probably will not have the time or the capacity!

Let us use the question we constructed from Case scenario 2.1. We need to break this down into concepts. This need be no cause for concern – the language you currently know will do for the time being.

We can break our question down into three parts:

- the *intervention* part: assistive technology
- the *outcome* part: effectiveness and safety
- the *topic* part: dementia.

We need to think of the variety of vocabulary to describe our parts, which we will call our 'keywords' when we start the search. I would suggest that you approach this by, first, brainstorming all the terms you know off the top of your head to describe your parts and write a list.

Here is an example of the terms I know about the three parts of our question:

- *Intervention*: assistive technology, devices, technology
- *Outcomes*: effectiveness, safety, security
- *Topic*: Alzheimer's, dementia.

Do not worry if you do not get all the terms and the variety of language right at this time. We will learn more about how the terms for our topics are used in the literature, internet and individual databases as we conduct the preliminary search. Record this on your search record (Box 2.2), as you will be retuning and adding to it later.

We now need to undertake some preliminary investigation into our enquiry. The internet is a good place to start, but there are a variety of other sources which are just as important, such as discussions with your peers, e-books and using the library.

The preliminary search

Just before we open the search engine to start the preliminary search stage, we have to do something to our thought process about personal bias. As a practitioner, you will know a great deal about your area of practice and may use this to make assumptions about what you are going to find – which is perfectly natural. However, these assumptions can bias a search from the outset. Your professional view, experience and judgement will be needed to compare evidence *against* and *evaluate* your enquiry at later stages of the searching and appraisal process. It is therefore best to pretend you know nothing until after the preliminary searching stage.

The preliminary search stage is generally a broad search approach using our terms across a variety of sources. This 'quick and dirty' stage across a broad set of selected sources should enable you to have an overview of the topic area, an ability to see how your original question works, or whether you need to change it, and should provide you with some key resources on which to build future searching.

With our search record open, you need to record the date and the database name, then put the following example into a search engine (e.g. Google) search box:

Dementia technology
(search tools: *Limit to UK*)

The reason why we are inputting the search term in this way is because Google looks for those specific words within the full text of each webpage. However,

Google (like many other search engines) will not provide you with a neat ordered set of results. Your search terms could appear in any order, or some of the results may only contain one part, or a variety, of the terms, rather than the exact collection of associated terms in the order you wanted. You may additionally want to add a date period, or focus your results by using the *search tools* tab and select the *country:uk* tab, to make your results more specific to your local needs. Additionally, you may wish to add *filetype:pdf* at the end of your terms to retrieve PDF content only (Blakeman, 2014). Just remember to record the exact terms you used and any additional limits in your search record.

At this stage, we need to scan the results and investigate which are relevant to our enquiry. It is worth remembering that no individual search will be the same, so it is highly likely that when you re-run this search the results may have changed. It is also likely your results will contain a variety of both grey and research literature, and you will need to find those relevant to dementia and technology, and discard or ignore those that do not fit your specific need.

When I completed the search, I scanned the first 15 results which contained a mixture of organisation and academic websites, journal articles and reports. The first result came from the Alzheimer's Society and the link took me to a factsheet (Alzheimer's Society, 2012), which I saved for consideration in my search record. The second was an organisation which focuses specifically on assistive technology and dementia. The third was a blog about how technology is supporting people with dementia. The fourth was about technological innovation in dementia. The fifth was an academic literature review on the cost-effectiveness of assistive technology in supporting people with dementia (Bowes *et al.*, 2013). The remaining ten results contained a mixture of news articles, reports, journal articles and presentations. I added the literature review and another about designing technology for people with dementia to my search record. Why? Because all three came from well-known trusted sources, two from universities and one from an organisation considered to be the UK leader in dementia evidence and research.

I scanned the index of the literature review to see whether it contained an executive summary. If it had, I would have scanned this and the conclusion, but this review had a 'background and purpose' section instead of an executive summary, which I read. I then searched for '*safety*' within the document using the *Find tool* and this highlighted the sections referring to '*safety*', which I checked for relevance to my enquiry. I copied and pasted these references into my search output to investigate later. This task is *searching* and *growing* from a key document, and I did this for the other report and the factsheet.

I also noted the language used in relation to dementia, technology and safety by recording any terms I felt useful or interesting in my search record. In reading the factsheet, I discovered a section about devices that enable safer walking using tracking devices, which referred to the Alzheimer's Society position statement on safer walking technology (Alzheimer's Society, 2013). In reading this, I noticed the term 'wandering', together with an explanation of the types of assistive technology which are relevant to safer walking and wandering for individuals with dementia, such as tracking devices and alarms. The statement also highlighted other issues I had not yet considered in relation to ethics, privacy and consent. The position statement and the literature review had references which looked relevant to my topic and I noted 'reference harvest' next to them on my search record for later.

So far, I have collected four pieces of evidence and used these to build on my vocabulary and my overall knowledge of the topic of wandering, technology and dementia; yet, some may contain bias and may not tell the whole story. I will need to search broadly to capture a wide range of literature to test whether my question is fit for purpose before I complete a systematic review. I need to test the assumptions I have made from the limited set of sources I already have, and will need to complete more searches translating the language and vocabulary across a variety of sources (see Box 2.3 for examples of diverse sources of social care information).

It would also be advisable to search organisations that are specific to your enquiry; in the case of our scenario, this would be those with expertise and interest in dementia, technology and wandering. If your enquiry is just to advise service users, or if you do not have the time or financial ability to access bibliographic databases, then the information gained from this preliminary searching may be sufficient for building an information collection, but not an evidence base. I would suggest that you pull all the information together in the form of a report detailing what you have found. Alternatively, you could use a mind mapping software such as *freemind* to arrange and identify which pieces of the information you think best answer your enquiry. This, however, would just be information and not a source to advise on evidence-based options; you will have to complete a systematic search to provide this. I would also suggest that you discuss your findings with fellow professionals, both for their information purposes and for them to share their own knowledge with you. This can be helpful, if you intend to take your enquiry further. The basic rule is to record everything you do, as this will always be the foundation on which to build as you undertake a systematic review.

The systematic search

From my preliminary search, I now have a small selection of key evidence from a variety of trusted sources. After selecting those that are most relevant to my enquiry, I read and note similarities and differences in the narratives and the points of view contained. However, the information gathered through the preliminary stage needs to be put into context. It may contain bias in its content, its argument, in my collection and in my decision-making about the information I have selected. If I used this information to make any evidence-based conclusion, it could be inaccurate, or even wrong. This would mean that all my hard work in formulating my process accounted for nothing, because I have not yet tested the question across a broad range of bibliographic sources.

I need to return to my question and refine it, with the newly acquired information from our preliminary stage. My preliminary search also provided me with specific knowledge on the types of device available in connection with the issue of walking and wandering, and other issues about ethics and consent. I therefore rephrased the question to:

BOX 2.3 SOURCES OF SOCIAL CARE INFORMATION

Search engines
Google, Google Scholar, Bing, Yahoo, Alta vista

Databases (free)
Social Care Online (SCO), NICE Evidence Search, Cochrane Library, Campbell Collaboration, AgeINFO, Centre for Reviews and Dissemination Database (CRD), TRIP database, PLOS ONE

Policy and legislation
UK Government, UK Legislation, UK Parliament, UK Department of Health, UK Department of Education, UK Department for Communities and Local Government, UK Department Home Office, Government Equalities Office (GEO)

Local and national government organizations
Local Government Association (LGA), County Councils Network (CCN), National Association of Local Councils (NALC), The Knowledge Hub, National Audit Office (NAO)

Charity, third-sector organization or user-led group
Social Care Institute for Excellence (SCIE), Think Local Act Personal (TLAP), Shaping Our Lives, National Council for Voluntary Organisations (NCVO), Third Sector Knowledge Portal, National Voices, Joseph Rowntree Foundation (JRF), Kings Fund, Social Services Research Group (SSRG), Picker Institute Europe, Institute for Research and Innovation in Social Services (IRISS), Age UK, Institute for Public Policy Research (IPPR), Nuffield Foundation, Research in Practice for Adults (RIPFA), Research in Practice (RIP)

Public bodies
National Institute for Health and Care Excellence (NICE), NHS England, Evidence Into Practice (NHS Scotland), Equality and Human Rights Commission (EHRC), National Institute for Health Research (NIHR), Economic and Social Research Council (ESRC)

Private organisations
Skills for Care, PricewaterhouseCoopers, Deloitte, OPM, Centre for Workforce Intelligence ➜

How ethical and effective are tracking devices in keeping individuals with dementia safe and secure?

I now have my research question, using relevant language to describe my new and improved enquiry using the knowledge I had obtained from a variety of trusted sources. I now need to break this down into groupings, just as I did in the preliminary stages:

- *Diagnosis*: dementia, Alzheimer's Disease

Academic and research centres
Quality and Outcomes of Person-centred Care Policy Research Unit, Personal Social Services Research Unit (PSSRU), Social Care Workforce Research Unit (SCWRU), Evidence for Policy and Practice Information and Co-ordinating Centre (EPPI-Centre), Royal College of General Practitioners, NatCen, Social Policy Research Unit (SPRU), Poverty and Social Exclusion, Research Information Network, Evidence Network (Kings College), Institute of Public Care

Regulators
Care Quality Commission (CQC), Health and Care Professionals Council (HCPC), Monitor, General Medical Council (GMC)

Statistics and data sources
Health and Social Care Information Centre (HSCIC), Office of National Statistics (ONS)

Member organizations
College of Social Work, British Association of Social Workers, Association of Directors of Adult Social Services, Local Government Information Unit

Clearing houses*
California Evidence-Based Clearinghouse for Child Welfare, National Registry of Evidence Based Programmes and Practices

Think tanks and market research
New Economics Foundation (NEF), Demos, Nesta, Centre for Social Justice, Social Market Foundation, Reform (Research Trust), IPSOS Mori

News sites (trade)
Guardian, Times, Mail, Community Care Magazine, BBC News

Social media
Twitter, Youtube, blogs, communities of practice

Key: * American sources.

- *Tools*: tracking devices, alarms, assistive technology
- *Outcomes*: independence, effectiveness, ethics, safety, security.

I need these to structure the systematic and final stage of searching, which is across databases specific to social care evidence. I recorded these in my search record, as I will need them repeatedly throughout the next stage. I also ran a few more search engine enquiries to reflect my newly-created question and to supplement those already contained within the search output from the preliminary searching stage.

These terms will be used to construct a search strategy across a variety of databases and they will form the basis of our free text and taxonomic terms. However, before we search we have to turn the unrelated parts of our question into a valid search string using a formulation called Boolean logic.

Another science bit ...

Most databases and journal sources use Boolean logic (see Box 2.4), which allows you to combine search strategies in a variety of ways; some automatically as a query-building device, or some will allow you to insert a whole prepared search string. This is helpful because they can make your enquiry as specific as you require. Boolean logic brings a mathematical equation to language and helps us to interface with online databases in a relevant way.

BOX 2.4 BOOLEAN LOGIC OPERATORS

AND ~ OR ~ NOT ~

'EXACT' ~ * TRUNCATION

AND

(dementia) **AND** (tracking devices) **AND** (effectiveness)

Our results will contain a collection of information that includes dementia, technology and effectiveness. **AND** will return findings that include the combination of the search terms you entered

OR

(independence **OR** effectiveness **OR** ethics **OR** safety **OR** security)

Our results in this combination will be for all the search terms we have defined. Using **OR** broadens a search to include a variety of terms and synonyms but will usually result in more hits

NOT

(dementia) **AND** (technology **NOT** computers) **AND** (safety)

Using **NOT** is a way to reduce unwanted terms and related results

Truncation (*)

(dementia) **AND** (tracking device*) **AND** (effectiveness)

Truncation (*) increases the variety of your term from a single word to multiple words. Our results using truncation will include both 'tracking device' and 'device/*=s'

Exact ('quotation marks')

('dementia') **AND** ('wandering') **AND** ('ethics')

Using **'Exact'** makes your terms specific to that phrase of spelling only

---

BOX 2.5 EXAMPLE BOOLEAN SEARCH STRING

(dementia **OR** alzheimer's disease) **AND**

(tracking devices **OR** alarms **OR** assistive technology) **AND**

(independence **OR** effectiveness **OR** ethics **OR** safety **OR** security)

The last two examples in Box 2.4 are particularly helpful if you have too *little* or too *much* data when you search, but it is best to test the impact of these operators before you run the full search. You will notice that brackets are used to separate the formula out. Brackets compartmentalise each term so that the computer system understands which terms are being combined. This becomes even clearer when a full search string has been constructed (Box 2.5).

The overall use of Boolean is to control the way you structure your question and how you translate this into a relevant formulation for a technological device in the pursuit of evidence. Boolean can help to retrieve more relevant results by adding **AND** to your original enquiry. It can also widen your search by using **OR**, or even limit your results through the use of **NOT**. The main gain from this arrangement is that we now have a search question template – in the form of our Boolean search string – to run across a variety of online databases and journal sites which search using this type of Boolean search formula.

Your access to a wide range of online bibliographic databases may be limited as a practitioner. University libraries provide a selection of databases for their students. The NHS currently offers access to a specific set of databases through Athens Access, but funding is unstable and this free access for staff may change over time. Some local libraries are also slowly disappearing as the internet and e-publishing are starting to dominate the commercial and public marketplaces. However, if you have one, a local library, or one of the national libraries, should have access to a wide range of online bibliographic databases. If you have no access at all, you should investigate free sources such as Social Care Online, the Cochrane Library, or TRIP and online journals sites such as Palgrave Macmillan, Taylor & Francis or Oxford journals.

Before you start the systematic search, I would advise you to open a clean search record, as you will want to know exactly what you have gathered and how you have gathered it from each specific location. You will also need your reference management system open. The number of databases to search is dependent on your time, access and knowledge, but somewhere between six and eight online bibliographic databases should suffice. My advice would be to use as many as you can through your access points and to search across as wide a variety of sources as possible. You can be broad in your selection, but be precise in how you use your question in each source each time. Some of the key social science databases can be found in Box 2.6.

Let us run our Boolean search strategy on one of the free databases (the process will be same for each database you search). Some may already contain search boxes with an ability to click and select **AND, OR** and **NOT** and some

BOX 2.6 KEY SOCIAL SCIENCE DATABASES

- Applied Social Sciences Index and Abstracts (ASSIA)
- International Bibliography of the Social Sciences (IBSS)
- Social Science Citation Index (SSCI)
- Social Work Abstracts (SWA)
- Social Policy and Practice (SPP)
- Social Services Abstracts (SSA)
- SocINDEX
- PsycINFO
- Scopus
- Social Care Online (SCO) (free)
- Cochrane Library (free)
- Campbell Collaboration (free)

will simply provide you with a search box into which you can copy and paste your search string. Some databases will allow you to build in stages, or to combine complex singular searches after they have been run using **AND, OR** and **NOT**.

Our process within each source should be the same:

- a Boolean 'free-text' search;
- a Boolean search using the database's taxonomy, thesauri or MeSH descriptors.

We will need to use a variety of methods to limit and control the number of records we obtain. To control our sources, we should define a date period that covers a wide and relevant period of time in social policy and social work research (ten years is usually sufficient). Inside each database will be search filters to help with being more specific in the type of research we want in our results. Some disciplines, such as health, limit their searches to the highest elements of the evidence hierarchy searching for RCTs, systematic reviews and meta-analysis, followed by other quantitative and qualitative studies. We could do the same, if we had little time to wade through all types of evidence and a desire for a limited set of results that use similar high-quality methodological standards in their production and are highly valued in relation to health and social care. However, this is the case only if they exist on the topic of your enquiry 'since research evidence for social care practice is far more limited in scope than it is for healthcare' (Rutter and Fisher, 2013: 4).

I ran my free-text search string *all fields* in the advanced search section of Social Care Online, noted the search on my record and the number of results (see Box 2.7). Then, I selected the results and inputted them into my reference management system. I returned to the records and named and saved the search. Next, I explored the first couple of results and checked how they were classified as subject terms and retained those I thought relevant to my enquiry. Ideally, time permitting, I would search the electronic version of the thesaurus and check for all the words that described my parts and search for those using

BOX 2.7 EXAMPLE-FREE TEXT AND THESAURUS SEARCHES

Databases

Date	Name	Search terms	Results	Classification terms
18/03/14	**Social Care Online** FT	**Advanced search:** All fields (dementia OR alzheimer's disease) AND (tracking devices OR alarms OR assistive technology) AND (independence OR effectiveness OR ethics OR safety OR security)	221 (221)	Dementia, alzheimer's disease, assistive technology, alarm systems, risk assessment, wandering, cost effectiveness, ethics **Saved: SCOThes1.RIS**
18/03/14	**Social Care Online** TH	**Advanced search:** Subject terms (dementia or alzheimer's disease) AND Subject terms (assistive technology or alarm systems) AND Subject terms (risk assessment or wandering or cost effectiveness or ethics) AND Publication Date (2004–2014)	2037	1
18/03/14	**Social Care Online** TH	**Advanced search:** Content type (systematic review or research review)	689 (689)	2
18/03/14	**Social Care Online** TH	1 AND 2	101 (101)	**Saved: SCOThes1.ris**
19/03/14	**ASSIA** FT	(dementia OR alzheimer's disease) AND (tracking devices OR alarms OR assistive technology) AND (independence OR effectiveness OR ethics OR safety OR security) Additional limits: 2004–2014 English	13 (13)	Electronic monitoring, dementia, technical aids, personal safety, tracking, alzheimer's disease S1
19/03/14	**ASSIA** TH	SU(dementia) OR SU(alzheimer's disease) AND SU(technical aids) OR SU(electronic monitoring) AND SU(personal safety) OR SU(tracking) Narrowed by 2004–2014 and Narrowed by Peer reviewed	2041 (2041)	S2 **Saved: ASSIAThes1.ris**

the *subject term field*, and I would use **AND** to combine them using the inbuilt query-builder.

Using the information from both the thesaurus and the subject headings identified by the free-text searches, we have a collection of results that are broader than our first enquiry and specific to the classification of the database. Some databases will limit the amount you can export at one time and my results are over the 500 limit of the database. A good tip is to look for ways to divide the data up into smaller chunks by using date ranges or content types; in my case, I limited them to systematic and research reviews. I would advise you to test the impact of these limits when you apply them and see whether the limitation is what you want, because, as I have mentioned, neither the human nor the computer that created and classified the data is infallible!

I copied and pasted the search string from my SCO free-text search and entered it into the first box in the advanced search section of ASSIA and kept the default *in* field as *anywhere*. I then selected the *publication date* drop down box and clicked *specific date range* and entered my date range. I selected *English* articles as my language of relevance and selected the items per page box to 100 and then clicked the *search* button. My search returned 13 results (Box 2.7). As before, in my SCO search, I read the results on the first page, checking how relevant each record was to my need and looked at how each record had been classified, called *subject heading* terms in ASSIA, and I noted these in my table. I then built and ran the subject (SU) search using the *command line search*. I could, however, have clicked into the thesaurus and searched for each term individually and combined those. Even though I found a large number of results, I tested the subject heading for systematic reviews but I felt that it did not work sufficiently well. Therefore, I limited it by two-year date periods and decided to take the full list of results into my reference management system for sorting later.

Each enquiry should be the same across all databases. Start with a free-text enquiry and investigate the results and their classification. This informs the next type of search, a specific enquiry using the database's classification. Investigate these results for relevance and then repeat this process precisely on all other sources.

Both subscription databases such as ASSIA and some freely available databases provide the facility to save searches and print, or save search strategies.

BOX 2.8 EXAMPLE INCLUSION AND EXCLUSION CRITERIA

1. Exclude date
2. Exclude publication type
3. Exclude location
4. Exclude population
5. Exclude scope
6. Query
7. Include.

BOX 2.9 LITERATURE SEARCHING

Now it's your turn to practice searching for research papers that may help you to answer the practice question(s) you wrote down earlier in the chapter. Re-read the chapter and then:

Brainstorm and discover

1. Write a list of all the words you know that you could use as search terms to find information on your topic.
2. Open a search engine and enter your terms. What comes up? See how others have classified your terms.
3. Do this for each term so that you produce a list for each.

Combine and formulate

1. In preparation for searching, you will need to formulate and combine your lists of terms using Boolean operators (AND/OR/NOT/*/' ') into an overall search strategy, e.g. ('dementia') AND ('assistive technology' OR 'tracking device').
2. Record these terms in your search record.

Search and test

1. Open a database and investigate the 'help' and 'searching' sections. Find answers to questions such as how this database differs from others; how it uses Boolean operators; whether it uses UK English or American English; or whether it contains an index or taxonomy.
2. Run your first free text broad search and scan the results. Are they what you expected? Too many? Too few? Try the moderate search using truncation (*) or exact (' '). How does that affect your results?
3. Investigate the taxonomy and create a search using that. Scan the results. You might need to run a few free text searches on just one term if you find your results are off topic to see how the particular database uses that term, as you may be using the wrong one!
4. When you feel you have found the right term, run or combine your searches to give you a set of results.
5. Record the terms, the results and the number of those you think are relevant.

Collect and evaluate

1. Input your results into your reference management system.
2. Create inclusion and exclusion criteria, and screen your results against them.
3. Put all of the 'includes' together in preparation for evidence assessment.

They can also, as in the case of ASSIA and SCO, enable RSS feeds for your search strategies that email you when relevant content is indexed in the database system.

Each database is different, so take some time to consult the 'help' section, which will provide you with details about how to search within the database and how it uses Boolean terms within it. I advise you to sign up to each database's internal storage (which is free) such as ASSIA's 'my research' section, or to use SCO's advanced search. However, I would advise against using this as the only place you save your searches as, if you leave a database for any period of time and have not saved your search strategy, it may be lost. Always remember to record it in your search record as the master copy.

After completing searches across a variety of sources, which may have entailed additional searching such as reference harvesting (where you find an article on topic and you source the references contained within it), you will now need to create inclusion and exclusion criteria (see Box 2.8, for an example) to ensure that you obtain the data you want in relation to your original question.

You can create inclusion and exclusion criteria relevant to your enquiry, but this must be tested against some of your abstracts to see if they are fit for purpose. Whatever format in which you decide to have your inclusion and exclusion criteria, you must carry out exactly the same process for each abstract, starting at (1) through to (7). Of course, you may exclude at (1) and have no need to carry on with the whole set because it is excluded. However, if you do not exclude at (1), you should continue until either you exclude at (2), (3), (4), (5) or (6) or select for inclusion those studies that are deemed appropriate (7) for full text retrieval at the end of the process.

'Exclude scope' (5) is usually the section to be specific about the type of content you want from your studies and in relation to our scenario. I would exclude studies if the abstract did not contain dementia, technology and wandering. The best way to do this in your reference management system is to use one of the unused fields to enter your decision on each record using your seven points. It might be best to run a quality assurance test on the inclusion and exclusion criteria to see whether they are fit for purpose and, if this is not the case, then revisit (5) and amend them accordingly.

When I have screened all of my results by abstract and title, and coded them using my inclusion and exclusion criteria, I should have a final set of 'includes'. There is no industry standard to an ideal number of includes, but around 30–40 is the most manageable amount for a student or a practitioner to handle. Any larger and you will be overwhelmed in the next part of the process, where you will need to judge each piece of evidence against a set quality criteria, which is discussed in Chapter 3.

Conclusion

Searching social care data can be overwhelming due to its complexity. However, it may help if you remember the following rules:

- Lack of standardization in classification within social care databases means you have to approach searching in a standardised way. You should test what databases are doing and why they are doing it, especially in relation to results using combinations or limiters.
- You can utilise two types of searching for social care evidence:

◎ *broadly* – across a variety of sources (*preliminary search*);
◎ *focused* – systematically search across bibliographic databases using relevant classification (*systematic search*).

- As an evidence-based social worker, you will need to be aware of bias within your search, the results and your own thoughts.
- You need to consult a wide variety of sources, follow a structured process and record it every step of the way. Also, do not forget to report this process within the methodology section of your final report.

FURTHER READING

Aveyard, H. (2014) *Doing a Literature Review in Health and Social Care: A Practical Guide*, 3rd edn (Maidenhead: Open University Press). This practical guide takes you through the process of a literature review in health and social care, and provides many helpful definitions and tips for searching health and social care evidence more broadly.

Clapton, J. (2010) *Bibliographic Databases for Social Care Searching. Knowledge and Research Report 34* (London: Social Care Institute for Excellence). This research report evaluates the sources of social care data, and describes search techniques and approaches in locating good-quality social care evidence.

Grayson, L. and Gomersall, A. (2003) *A Difficult Business: Finding the Evidence for Social Science Reviews*, ESRC UK Centre for Evidence Based Policy and Practice Working Paper 19. This working paper highlights the complexities of searching for social science data, and the differences in health and social care evidence collection.

Webber, M. (2011) *Evidence-Based Policy and Practice in Mental Health Social Work* 2nd edn (Exeter: Learning Matters). This book provides comprehensive information on searching for mental health data and the use of evidence-based approaches for mental health social workers.

CHAPTER 3

Appraising the Quality of Evidence

Sarah Carr and Lisa Bostock

Introduction

Appraising the quality of research evidence is not simply an academic exercise for scholars undertaking research reviews; it genuinely matters for social work practice. As Macdonald (2003: 12) has argued: 'This is not just a sterile academic debate. It matters. When we intervene in people's lives we have a responsibility to try to get it right'.

Social workers need to know about the quality of research to ensure it is reliable to use to inform their practice. They also need to engage critically with research to ascertain whether it is relevant for the practice issue with which they are dealing, or the question they need answers to. Gough (2007: 213) is clear that practitioners need to make 'judgements of the quality and relevance of the research evidence considered' when using it to inform decision-making, or to answer a particular practice question. Elsewhere, it has been said that 'critical appraisal skills are about making sense of research, and recognising its strengths and weaknesses in order to decide whether it is trustworthy and relevant enough to use within practice' (Research in Practice for Adults, 2013).

In order to understand some of the background to this activity, we will start by briefly exploring some critical perspectives on knowledge, evidence and research in social work, and then go on to look at some of the practical frameworks and a detailed case study of critical appraisal practice.

Knowledge, evidence and research in social work: a broader critical picture

As discussed in Chapter 1, research needs to be recognised as a resource that is produced, appraised and applied in particular contexts. Research evidence also interacts with other factors and influences the overall decision-making process; it is not just about finding out 'what works'. Although they may suggest different ways of appraising research evidence, most experts agree that evidence and knowledge in social work is complex and needs some form of classification to sort it into different types, many of which will combine with each other to indicate 'what works, for whom, in what circumstances, in what respects and how'. In their work on developing a collective consensus on what counts as knowledge for social work, the Social Care Institute for Excellence (SCIE) mapped out the following five types of knowledge source for social work (Pawson *et al.*, 2003):

- organisational;
- practitioner;
- policy community;
- research;
- user and carer.

The interplay of these different knowledge sources is important for evidence-based practice in social work, as Sackett *et al.* (1996) noted for the equivalent in medicine. For example, Long *et al.* (2006) argued that social work policy and practice is 'informed and influenced by multiple sources of knowledge. These range from the tacit, experiential knowledge arising from everyday practice, to the knowledge embodied in rules and regulations, to the formal, codified knowledge arising from research into social work issues' (p. 208). Elsewhere, Lewis (2001) contests that 'researchers, practitioners and service users need to find ways of working together in order to strengthen the way in which [research] findings are interpreted' (p. 6). Sometimes, it is necessary to draw on many sources of knowledge because there may be no sufficiently relevant and good-quality research evidence about 'what works'.

Given the complexities, it is acknowledged that evidence-based approaches to social work can be challenging to achieve (Macdonald and Sheldon, 1998). Lewis outlined the following broader issues to bear in mind when appraising research as part of evidence-based social work:

- The nature of social [work] interventions makes it difficult to obtain clear evidence.
- The difficulty of knowing what evidence to look for – evidence of what? – makes understanding of causal relationships important.
- Much research is 'of the wrong kind' – that is, it focuses on problems not on evaluating solutions.
- Facts do not speak for themselves – findings have to be interpreted to produce evidence.
- Research evidence needs to be combined with practice wisdom and user experience to create knowledge. (Lewis, 2001: 5–6)

The social work frontline, particularly people who use services, have made important contributions to the critical debates about appraising and using research in practice. One of the main problems has been summed up in this way:

> Historically ... the knowledge base of social work has been derived from social research conducted using traditional methods of inquiry which claim to be 'objective', 'neutral' and 'value-free' and to produce knowledge which is independent of the persons carrying out the research. (Beresford, 2000: 499)

Beresford and others argue that not only does this devalue experiential knowledge, but also that research cannot be truly objective because it is undertaken by individuals who have values and opinions which may influence their work without being transparent (Beresford, 2003; Tew *et al.*, 2006). For this and other reasons, transparency and explicitness are important aspects of research reporting, and are crucial for engaging in the appraisal of and making judgements about the relevance and reliability of the evidence:

> Different people will make different decisions. This is fine as long as it is clear to the reader what decisions have been made ... so that they can make an informed decision about relevance. (Macdonald, 2003: 5)

Assessing and appraising research studies: principles, frameworks and techniques

Despite the critical debates, experimental research methodology used in (quantitative) clinical studies, such as the randomised controlled trial (RCT), is still thought to be the most rigorous and robust way to produce the most reliable findings. Systematic reviews, which are positioned at the top of the evidence hierarchy (see Chapter 1), are systematically conducted and replicable reviews of experimental studies such as RCTs (see Macdonald, 2003). Classic critical appraisal hierarchies in medicine are based on study designs derived from ways of appraising research for systematic reviews (Crombie, 1996) generally appear in the following order:

1. systematic reviews and meta-analyses;
2. RCTs;
3. cohort studies, case-controlled studies;
4. surveys;
5. case reports;
6. qualitative studies;
7. expert opinion;
8. anecdotal opinion.

(Aveyard, 2011: 62)

The nature of social work research does not always lend itself to a hierarchical approach based on research design. It is possible that a study with a design lower down the hierarchy has findings that are more reliable or relevant than a poorly-conducted RCT:

> Research methodologies high up the hierarchy will not be the best way to approach every research question and it is not right to denigrate research methodologies lower down the hierarchy if they are the best way to answer your research question. (Aveyard, 2011: 62–3)

PRACTICE REFLECTION 3.1

Research appraisal

Social work students and practitioners should begin research appraisal by determining the question they need answering and then seeking the right research to answer that question, as Aveyard (2011: 67) recommends:

- You are likely to encounter a wide range of information that is relevant to your research question.
- It is important to identify types of information that you will need to answer your research question.
- It is useful to develop your own hierarchy of evidence to determine what evidence is most relevant to your ... question.

If you have not already done so in Practice reflection 2.1, reflect on your practice and create a practice question that you wish to answer through existing research.

In order to help students and practitioners appraise research and develop question-specific hierarchies, experts have developed assessment frameworks and sets of questions to support the critical appraisal of studies. In response to some of the challenges involved in appraising research evidence for social work, SCIE developed an assessment framework based on a set of generic standards, rather than conforming to a particular evidence hierarchy based on study design. The purpose is:

> The enablement of constructive reflection of the quality of a particular piece of evidence ... critically, it is not about privileging one source of knowledge over another. ... Methodological quality, which is the dominant consideration in the research community, cannot be the only criterion. (Long *et al.*, 2006: 209–10)

It sets out the following standards for research quality assessment:

- transparency: Is it open to scrutiny?
- accuracy: Is it well-grounded?
- purposivity: Is it fit for purpose?
- utility: Is it fit for use?
- propriety: Is it legal and ethical?
- accessibility: Is it intelligible?
- specificity: Does it meet source-specific standards?

(Adapted from Pawson *et al.*, 2003: 67)

These standards form questions which practitioners can use to engage critically with relevant studies. They are based on standards set out for the appraisal of education evaluation research in the United States, the main headings of which are described as: 'utility ... feasibility ... propriety ... accuracy' (Long *et al.*, 2006: 209).

BOX 3.1 APPRAISAL QUESTIONS

Area for assessment	Appraisal question
Findings	How credible are the findings?
Findings	How has knowledge/understanding been extended by research?
Findings	How well does the evaluation address its original aims and purpose?
Findings	Scope for generalization: how well is this explained?
Findings	How clear is the basis of the evaluative appraisal?
Design	How defensible is the research design?
Sample	How well-defended is the sample design/target selection of cases/documents?
Sample	How clear is the basis of evaluative appraisal?
Data collection	How well was the data collection carried out?
Analysis	How well has the approach to, and formulation of, the analysis conveyed?
Analysis	Contexts of data sources – how well are they retained and portrayed?
Analysis	How well has the diversity of perspective and content been reported?
Analysis	How well has detail, depth and complexity of the data been conveyed?
Reporting	How clear are the links between data, interpretation and conclusions?
Reporting	How clear and coherent is the reporting?
Reflexivity and neutrality	How clear are the assumptions/theoretical perspectives/values that have shaped the form and output of the evaluation?
Ethics	How clear and coherent is the reporting?
Auditability	How adequately has the research process been documented?

Source: Adapted from Spencer *et al.* (2003): 9–15.

Elsewhere, quality assessment has been split into three concepts: validity (are the results true?); reliability (what are the results?) and applicability (can we generalise the results?) (Booth *et al.*, 2011).

A similar way to appraise research is to use a 'weight of evidence' judgement, which was developed by Gough and colleagues at the Evidence for Policy and Practice Information and Co-ordinating Centre (EPPI-Centre) in London (Gough, 2007). This approach was developed as part of their systematic research review process as a means by which individually to appraise a number of studies to see how they then collectively can answer a research question. It can be usefully applied to practice questions or problems, using the following weight of evidence appraisal criteria:

- the *trustworthiness* of the results judged by the quality of the study within the accepted norms for undertaking the particular type of research design used (methodological quality);

- the *appropriateness* of the use of that study design for addressing your research review or practice question;
- the *relevance* of focus of the research for answering your research review or practice question;
- judgement of *overall weight of evidence* based on the assessments made for each of the criteria A–C.

Another helpful related appraisal framework is that developed for qualitative research at the former Government Chief Social Researcher's Office (Spencer *et al.*, 2003). The framework has both guiding principles and appraisal questions. Similarly, the four central underpinning principles are that the research should be: 'contributory ... defensible in design ... rigorous in conduct ... credible in claim' (Spencer *et al.*, 2003: 7). These principles have been used to define 18 appraisal questions to help with assessment and are reproduced in Box 3.1, together with the part of the study report where they need to be applied.

Overall, quality assessment prompt questions which can be used to interrogate a study have been summarised by Dixon-Woods *et al.* (2006) as follows:

- Are the aims and objectives of the research clearly stated?
- Is the research design clearly specified and appropriate for the aims and objectives of the research?
- Do the researchers provide a clear account of the process by which their findings were reproduced?
- Do the researchers display enough data to support their interpretations and conclusions?
- Is the method of analysis appropriate and adequately explained?

PRACTICE REFLECTION 3.2

Assessing research evidence

Making an assessment of the quality of research evidence is essential for social workers, whether using it to inform decision-making or to answer a particular practice question but, as with other skills, takes time and practice to develop. Frameworks and assessment questions are very important for successful critical appraisal of research studies to inform social work practice, but, as Sackett *et al.* (1996) and others have argued, practitioners will also apply their own judgement about research. The practitioner's or student's critical relationship to, and interpretation of, research studies being used to inform their work is arguably a contribution to making evidence (Lewis, 2001).

Reflect on the skills you have that can be utilised in the critical appraisal of research. As you read this chapter, consider what extra skills you may require and think about how you can develop them.

Assessing and appraising research to inform practice: a case example of evaluating joint working between health and social care

This section presents a case study example of research evidence appraisal for a SCIE research review that was undertaken by one of the authors of this chapter in partnership with two academic experts. If you are undertaking a literature review for a research project, either as part of a social work programme or as a piece of practice research, this example will show you the processes for critiquing and combining literature to identify a gap in the existing research evidence base, and help you to justify your proposed research question. It also demonstrates the application of critical appraisal frameworks (pp. 47–9) in practice and how they are used to interpret the strength of the evidence base.

Each stage of the review was developed in line with systematic review methodology established by SCIE (Rutter *et al.*, 2010). It shows how studies were selected and appraised using a framework designed by the authors, and the technique used to extract data as relevant to the review questions. In a literature review, all the available evidence on any given topic is retrieved and critically appraised, so that an overall picture of what is known about the topic is achieved (Aveyard, 2011). The value of an individual piece of research is greater if seen in the context of other literature on the same topic and so can potentially be recognised as more relevant to practice development.

SCIE produces literature reviews ('research briefings') in order to inform policy and practice. This case study is based on a research briefing reviewing the evidence on integrated working between health and social care services (Cameron *et al.*, 2012). Given the importance of integrated working between health and social care for outcomes for service users, the aim of our research briefing was to give people who provide and use social care services an overview of the research evidence for integrated working by identifying and systematically describing the following:

- different models of working between health and social care services at the strategic, commissioning and operational levels;
- evidence of effectiveness and cost-effectiveness;
- factors promoting and obstacles hindering the success of these models;
- the perspectives of people who use services and their carers.

The briefing updated an original systematic research review by Cameron and Lart (2003) that reported on the factors that promote and hinder joint working between health and social care. In line with the original review, papers were only included in this briefing if they referred to an actual, rather than proposed, model of joint working, which had been evaluated, and included primary data in the paper.

Papers reported evaluations published before 2000 were excluded from this briefing but papers published before are reported in Cameron and Lart (2003). Taken together, the findings provide a 30-year overview of UK-based evaluations of joint working in health and social care, thereby providing a robust assessment of what works best from the perspectives of frontline staff and their managers and, where evidence is available, people who use services.

Forty-six papers were identified, reporting 30 separate studies. The majority of studies (n = 22) evaluated services for older people, while six looked at mental health services and two papers looked at services for both older people and people with mental health problems.

Models identified were focused on frontline practice, with the majority of papers reporting evaluations of multi-agency teams, placements of individual staff across agency boundaries, single assessment processes (SAP), provision of intermediate care and use of pooled budgets.

Appraising the research studies

Critical appraisal is the structured process of examining a piece of research in order to determine its strengths and weaknesses and, therefore, the weight it should be given. SCIE undertakes evidence assessments when the research briefing includes policy and practice questions about the effectiveness of a specific intervention and where there is evidence from research studies of effec-

BOX 3.2 EXAMPLE OF EVIDENCE TABLE ON INTEGRATED WORKING

Data extraction headings	Explanation
Data extractor	If more than one reviewer, name of person extracting the data from the paper
Study reference details	Author, date, title and reference details
Summary	A brief description of the study, including study type and aims; sometimes, the abstract from the study is recorded here
Evaluation method	Describe the study methods, including setting or population; was there a control group; what length of follow-up for impact; any sense of including service user as well as professional/provider perspectives
Model of joint working	Identify and describe the model of joint working, e.g. multi-agency working, care management
Effectiveness evidence	Identify and describe what outcomes were measured
Costs and cost-effectiveness	Identify and describe costs and cost-effectiveness of service, where data available
Factors that promote integrated working	Identify and describe the factors that promote integrated working
Factors that hinder integrated working	Identify and describe the factors that hinder integrated working
Service user and carer views	Identify and describe the perspectives of people who use services and their carers
Quality appraisal	See note below
Reviewer notes	Any observations by the reviewer

tiveness. Effectiveness studies are those which use a recognised measure of outcome and, ideally, include comparison with a population who did not receive the intervention. In the hierarchy of evidence discussed earlier and in Chapter 1, such research might include cohort studies or case-controlled studies. The most useful intervention studies will include an economic evaluation (based on these outcomes) and evidence (often qualitative) on the accessibility and acceptability of the intervention.

In order to achieve the systematic appraisal of the evidence, evidence tables are developed with an agreed set of appraisal questions to guide assessment of the evidence. Evidence tables are designed to extract information about the study in line with the research review question (see Box 3.2). The aim of the evidence table is rigorously to record and appraise the strength of evidence from across a wide range of papers. It is a systematic way of posing questions about each piece of research and capturing it in tabular form for future data synthesis, as well as allowing for future replication of the research review. Box 3.2 outlines the headings used in our review of integrated working, reflecting the aims and objectives of the review. Data extraction involves systematically working through the headings, extracting data from each study included for review.

Quality appraisal

For the requirements of this research review, the authors agreed generic quality assessment criteria as described in SCIE's guidelines on systematic reviews (Rutter *et al.*, 2010). These criteria are similar to Dixon-Woods *et al.*'s (2006) summary of quality assessment prompt questions, but also include questions on outcome measures, ethics, research findings and service user and carer perspectives as set out in SCIE guidance. The prompt questions are designed to assess both the trustworthiness of study findings and their relevance to the aims of the review itself. Questions include:

- Are the aims and objectives of the research clearly stated?
- Is the design appropriate to the aims of the research and methods clearly explained?
- Have research ethics issues been considered?
- Is there a clear explanation of the outcome measures? For example, what outcomes have been defined and by whom?
- Is the method of analysis appropriate and adequately explained?
- Do the researchers discuss their interpretations and conclusions?
- Has the study captured service user and carer perspectives?

Example of using an evidence table in practice

Extracting data from research papers can be time-consuming. This is because the aim of the evidence table is to provide a systematic overview of the evidence, extracted around themes that are relevant to the objectives of the review being conducted. They are designed to be comprehensive, meaning that the reviewer should not need to return to the original paper at analysis stage. While the data extraction stage can feel quite lengthy, analysis is greatly enhanced by the accessible nature of the data, allowing themes to be identified and synthesised quickly. Making an assessment of the methodological trustworthiness of individual research studies ensures transparency and allows the reviewer to make an overall assessment of the quality of the evidence base.

Box 3.3 is a short summary of one evidence table used for our review of integrated working. The study by Le Mesurier and Cumella (2001) is a comparative evaluation of a social worker based in a primary care setting with her equivalents in an area team. It is a valuable example of one model of integrated working that we described as a 'placement scheme', because the social worker was attached to a GP practice. Unusually, this study compares costs of the different types of service. The study provides useful insights into the effectiveness of the placement scheme across a series of areas, highlighting improved access to social care for older people via the GP-attached social worker compared with referrals via the area team, as well as offering explanations about the factors that promote and hinder this model of joint working. However, trustworthiness of findings is compromised by poor reporting of the methods. The reporting methods found in this paper are not untypical of the types of small-scale, local evaluations identified in the review.

Arriving at an assessment of methodological trustworthiness is necessarily interpretative, meaning that judgements are based on 'evaluating the quality of this type of evidence by those who generally use and produce it' (Gough, 2007: 222). In order to make such judgements, the series of questions described above (p. 52) were worked through to interrogate the methodological soundness of the evidence presented. The assessments were based on what one would expect to see explained about how a study was conducted. In other words, assessment of quality is based on knowledge of research methods as appropriate to the aims of the study being reviewed. It is also based on the extent to which the study addressed the aims of the review itself.

Given the interest in evaluation studies, first, a specific question on outcome measures was agreed. This focused on who defines the outcomes (researchers, practitioners or service users) and what difference this makes. Second, our question on interpretation of findings was designed to assess whether authors discuss their results and attempt to explain the factors that promote and hinder integrated working. Third, and very importantly, we wished to understand the extent to which evaluations collect the views of service users and carers, something that we considered crucial to the understanding of the effectiveness of joint and integrated working. Having identified a lack of intervention studies, the aim of critical appraisal in this review was not to exclude papers on the basis of quality. Rather, the systematic review of methodological soundness and relevance of research findings to the aims of the review enabled us to draw conclusions about the overall picture of the quality of the research evaluation evidence in this significant area for policy and practice.

BOX 3.3 EXAMPLE EVIDENCE TABLE

Data extractor: Lisa Bostock

Study reference: Le Mesurier, N. and Cumella, S. (2001) 'The Rough Road and the Smooth Road: Comparing Access to Social Care for Older People via Area Teams and GP Surgeries', *Managing Community Care*, 9(1): 7–13.

Summary: Small-scale evaluation of a local initiative that compares the process of accessing social care for older people via a social worker attached to a GP surgery with access via a duty service and area team.

Evaluation method: Study based on comparing data from social worker's log with computerised and other records of activity of social workers in the area team. Interviews with staff but not service users and carers.

Model of joint working: Placement scheme.

Effectiveness evidence: Placement scheme described as more effective in outcomes for staff including more manageable workload and improved inter-professional contact; improved outcomes for service users included rapid referral and assessment and improved service quality.

Costs and cost effectiveness: GP-attached social worker made less use of permanent residential or nursing home, and greater use of respite facilities for older people with more severe disabilities than local area team.

Factors that promote joint working: Improved strategic support; clarity of roles and responsibilities; strong frontline management and professional support, and improved information-sharing and access to IT systems.

Factors that hinder joint working: Some concerns about loss of social work identity; and lack of cover when social worker on leave.

Service user and carer views: Not included.

Quality appraisal:
Aims and objectives are clearly stated. The study aimed to assess the effectiveness of a single social worker attachment to a GP surgery compared with 'usual care' provided by an area team.

The *comparative design* is appropriate to the aims of the research, but study design description limited to one paragraph. No response rate is reported.

Study predates requirement for *Research Ethics Committee* (REC) approval. Ethical issues are not discussed.

Outcome measures are not articulated within the methods section.

There is no explanation of *data analysis* within the methods section.

There is a *good discussion* of the factors contributing to the success of the placement scheme, with more limited comment on the factors that hinder this model of joint working.

Service user and carer perspectives are not included.

Reviewer notes: Study suggests that placement schemes are a more effective means for older people to access social care. However, methodological trustworthiness undermined by poor reporting of methods and lack of clear outcome measures. Small-scale nature of the study limits generalizability but authors recognise that an in-depth programme of research is needed to compare schemes across different locations and identify more clearly the mechanisms inhibiting access to social care for older people via local teams as well as factors that contribute to successful GP practice-based social work.

Source: Le Mesurier and Cumella (2001).

PRACTICE REFLECTION 3.3

Evidence tables

When conducting reviews of the evidence to support policy and practice development, evidence tables are an effective way of extracting and organizing the data that is relevant to your question(s). They provide a systematic method for summarizing, interpreting and appraising findings. Have you used an evidence table before when conducting literature reviews? If not, why not find a piece of research relevant to your practice question and use an evidence table to extract data from it systematically. How useful did you find this process? What difficulties, if any, did you encounter?

The research review findings and implications for practice

Having completed data extraction, the next stage was to bring these together from all the papers in order to address the review question(s). While part of this process is to summarise the findings into manageable amounts, the aim is to interpret the results. According to Fingeld (2003), the goal is to 'produce a new and integrative interpretation of findings that is more substantive than those resulting from individual investigation' (p. 894). This is why critical appraisal is so important; it enables us to interpret the strength and limitations of the evidence base to produce an overall view of a particular topic and thereby support practice development.

Using the data extraction template (Boxes 3.2 and 3.3) in our review of integrated working, we were able to appraise the research evidence and identify the findings that now follow.

Evidence of effectiveness

Assessment of effectiveness is based on the evaluation of how a policy or intervention is implemented, the effects it had, for whom, how and why (Her Majesty's Treasury, 2011). However, not all evaluations included in the review reported data in this way. Some studies were descriptive, providing no clear data on effectiveness, and others did not define outcome measures, or reported outcomes that were unrelated to the evaluation. Few studies were comparative in design, or offered a before and after analysis, making it difficult to assess whether an intervention had been a success. This difficulty is compounded by differences in the models of joint working and the range of working arrangements identified, differences in study design, as well as the complexities of comparing services for two large and heterogeneous service user groups (older people and people with mental health problems).

Despite these limitations, trends in the data were evident. For example, improvements in quality of life, health, well-being and coping with everyday living were reported for users of services in a number of studies (e.g. Banerjee *et al.*, 2007; Clarkson *et al.*, 2011). However, in studies using a comparative design, assessing different types of integrated and non-integrated care, no significant differences, or only marginal differences, were reported (e.g. Davey *et al.*, 2005; Trappes-Lomax *et al.*, 2006). Studies evaluating initiatives designed to avoid inappropriate admission to acute or residential care found that they did reduce inappropriate admissions (Beech *et al.*, 2004; Kaambwa *et al.*, 2008), while a study of rapid response teams suggested that such services can have an important role in supporting people to remain in their own home (Brooks, 2002). Despite these positive findings the evidence suggests that the organisation of service does not appear to improve the likelihood of living in the community. Instead, need and access to support at home are key factors (Clarkson *et al.*, 2011).

Costs and cost-effectiveness evidence

Some evidence on the cost of services was identified, but no evidence on cost-effectiveness was found in our searches. This meant that we had no means of assessing the costs and benefits to service users and carers of integrated care versus standard care, or different types of integrated services.

Factors that promote and hinder joint working

Three broad themes were used to organise the factors that support or hinder joint working: organisational issues, cultural and professional issues, and contextual issues. There is significant overlap between factors, with many of the organisational factors that promote joint working hindering collaboration when insufficient attention is paid to their importance. Key factors include: clarity of aims and objectives, communication and information sharing, and roles and responsibilities. Studies exploring the establishment of integrated services or systems consistently report operational difficulties that originate from a lack of appreciation of the intentions of these initiatives, particularly among health professionals.

Service user and carer views

The voice of service users and carers remains largely absent. Their views are not routinely collected in the evaluations reviewed, which makes it almost impossible to comment on the outcomes that matter to the people who use services, users and carers, who are frequently treated as a homogeneous group. This makes it difficult to understand the impact of integrated services on groups who may have different and sometimes competing needs.

Study limitations and conclusions

Studies largely focus on small-scale evaluations of local initiatives that are often of poor quality and poorly reported. Details about working practices and arrangements are often limited and/or the authors fail to discuss the factors that promote and hinder joint working. Few studies are comparative in design, so differences between 'usual care' and integrated care are not assessed. Small-scale, 'boutique evaluations' of joint working make it difficult to draw firm conclusions about the effectiveness of UK-based integrated health and social care services.

> PRACTICE REFLECTION 3.4
> **Research studies**
> The practitioner's or student's critical relationship with, and interpretation of, research studies being used to inform their work is arguably a contribution to making evidence. Critically appraise the study from which you extracted data and consider how it can be used to inform your practice.

Conclusion

This chapter has introduced some of the frameworks and techniques for critically appraising research studies for research reviews and for supporting evidence-based practice. It has also presented a detailed account of a real-life case example of assessing and appraising studies for a research review aimed at answering practice questions. The discussion has shown that it is important to examine both the quality and relevance of the research in relation to the question or problem in hand. Research studies may be important for evidence-based practice, but they are only one social work knowledge source, and critical engagement by practitioners and students with research can ensure a vital relationship between research and practice.

FURTHER READING

Below is a list of the key websites and online resources for critical appraisal and evidence-based social care and health that can help to extend your understanding of the ideas presented in this chapter.

The Evidence for Policy and Practice Information and Co-ordinating Centre (EPPI-Centre), Social Science Research Unit, Institute of Education, University of London:
http://eppi.ioe.ac.uk/cms/

National Institute for Health Research (NIHR) School for Social Care Research:
http://www.sscr.nihr.ac.uk/

London School of Economics and Political Science Personal Social Services Research Unit (PSSRU):
http://www.lse.ac.uk/LSEHealthAndSocialCare/aboutUs/PSSRU/home.aspx

Centre for Evidence Based Medicine, Oxford University, resource directory:
http://www.cebm.net/?o=1016

University of York Centre for Reviews and Dissemination:
https://www.york.ac.uk/inst/crd/index.htm

The Campbell Collaboration Resource Centre:
http://www.campbellcollaboration.org/resources/research.php

The Cochrane Collaboration:
http://www.cochrane.org/

Social Care Institute for Excellence (SCIE) Managing Knowledge and Research Resources:
http://www.scie.org.uk/topic/developingskillsservices/managingknowledgeresearch

Research in Practice for Adults:
http://www.ripfa.org.uk/

Research in Practice (Children and Families):
http://www.rip.org.uk/

National Elf Service Evidence-Based Health and Social Care:
http://www.nationalelfservice.net/

British Library Social Welfare Portal:
http://socialwelfare.bl.uk/

CHAPTER 4

Using Evidence to Inform Assessments

Mark Hardy

Introduction

Assessment is a crucial 'sense-making' activity which sets the parameters for subsequent stages of the social work process, including decision-making, planning and direct intervention. However, how practitioners ought best *undertake* assessment – how they should go about it – is not necessarily straightforward. There are ongoing debates regarding whether assessment is best conceived of according to a broadly 'artistic' or 'scientific' logic. Consequently, the role that research evidence might play in the process of assessment can sometimes be unclear.

This chapter will review these issues as they apply to needs and risk assessment, particularly in statutory social work settings such as child protection and mental health. I will explore what assessment is; differing approaches to assessment, including both subjective clinical approaches and objective actuarial and structured approaches; their respective strengths and limitations; their association with evidence-based practice and 'the rise of risk', as well as claims that recent developments in practice have fundamentally affected the nature and function of assessment, and so change the nature of social work itself.

I will also specify what the integration of research evidence into practice actually involves. Research represents a crucial source of knowledge that practitioners might draw on to inform their assessments. Traditionally, however, formal sources of knowledge, such as research evidence, have been accorded relatively little significance in assessment practice. There is a strong case for encouraging better integration of evidence from research with other important sources of knowledge, and a specific skills base for doing so. Arguably, there are benefits for both social work and wider society in conceiving of and practising social work in ways that are more 'scientific' than has traditionally been the case. However, research findings represent just one of many sources of knowledge that social workers must synthesise when undertaking assessments, alongside service user and practitioner knowledge, as well as organisational and policy frameworks. I will therefore outline the basis for a 'knowledge-based' approach to assessment practice in which evidence and understanding from multiple sources are synthesised. I will conclude by making the case for critical pluralism, a pragmatic approach to assessment practice which offers potential in enabling practitioners to reconcile some of the tensions between traditional approaches and contemporary expectations.

Background

Social work is under sustained scrutiny. High-profile service failures across the 'domains' (Shaw *et al.*, 2010a) of social work have led to demands that professional assessments, and the judgements and decisions that follow on from these, be both as transparent and accurate as possible. These 'failures' are hardly novel, certain iconic 'cases' being known well beyond the distinct professional domains in which they arose (Butler and Drakeford, 2005). Neither are they necessarily limited to social work, as similarly high-profile and influential cases have occurred in criminal justice and health care (Fitzgibbon, 2011; Heyman *et al.*, 2010). However, the challenges which they pose for the legitimacy of social work agencies, whose failings often seem to be perceived as of a different nature and gravity to those of other agencies, are arguably distinct. Rightly or wrongly, service failures are regarded as indicative of a more generalised problem with the quality of judgements and decision-making by practitioners.

The case of Baby Peter in England represents perhaps the most potent recent example of what Epstein (1996) refers to as 'extreme failures' (p. 114) in social work (naturally, there have already been similar failures, and such failures continue in the future). It led to the establishment of the Social Work Taskforce to reform social work training and practice, which dovetailed with the Munro Review of Child Protection practice (Munro, 2011) and contributed to the establishment of the College of Social Work. Central to these developments are concerns over the status of the knowledge base on which the judgements and decisions of social workers are made regarding vulnerability and harm to others.

The expectation is that competent, well-trained professionals ought to be able, consistently and accurately, to identify and address need, and to differentiate between, and predict, low- and high-risk eventualities. But service failures suggest they do not always manage to achieve this. Munro concluded that the ability of social workers to make accurate judgements is hampered by the burdensome degree of both scrutiny and administration to which they are subject, which impact on the time available to spend with children and families gathering accurate information and developing potentially protective relationships. Consequently, practitioners often have to make judgements in far from ideal situations, based on less than full knowledge, compounding rather than alleviating the uncertainty that characterises the complex assessments they must undertake. Subsequent reforms have sought to strengthen the status of social work by equipping it to deal with the related issues of the quality of day-to-day practice, and the legitimacy of the profession.

PRACTICE REFLECTION 4.1

The challenges of decision making

Social workers are sometimes criticised for making poor-quality decisions. Do you think these criticisms are fair? Reflect on your practice and consider some of the challenges you encounter when making decisions.

Assessment

Assessment represents a key part of the social work process. But what does assessment actually mean and entail? There are book-length accounts defining and exploring assessment which seek to describe and proscribe the meaning and process of assessment in various areas of social work (e.g. Baker *et al.*, 2011; Beckett, 2010; Pincus and Minahan, 1973). Additionally, the precise format and contents of assessments vary by specialism, context, agency and function (useful overviews can be found in Barlow *et al.*, 2012; and Milner and O'Byrne, 2009).

In most social work agencies, practitioners are required to provide written assessments of service users. These assessments generally involve the identification and description of key social, individual and psychological factors at play in a particular situation in which a service user finds themselves, as well as analysis of, and an attempt to formulate an explanation for, what is going on and why. They represent attempts to make sense of particular situations and provide a basis for deciding whether and how best to intervene.

Since its inception, there have been debates within social work about the relationship between 'cause' and 'cure' (Cree, 2002; Wilson *et al.*, 2008), with assessment representing the means by which these causal relationships are identified, described, elaborated and untangled. As well as representing a discrete stage within the social work 'process' (Parker and Bradley, 2010), assessment itself comprises a number of elements, including information gathering, analysis, judgements and decision-making.

In social work, practitioners must make judgements and decisions constantly regarding all sorts of issues and problems, some commonplace, some more serious. When explicitly engaging in assessment, however, there are a number of related issues that their attention is focused on. First, what is going on in this particular situation? Second, what should be done about it? And underpinning each of these, what sources of information must be gathered, what processes should be followed in arriving at judgements, and what are the implications of those judgements for decisions regarding whether and how to intervene? These generic issues resonate across the practice-based disciplines. In psychology and medicine, for example, the terms 'case formulation' and 'diagnosis' are used to encapsulate similar processes. In social work, though, it does seem that the consequences of fallibility are regarded through a less sympathetic lens.

Assessment, then, is the process by means of which practitioners make sense of people and their environments, and the intersections between them. Crucially, although often portrayed as a particular stage, it ought to be conceived of as continuous. It is while they are engaged in the analysis of information that practitioners form views and opinions about the situation, character, motivation, responsibility and – sometimes – blameworthiness of those they are assessing. Consequently, it plays a very influential role in framing the extent, nature and content of future contact with potential service users. It is crucial that the basis on which these judgements, and the decisions which flow from them, are made are as accurate as possible, if what follows (intervention) is to be effective. But how do practitioners actually 'do' assessment? What information should practitioners gather? How should it be filtered, analysed and integrated in arriving at a conclusion? And how should the relationship between 'cause' and 'cure' be formulated in the less than straightforward sets of circumstances of which social work assessments seek to make sense?

PRACTICE REFLECTION 4.2

Information sources

When you have undertaken assessments, either at work or on placement, what sources of information did you draw on? How did you access these? And what did you do if, for whatever reason, there was a source of information that you were unable to access?

Although it is a crude dichotomy, here I will use the recognised distinction between 'artistic' and 'scientific' approaches to assessment (Holland, 2011) as a framework for illuminating various ways in which assessors might address these issues.

The 'art' of assessment

The idea that 'art' might function as a useful metaphor for understanding the nature of social work practice is enduring (Hudson, 2009; Martinez-Brawley and Zorita, 1998). Key to understanding its utility is its emphasis on the creative interaction between worker and service user as a necessary prerequisite for meaningful judgements regarding what is going on in a particular scenario, and how best to intervene. Priority is attached to the significance of the relationship between worker and client, and the creative, inter-subjective process in which they engage when they interact as the basis for the co-construction of meaning. Here, formal knowledge is accorded secondary status to that derived experientially through contact with, and a developing understanding of, the service user and their situation.

The idea of assessment as a form of subjective interpretation has been influential in social work. There is stress on the value of self or what the practitioner – and more recently, the service user – brings to this interaction. Creativity is privileged as a basis for the holistic interpretation of individuals and their circumstances and problems. Holism entails attention to all aspects of an individual's circumstances and functioning, both past and present, rather than to discrete elements of it. Assessments, then, are co-constructed via communication within relationships between practitioner and service users. Rather than representing an incidental add-on, knowledge derived through lived experience is privileged, a necessary precursor for what follows.

Although this is a seductive vision, 'artistic' approaches have inherent limitations. A lack of precision regarding processes of reasoning – how particular judgements are reached – leaves social work decision-making 'shrouded in mystery' (Sheppard, 2006: 170). Logically, judgements which are not founded on transparent processes of reasoning are difficult to justify and so do not lend themselves to defensible decision-making (Kemshall, 1998). Attempts to specify means by which accurate assessments are formulated are thus hampered, with implications for practitioners if and when something goes wrong, and, as a corollary, the credibility and legitimacy of agencies. As a result, there have been concerted efforts since the 1990s to shift social work away from its subjective 'artistic' bearings to approaches to assessment which are more objective, evidence-based and scientific.

The 'science' of assessment

Science represents a means of generating knowledge according to a particular method, entailing the generation and testing of theories in the form of hypotheses. The production of knowledge fills gaps and reduces uncertainty. Kirk and Reid (2002) argue that numerous historical innovations in social work can be regarded as low-level efforts to 'scientise' social work by shifting the basis of knowledge claims from informal to formal knowledge sources and therefore reducing uncertainty of prognosis, prediction and outcome. Examples include the use by nineteenth-century Charity Organisation Society caseworkers of home visits and interviews to generate knowledge which would enable them to differentiate between the 'deserving' and 'undeserving' on the basis of an evaluation of moral character (Cree, 2002).

Similarly, Mary Richmond's specification of the key principles of casework for practitioners to utilise in their practice represented a move towards the formalization of approaches to practice based on the application of empirical principles – those deemed to have been confirmed by experience as contributing to the achievement of positive outcomes. These were outlined in her influential *Social Diagnosis* (Richmond, 1917), which Soydan referred to as 'a scientific manual of methods' (1999: 90). The integration of psychoanalytic theory into casework, whereby social problems came to be seen as being underlain by the psychological needs of the individual, a contemporary 'acting out' of the enduring effects of experiences in early life which impacted on the establishment of bonds with primary care-givers, can also be regarded as a shift towards ensuring that social work practice is premised on a 'scientifically' derived knowledge base, albeit according to a formulation of science which is now outmoded.

Approaches to practice which draw on behavioural and cognitive psychology are more overt in their emphasis on the merits of scientific method; namely, 'rigour ... replicability and transferability' (Sheldon and Macdonald,

2008: 52). Relatedly, the ascendency of evidence-based practice reflects a belief that the methods of science represent a more appropriate means of determining whether and how to intervene than the 'vagaries' of practitioner preference (Shaw, 1999).

Although, then, there have clearly been efforts to place the judgements and decisions of social workers on a more scientific footing, at the same time there have been parallel, alternative approaches to sense-making in social work which privilege less prescriptive, more holistic approaches to assessment. For many decades, Biestek's (1957) version of 'casework' was arguably more influential as a framework for understanding human behaviour than any scientifically derived knowledge. This essentially humanist approach privileged the relationship between practitioner and client as the essence of casework, and the practice manifestation of social work's essential values, including acceptance, non-judgementalism, respect for the individual, confidentiality and self-determination. Here, the emphasis is on judgements and decisions as 'value driven', rather than knowledge-based (Hollis, 1964).

Later, efforts to develop unitary and integrated approaches to practice – in the wake of the Seebohm reforms in the early 1970s based on systems theory – highlighted the complexity of inter-relationships between variables in the social world which do not lend themselves to routinisation (Payne, 2002). The 'radical' social work of the late 1970s, meanwhile, drew on those early 'versions' of social work which argued that problems in particular communities were indicative of social disadvantage and that, as such, the resolution of social problems lay not in some form of individualised treatment based on the imprecise 'appliance of science' but, rather, in social reform, whether piecemeal – 'I give them money', as Parkinson (1970) put it – or more wholesale.

The discourse and practices of anti-discriminatory and anti-oppressive practice, which broaden out this structural critique to include more diverse aspects of difference than class, have become increasingly significant from the 1980s onwards. They are based on a principled commitment to emancipation and empowerment – rather than abstract, neutral formulations – and remain influential today (Dominelli, 2002; Lavalette, 2011). More recently, novel approaches informed by postmodern perspectives, such as solution focused approaches (de Shazer, 1985; 1988) and constructive social work (Parton and O'Byrne, 2000), subvert the traditional insistence that solutions are not possible without some causal formulation of the aetiology of the problem developed by empirical means. The future is not determined – and thus predictable – by the application of science, but can be co-constructed through a process of 'meaning-making' in which service user and practitioner explore strengths and possibilities.

Whereas conceiving of assessment as 'art' entails autonomous, individualised, relationship-based meaning-making, scientific approaches involve more objective processes, drawing on pre-defined sources of knowledge in accordance with consistent processes, rather than individual creativity. Whereas, traditionally, assessors utilised informal forms of knowledge as a basis for assessment, more structured approaches integrate other sources of knowledge. Clinical judgement entails practitioners arriving at a decision regarding what is going on and how to intervene on the basis of their knowledge of this 'case' or 'patient' gleaned from their own involvement in the case and interaction with the service user(s). Structured assessment tools, pro formas and actuarial scoring tools, by contrast, entail assessment according to pre-specified criteria, and the making and using of generalisations based on the accumulation of statistical data regarding other – albeit similarly categorised – people. In such circumstances, some feel, the centrality of the relationship between service user and worker is devalued, and in the process the professional endeavour takes on a wholly different nature. The ability of the practitioner and client to co-construct meaning on the basis of empathy and understanding is inhibited by an emphasis on compliance with pre-proscribed assessment frameworks involving form filling and tick boxes. None of these is a professional task, properly understood, and so lay the ground for a process of de-skilling in which unqualified staff increasingly undertake roles and responsibilities which previously were firmly within the province of the professional practitioner.

Of course, proponents of scientific approaches are unconvinced by arguments that assessment either ought or must be a subjective endeavour (Sheldon, 2001). They claim that emphasis on social work as art or craft has not served the profession or its users well. Generally, over time, and at the level of general populations, more systematic and procedurally led assessments would be more accurate in their appraisal of need and risk, and crucially, the intersection between the two. As I suggested earlier, this is an enduring debate, which has not, as yet, reached its conclusion. However, it is worth noting that it has also been suggested that assessment is neither art nor science. Instead, art and science, intuition and analysis, subjective and objective, are best represented as points on a continuum, with 'good enough' assessment practice as a hybrid amalgamation located somewhere towards the mid-point (Corby, 2006). This is a helpful way of thinking about these issues, which transcends undue polarisation of positions, and is increasingly recognised as a valuable component within assessment practice, particularly where concerns regarding risk are to the fore.

PRACTICE REFLECTION 4.3

Discerning the types of knowledge

Earlier, you identified various sources of information that you draw on in completing an assessment. Think about the different types of knowledge you have noted down. Consider which are informal and 'subjective', and which are formal and 'objective'. How easy is it to make this distinction? How does this distinction inform your social work assessments?

Risk assessment

While assessment itself, especially the assessment of need, has been a central activity of social work since its inception, risk assessment is arguably a relatively novel undertaking. Although the notion of 'risk' originally referred to the probability of any particular event occurring, in social work – and society more generally – it has come to refer to the likelihood of a negative outcome; for example a child death, a suicide, harm to a vulnerable adult, or the commission of a serious offence by a service user. While there are debates about whether 'the rise of risk' is a beneficial or detrimental development in social work (Warner and Sharland, 2010; Webb, 2006), social workers – particularly those working in statutory settings – are nevertheless required to assess the likelihood of such outcomes occurring in particular cases, and take appropriate action to prevent harm from occurring. How they might best do this remains contentious.

Histories of the development of approaches to risk assessment posit a shift from first-, through second-, to third-generation approaches. First-generation approaches are sometimes referred to as 'clinical' approaches. Clinical approaches to risk entail a practitioner making a judgement as to whether a particular service user poses a risk to themselves or others on the basis of their understanding of that person and their situation gleaned from the relationship they have established with that person and case records. These approaches have their roots in holistic, needs-based approaches to assessment, and links with those theories and models which emphasise the value of self and the relationship.

Second-generation actuarial approaches to risk assessment are very different. They utilise statistical analysis of relationships between social and psychological variables as the basis for the calculation of probabilities at a population level. They developed partly in response to the limitations of first generation approaches, particularly the potential for both bias and injustice inherent in wholly subjective processes.

Third-generation tools, meanwhile, seek to incorporate both clinical and actuarial information, on the basis that the advantages of each potentially outweigh their respective limitations when combined in this way. Although often represented as a natural progression from first- to third-generation, in reality these approaches have been used variably depending on the context in which practitioners are required to undertake risk assessments. Arguably, in UK settings, clinical approaches remain generally dominant. Occasionally, in some contexts, there are initiatives which seek to formalise the process of assessment – the Common Assessment Framework for Children and Young People (Department for Education, 2013a) and Care Programme Approach (Department of Health, 2008) in mental health services are notable examples. However, it is rare that these would go as far as to include an actuarial component. These are, however, present in areas of practice involving work with known offenders – domestic violence, youth justice, the probation service, forensic mental health and work with perpetrators, for example. Perhaps the most developed attempt to integrate the two is 'hybrid' needs/risk approaches which are used in work with offenders, especially in youth justice and the probation service. Outside of these settings, in more 'mainstream' social work – local authority children's and adult services, for example – risk assessments are commonly undertaken according to the format and expectations of structured assessment tools. To variable extents, these proscribe the format and content of assessments, and prompt practitioners to identify and draw on particular information. Generally, however, practitioners retain discretion regarding how much substance they attach to these, and the weight they attribute them in the process of analysis.

This shift away from first-generation approaches has attracted pointed criticism. Parton (2008), for example, has suggested that structured approaches, especially those which are IT based, herald a shift 'from the social to the informational', whereby assessments are based on spurious connections between disjointed fragments of data, rather than true knowledge or understanding gained via 'depth level' engagement with service users and their situations. Similarly, in relation to mental health, Rose (2005) highlights the potential in practice for risk 'factors' to mutate into markers of dangerousness as service users become bearers of immutable pathological dispositions. The work of Pithouse *et al.* (2012), meanwhile, points to systemic difficulties in work with children and families, where measures introduced to improve the quality of practice paradoxically distract practitioners from their principal tasks. Although academic critiques of this nature are now common, they are often polemical, based on a misunderstanding of what actuarial logic entails, disregard the role that clinical override plays in hybrid assessment tools and, consequently, do not necessarily reflect the views and perspectives of practitioners (Hardy, 2012; Stanford, 2008).

Notwithstanding the quite significant changes to assessment practice associated with a shift from 'art' to 'science', demands that social workers improve their practice have not receded. Service failures have highlighted the apparent inadequacy of social work decision-making and the seeming inability of practitioners to make correct judgements on some occasions. Cumulatively, such failings suggest a lack of professional competence, with a consensus that further change is required to improve the quality and accuracy of assessment practice. Central to this is renewed emphasis on the ways in which assessors' judgements and decisions might improve if the knowledge on which they were based was more substantive. There are longstanding debates concerning the nature of knowledge (see Evans and Hardy, 2010, ch. 1, for a flavour). Several 'varieties' of knowledge are generally acknowledged, broadly divided into informal and formal, with the latter including research knowledge. The incorporation of research knowledge into judgements and decision-making is increasingly seen as a means of potentially enhancing the quality of social work assessment practice. Both the Munro report (Munro, 2011) and curriculum guidance issued by the College of Social Work emphasise the need for social workers to develop and utilise skills in reasoning, making judgements and decisions, and the application of knowledge as a basis for good practice.

Research-minded assessment

Research-mindedness entails practitioners 'informing themselves of research findings and applying them to practice, and undertaking their own research where appropriate' (Humphries, 2008: 2). The success of research-mindedness as a strategy for improving assessment practice is dependent on various related components.

First, a commitment to embedding both research and evaluation within practice is required (see Shaw (2011), for an elaborate account of how individual practitioners might actualise this), which is dependent on rejection of the primacy of the 'decision-maker as expert' model.

Second, an awareness of ontological and epistemological perspectives is needed, so that the paradigmatic affiliations underpinning a knowledge claim can be taken into account when making sense of and integrating competing knowledge claims.

Third, critical appraisal skills (see Chapter 3) are required, which entail practitioners actively seeking, identifying and integrating research findings during the various stages of assessment (information gathering, judgement and decision-making) based on explicit recognition that research represents one of various sources of knowledge that need to be taken into account in decision-making. Critical appraisal 'is about deciding whether or not to use particular research findings to inform decision making within practice' (Newman *et al.*, 2005: 56). It is therefore of key importance in determining *whether* and, if so, *how* research is relevant and useful to practice, as the intention is that research findings should inform assessment, rather than determine its outcome.

Additionally, there is also merit in recognising the potential utility of assessment skills to social work research – and vice versa, as the skills which social workers utilise in their day-to-day practice (information collation, interviewing, critical thinking, analysis) parallel those which are important in social enquiry. Gilgun (1994) argues that research and practice fit each other like 'hand and glove' and that, consequently, social workers themselves are well placed to undertake practice-based research so as to further enhance knowledge and understanding. Practitioners who are 'research-minded', then, will not only contribute to their own professional development by continually engaging with and appraising research literature, but will also ensure that an up-to-date and evolving understanding of how knowledge in their area of practice is developing over time informs the ongoing development of the disciplinary knowledge base. Consequently, 'research minded practitioners are likely to be excellent social workers' (D'Cruz and Jones, 2004: 81).

> ## PRACTICE REFLECTION 4.4
> **Are you research-minded?**
> Reflecting on social work assessments you have undertaken, to what extent have you been 'research-minded'? How can you be more 'research-minded' when undertaking assessments?

Using research evidence in risk assessment

There is a clear logic to the account provided in Case scenario 4.1. However, although the potential that research might play in illuminating the causes and consequences of social problems is seductive, this should not be overstated. Research has real limitations, which undermine the ambitions of strong advocates of 'research-based' practice. The knowledge generated through research,

CASE SCENARIO 4.1

Karl

Karl has a diagnosis of bi-polar disorder. Since Karl was discharged from hospital 18 months ago, after being detained under the Mental Health Act following a suicide attempt, his care coordinator has been Charlie, a mental health social worker and Approved Mental Health Professional. Karl is currently stable, subject to the Care Programme Approach (CPA) and has ongoing contact with various professionals within the community mental health team (CMHT), including Charlie, who feels they have developed a good working relationship.

Previously, when he has become ill, Karl has drunk alcohol quite heavily. Although this does not cause his disorder, it sometimes appears to accentuate it. Karl's wife recently rang Charlie and told him that Karl's drinking has increased over the last few weeks, and that he is being defensive when asked about this, and sometimes quite verbally aggressive. She is clearly worried that Karl may deteriorate. When Charlie meets with him, however, Karl claims that his wife is over-reacting to very normal levels of recreational (rather than habitual) drinking, misinterpreting disagreement as aggression, and that their disagreements on this are indicative of issues within their relationship, which has not been wholly content for some time. He also says that his mood is stable. This seems plausible to Charlie, who is hardly abstentious himself.

As Karl's care coordinator, however, Charlie is required to make routine assessments of the risk that Karl may pose to himself or others. Intuitively, Charlie thinks that there may well be merit in Karl's view on this issue. However, he is also aware that there is research evidence that suggests there is a relationship between alcohol use and depression, and that alcohol use can precipitate incidents of mood disorder. He is therefore unsure whether or not this change of circumstances ought to lead him to alter Karl's risk status and/or the nature and extent of contact that the CMHT has with him.

In supervision, Charlie's manager suggests that he utilise a new piece of software that is being trialled by community-based forensic social workers in the office. Although a little unsure, Charlie uses the tool and inputs a range of information about Karl's history, current circumstances and psycho-social functioning. The assessment tool concludes that there is a medium to high risk of self-harm occurring in the next three months. It also makes clear that this is an estimation based on data drawn from other previous similar cases, and may well not apply in Karl's case. However, after discussion with his supervisor, another conversation with Karl and his wife, Charlie decides that there is enough new information to justify updating Karl's risk assessment to reflect this heightened risk.

At a subsequent multi-disciplinary meeting, it becomes clear that it was not just Karl's wife who has been concerned about his mood and behaviour. Their son's teacher had very recently made a safeguarding referral, having observed a couple of incidents that she described as 'drunken and abusive' behaviour around school drop-offs. As Karl routinely drove his son to school, this was clearly problematic. The corroboration of the outcomes of the assessment tool by the behavioural evidence provided by Karl's wife and their son's teacher provided Charlie with sufficient evidence to intervene and address Karl's drinking with him.

particularly research undertaken within the social sciences, including social work research, is rarely definitive and usually contested. In this, it reflects its subject matter – human beings – whose thoughts and feelings differentiate them from the more predictable variables that form the foci of the natural sciences. This applies irrespective of whether data is quantitative or qualitative, as neither is inherently sufficiently robust to render challenges to claims of quality redundant. Additionally, research criteria vary according to *inter* and *intra* disciplinary conventions. Consequently, when engaging in assessment, social workers concerned to do justice to the complexity of a client's reality, and to complete as accurate an assessment as possible, *of necessity* need not only to incorporate, but also to supplement research-based knowledge with that derived from other sources.

Knowledge-based assessment

Knowledge-based practice recognises that research knowledge is one of many 'sources' of knowledge that practitioners need to take into account in practice if they are to arrive at the fullest, and therefore the potentially most 'accurate' or 'truthful', approximation of a situation as a basis for determining how to intervene, as well as whether intervention is working. Pawson *et al.*'s (2003) taxonomy specifies that, when integrated, knowledge from practitioners, service users, organisations, policy and research helps to formulate as complete a picture as possible. Although there are sometimes tensions between these various sources, which crudely reflect the various stakeholders in social work, a genuinely knowledge-based approach to practice requires that the value of each of these sources be acknowledged and incorporated within key activities such as case formulation and decision-making.

This taxonomy emphasises not only that research has a crucial role to play in assessment practice, but also that there are strengths and limitations associated with all of these 'sources', including research. Complexity confounds knowledge because the precise specification of the relationships between multiple variables is by definition a difficult task; it is also one which, even where successful, does not necessarily lend itself to transferability of knowledge beyond the situation in which it was generated. Put another way, it does not tell us 'what works for whom, in what circumstances, and why' (Pawson and Tilley, 1997), thus rendering the generalisable application of evidence of possible effectiveness from one setting to another problematic (Kazi, 2003). Even high-quality research knowledge acquired through the development and application of well-formulated research design and robust methods, and which satisfies conventions and criteria for 'quality', such as validity, rigour and trustworthiness, cannot be assumed transferable (Hammersley, 2013), particularly within what Sheppard (2007) refers to as 'the practice paradigm'. It would therefore be foolish to suggest that research-based approaches to assessment, or any other strategy premised on certainty as a prerequisite, will directly impact on outcomes. Consequently, it is apparent that the difficulties assessors face in arriving at accurate judgements and making appropriate decisions have as much to do with the challenges entailed in synthesising diverse sources of knowledge as the perceived competence of either individual social workers or the profession as a whole.

Aware that research is one of several components of the wider knowledge base of the profession, each of which has strengths and limitations in specific situations or contexts, practitioners need to have two related skills. They require the ability, first, to assess relevance and utility in context; and, second, to synthesise knowledge generated from alternative sources according to fluid and variable conventions which nevertheless enable judgements and decisions to be both made and substantiated. This is a challenging task, by any standards, and helps us to understand the difficulties that practitioners sometimes face in seeking to undertake assessments which are timely, focused and accurate.

Rapprochement

It is potentially helpful to conceive of assessment as the analysis and synthesis of knowledge from multiple sources to inform judgements and decision-making in a useful manner. It emphasises that assessment is a complex, imprecise and difficult endeavour, not only in terms of what is entailed in the task, but also in doing it accurately. There are practical and theoretical challenges in integrating multiple sources of knowledge, particularly regarding how much weight should be attributed to each of these and on what basis. In social work agencies, there will be disputes at the 'borderlines', in differentiating the sorts of cases – people, situations, needs, risks – that ought to be dealt with 'scientifically' from those requiring a more artistic approach. Crudely, agencies will generally respond procedurally where knowledge is relatively certain by virtue of its 'scientific' status. Logically, this would imply that they would privilege 'artistic' approaches where knowledge is relatively uncertain. In reality, however, often they do not. But it is worth stressing that the case for *integrating* art and science is a strong one. This is because both actually rest on the same fundamental assumptions. By this, I mean that artistic processes mirror those that science – properly understood – also utilises. Scientists themselves utilise subjectivity, which arguably is built into scientific method itself. They use it in making decisions and they use it in theory development (Collins, 1985; Collins and Evans, 2007).

This understanding of science as something other than the objective production of incontestable knowledge is distant from the assumptions of evidence-based approaches to assessment, but congruent with those of knowledge-based practice. This recognition means that there is little merit in arguing that subjective and objective knowledge are in some way incommensurate, and much to be said for highlighting how reciprocal interaction between art and science necessarily complement each other and contribute to a knowledge base which has real practical impact. As Glasby puts it, there is:

> a need to move away from traditional models of 'evidence-based practice' … towards a more inclusive and broader concept of 'knowledge based practice'. Whilst this may be difficult, seeking to combine insights from theoretical, empirical and experiential sources may be one way of making different and better decisions about health and social care in the future. (Glasby, 2011: 96)

The dividing line between certainty and uncertainty represents a difficult balancing act, but the integration of art and science might go some way to enabling social workers to better navigate the complex terrain of practice. This might not guarantee certainty, but it increases the likelihood of assessments which are accurate, and thus practice which is effective.

All of which is easier said than done.

Independently of her work for government, Eileen Munro has sought to develop a model of social work practice which combines the strengths of both objective and subjective, or analytic and intuitive, approaches to judgement and decision-making, which are at the heart of assessment practice (Munro, 2005; 2008). This broadly systemic model privileges notions of complexity and seeks to specify not how to eliminate uncertainty but, rather, how to manage or engage with it. The assumption is that it is possible to improve and potentially standardise the quality of decision-making in practice where the appropriate style of reasoning informs particular judgements. Munro (2010) distinguishes between areas of practice which ought to be proceduralised and those which should be judgement based, but acknowledges the challenges entailed in establishing which areas of practice in which contexts and domains fit into each category, and in terms of establishing criteria which might be utilised as the basis for such differentiation. In the absence of definitive guidance regarding how such judgements can or should be made, then, the question arises: Are there *principles* which might helpfully inform how practitioners do this? It does seem that the ubiquity of uncertainty helps us to understand why studies of social work practice consistently highlight the *pragmatic* approach which practitioners describe when accounting for the decisions they make. The potential that pragmatism might hold as a philosophy for practice is little discussed in social work, perhaps because of misunderstanding of what it entails, itself related to lay usage of the term as meaning 'unprincipled'. Properly understood, however, pragmatism offers real potential as a framework which practitioners might use to inform assessment practice.

PRACTICE REFLECTION 4.5

Pragmatic social work practice

What does the term 'pragmatic social work practice' evoke for you? To what extent does it relate to the way in which you work?

Pragmatic principles

The pragmatic position on perennial philosophical concerns regarding the nature of knowledge and how we might 'know' is distinctive. Rather than being defined as some objective representation of reality, knowledge is primarily regarded as a means of problem-solving so as to achieve specific, practical and ethical ends (see Evans and Hardy, 2010, for a more elaborate account of what pragmatic thought entails).

Although philosophy tends to be an abstract discipline, the Harvard psychiatrist Brendel has elaborated on its practical implications for human services.

He specifies four pragmatic principles which ought to inform practice: *practicality, pluralism, participation* and *provisionalism* (Brendel, 2006). The suggestion is that where these criteria are adhered to, they have real potential to promote integration of art and science in practice-based disciplines.

Here, *practicality* relates to the notion that ideas should be judged according to their capacity to assist people in addressing the challenges with which they are faced. As these challenges are diverse, they require responses which are flexible and open-minded, or *plural*. Life is lived interpersonally, and so there is recognition that any approximation of 'truth' will include the views and perspectives of all of those *participating*, albeit with awareness that the uncertain, complex and ever-changing nature of people and the world they live in is such that knowledge is only ever *provisional* and will alter according to context and circumstances.

Thus, in social work decision-making, assessors will need to consider the extent to which their judgements, and the actions which follow on from these, will facilitate *practical* effects, rather than whether or not a particular theory or version of reality appeals to us at an abstract level, or resonates intellectually or aesthetically. Because pragmatists reject the notion of one single truth, or means of establishing it, they regard negotiation between *plural* perspectives as more appropriate than those approaches which seek to prove or disprove alternative approaches. Consequently, where knowledge derived from different sources is to some extent contradictory, tensions are addressed via the Hegelian approach known as 'dialectical reasoning'. This involves paying attention to the positions and arguments of varying approaches, and attempting to integrate the perspectives of all *participants* in a conciliatory way. It 'does not lead to the triumph of one approach over the other, but instead to a dynamic equilibrium between scientific and humanistic concepts' (Brendel, 2006: 13). In this way, assessments are more likely to lead to useful, workable solutions which have potential for achieving practical gains.

Pragmatists, then, are all too aware of the limitations of aesthetics (its relativity) and reason (its fallibility). Their assumption is that, whatever its source, knowledge is *provisional*. As a corollary, assessors need a provisional sensibility, characterised by open-mindedness and flexibility, although the value of a knowledge claim is assessed according to its practical merit. Decisions made according to pragmatic precepts, then, would be integrative, rather than based on singular sources. Judgements regarding whether and how to intervene will be on the basis of the 'balance of evidence' generated from multiple sources. It is unavoidable that such decisions will involve differentiating between competing claims based on less than full knowledge. This, however, is the reality in social work. As Evans and Hardy (2010) suggest, practitioners have little option but 'to make decisions and act as though these choices are objective, knowing full well that the knowledge upon which they are based is often contested and so their judgements and actions may be "wrong"' (p. 175).

Pragmatism in practice

Pragmatism, then, has real potential as a framework for assessment in social work. This is mainly because its underpinning assumptions correspond closely with those of social work, properly understood. This does mean, however, that its emphasis will differ from those of strong advocates of other, quite particular approaches to social work. Assessments undertaken according to pragmatic principles would, for example, be non-partisan. Partisanship – 'taking sides' – is incompatible with pluralism, here understood as a commitment to ensuring that assessments incorporate the views of the various stakeholders with a perspective on a case. 'Taking sides' is central to some understandings of the social work task, particularly radical and critical variants, and, to some extent, person-centred models, but pragmatism emphasises the need to avoid 'taking sides' and, instead, retain a concern with practical effects.

Additionally, in statutory settings there are all sorts of judgements and decisions which practitioners make with which one or more stakeholders may disagree, including service users. Service user perspectives have come to the fore in social work since the 1990s (Glasby and Beresford, 2006; McLaughlin, 2010), but tensions remain regarding the extent to which, in certain situations, partnership working is practicable, when it might be appropriate for practitioners to override service user views, and on what basis. Although useful work has been undertaken considering the inclusion of service user perspectives in risk assessment (e.g. Langan and Lindow, 2004; Ryan, 2000), this does not resolve the issue of whether and when the views and perspectives of 'experts by experience' should supplant, rather than inform, the judgements and decisions of practitioners.

PRACTICE REFLECTION 4.6

Considering the service user

In what types of situation do you think it is, or should be, appropriate for social workers to 'over-rule' the stated perspectives or preferences of a service user?

One clear benefit of approaches to assessment which are integrative stems from the tendency towards confirmatory bias that Munro (2003) identifies. In social work, this has manifested in, for example, the so-called 'rule of optimism' (Dingwall *et al.*, 1983) in child protection, or an uncritical acceptance of service user perspectives as representing the 'true' account of a situation. Knowledge synthesis has the potential to counter the bias that manifests in partisan decision-making by ensuring practitioners take into account sources of knowledge other than those which are based on gut instinct. Tacit knowledge is important in social work, but requires integration with more formal sources.

Finally, for many, reflection – critical reflection, reflexivity or critical reflexivity – is central to ensuring good practice in social work. Within a pragmatic framework, however, the emphasis would be on suspending undue reflection in favour of situated problem-solving and action. Pragmatists are aware of the potential for idealism to limit action and, thus, the achievement of practical effects. However, and contrary to the caricature of pragmatism as value-free, it is clear that pragmatic method supplements, rather than supplants, ethical deliberation in that, although its concerns may be situated rather than global, they occur within the context of a commitment to the notion of action as a means to a particular end, which is 'what is best in a particular situation for a particular person' (Polkinghorne, 2004: 123).

Towards critical pluralism

In the absence of certainty, we need to keep our options open, which is what the application of pragmatic principles to assessment enables us to do. It seems unlikely that we will ever be fortunate enough to have anything approaching definitive knowledge regarding 'what works for whom in what circumstances and why', and so it is essential that practitioners are equipped, and free, to utilise pragmatic principles as a basis for determining how to act to achieve their ends. In its commitment to practical action, pluralism, participation and provisionalism, pragmatism offers potential to do justice to the 'commonplace complexity' which characterises social work, without allowing awareness of the ubiquity of uncertainty to descend into relativism or anti-scientism. Pragmatists regard uncertainty as a starting point – a problem on which to work towards providing workable, practical solutions, rather than an insurmountable difficulty which we have no option but to celebrate. Of course, by definition, a pragmatic framework for practice is unable to offer prescriptive guidance to practitioners regarding how assessment 'ought' to be undertaken. It does, however, encourage practitioners to navigate the tensions between art and science according to criteria which have clear relevance and utility within the practice paradigm. The unavoidable process of *considered but tentative selection of the seemingly most appropriate strategy in a given situation* – critical pluralism – represents a robust defence of the necessity of professionalism to social work practice.

Conclusion

Emphasis on the value of research knowledge as a key element for social workers and its integration, based on shared assumptions and characteristics, offers potential to contribute gradually to the development of approaches to assessment which genuinely integrate art and science. There is no expectation that this approach would, in some way, lead to infallible decisions in social work practice. But it is my contention that this integrative, pragmatic approach offers a useful framework within which assessment practice can be undertaken. It is worth stressing, however, that this is not to be overly critical of established ways of undertaking assessment. At heart, the pragmatic approach to decision-making has both an empirical and a normative basis: it describes how practitioners actually work and suggests that this is as it should – or, maybe, must – be. We do not actually know how accurate social work assessments are. We do know that the number of child deaths per annum remain about constant, or are in decline (Corby, 2006), and that international reviews indicate high levels of satisfaction with social welfare services (Fraser and Wu, 2013). These facts are hardly suggestive of incompetence, unless competence is equated with infallibility. Nevertheless, social work will remain a demanding and challenging profession however it is conducted. Perhaps critics should remember that, when social work fails, this is because it is actually very difficult to get right. The fact that 'extreme failures' are so few is testament to the enduring professionalism of its practitioners.

FURTHER READING

Holland, S. (2011) *Child and Family Assessment in Social Work Practice*, 2nd edn (London: Sage). A very good overview of debates regarding the respective merits of artistic and scientific approaches to assessment in children's services.

Trevithick, P. (2012) *Social Work Skills and Knowledge: A Practice handbook*, 3rd edn (Maidenhead: Open University Press), see especially ch. 4. A very thorough overview of the various different ways of thinking about the nature of knowledge for practice.

CHAPTER 5

Using Evidence to Inform Decision-Making

Tony Evans

Introduction

Social workers cannot avoid making decisions. In working with service users and carers, they have to think about how they use their skills to communicate and to build a working relationship. They have to decide on the advice to give and the strategies they choose to employ in interventions with people, groups and communities. They are also involved in deciding how resources are allocated, and how sanctions and public powers are invoked to constrain problem behaviours and address risky situations.

Evidence is central to decision-making but there can often be confusion about the nature of evidence. I have been party to several discussions about evidence-based practice, and it has gradually become clear that the discussion has been at cross purposes: on one side, 'evidence-based' has been understood as grounded in the facts of the case; on the other, the term has been used to refer to research informing practice. Both these forms of evidence play an important role in decision-making in practice.

Decision-making implies discretion, in the sense of having some freedom to choose what to do. Discretion also implies judgement and discernment in making these choices. This idea of the relationship between freedom and judgement is central to how we understand professional practice. In looking at evidence and decision-making, I want to look at how professional judgement relates to broader frameworks of discretion within which decisions are made.

In this chapter, I will look at the idea of discretion in terms of a combination of freedom and standards of appropriate decision-making about how to use that freedom. In relation to legal decisions, for instance, social workers make decisions about allocation of sanctions and resources, which are limiting in the degree of freedom of choice and quite prescriptive in relation to how decisions should be made. On the other hand, decisions about how to intervene are much less limited (although there may be practical limitations of time, skills and so on); but any decision will need to demonstrate reason and professional rigour. I will explore these issues by looking at the idea of evidence-based decision-making. I will argue that this idea tends to present decision-making as a clinical process, and that legal and administrative processes and requirements in decision-making are given little attention, except as side constraints on professional decision-making. This, I will argue, reflects a tendency in evidence-based decision-making to play a 'one club game', and tends to denigrate other approaches and their contribution to decision-making. I will then look more closely at the process of evidence-based decision-making. After outlining the five steps in this approach to decision-making, I will argue that it pays insufficient attention to the role of theory in decision-making, and that it also tends to approach professional ethics as an authority, rather than engaging with ethics critically.

Social work expertise not only covers technical questions about what to do in a situation, but is also concerned with advancing certain ideas of fairness, well-being, and justice. The relationship between these ideas of freedom, expertise and ethical commitments is central to any consideration of professional decision-making.

Dimensions of practice and decisions in social work

Social workers, as most contemporary professionals, work in organisations (Freidson, 1994) where their work balances accountabilities – to people who use their services, to their employers, to broader society and to their professional identity. Local authority social workers are qualified and registered professionals making decisions about the allocation of resources. They deploy public authority and sanction, use professional skills to support people in difficult circumstances, and engage with individual and structural inequalities and discrimination through their work. Social work involves interpersonal skills of working with individuals, families and groups; drawing on and deploying technical knowledge and skills to help; and making decisions within the law and policy, and about organisational rules about meeting needs and controlling behaviour.

Decision-making assumes some freedom of action within the job to decide what to do. However, the idea of discretion in contemporary social work is contentious (Evans, 2010). Historically, local government bureaucracy and, more recently, the increasing influence of managerialism have been seen as significant constraints on professional decision-making and have led to scepticism about whether social workers actually have choices and make decisions. This is the view that policies and procedures limit and constrain practice in such a way that it is no longer possible to see professionals as having any freedom in deciding how they work or what they do in work. Some have even argued that professionals are, in effect, subject to remote control by management through procedures and policies that not only constrain behaviour, but also have come to dominate the ways in which professionals can think about their practice.

However, while it would be naïve to dismiss concerns about the increasing top-down control of practice and the constraining influence of volumes of procedures, checklists and timescale, it would be equally naïve to deny the extent of freedom social workers have to make decisions in between rules, in the interpretation and application of rules, or the ways in which policies and procedures often require social workers to exercise professional judgement

(Evans and Harris, 2004). Furthermore, we should not confuse procedural rules that embody services user rights and principles of fair decision-making with an undue constraint on professional decision-making. As Smith and White point out:

> procedural frameworks are useful in co-ordinating activity, clarifying methods and responsibilities, and contributing to consistency and fairness. They are not, and are not intended to be, a substitute for the discretion which has to be used in everyday encounters. (Smith and White, 1997: 291–2)

The point here is that social work decision-making occurs across a range of fields, such as administrative, interpersonal or risk/needs identification, for example. Furthermore, the degree of freedom in decision-making is more constrained in some areas (e.g. administrative decisions) than in others (e.g. professional judgement). Here, the work of Dworkin (1978) is useful in teasing out further the different dimensions of freedom and constraint contained within the broad idea of discretion. He explains that making decisions in your private life is different from making decisions in a public role, such as being a professional or in a public office. He argues that freedom to make decisions in a public role exists in a range of different situations, such as where we have to apply a standard or rule to a particular situation, where rules make us responsible for making judgements, and where we have to decide what to do. Across all aspects of decision-making, you are expected to act within rules of legitimacy; it always makes sense to ask: 'Discretion under which standards?' (Dworkin, 1978: 31). We talk not only about having discretion to act [freedom], but also exercising discretion [judgement]. Discretion is not the absence of principles or rules; rather, it is the spaces they create for decisions. Professional freedom is not autonomy: ' and does not exclude criticism. Almost any situation in which a person acts ... makes relevant certain standards of rationality, fairness, and effectiveness' (Dworkin, 1978: 33).

PRACTICE REFLECTION 5.1

Room for decision making

As a social worker, it can sometimes seem as though you have very little room in your practice to make decisions – you simply have to follow procedures. Looking at your practice and that of your colleagues, is it that uniform? For instance, does everyone in your team apply thresholds or eligibility criteria in the same way?

When you look at your organisational policies and procedures, what areas do they tend to cover? Are there any areas where policies and procedures are thin? In which areas of your work do you feel you have more freedom to make decisions and in which areas do you feel you have less?

Discretion is not about absolute freedom to choose, and to choose what to do on whatever basis you decide. The freedom implied by discretion is freedom set within two sorts of limits. First, the extent of your freedom to decide

– your room for movement, which can vary according to the particular tasks you are undertaking. As a social worker, you often have more freedom of movement in coming to a professional judgement about what theory or approach works best in a situation than you have in choosing how to allocate resources to a service user (where your decision will be more tightly circum-scribed by rules and procedures).

The second dimension of discretion is what is seen as the appropriate way in which you should go about making your decision, or what is seen as sound or valid evidence for making the decision. There is, for instance, wide-ranging acceptance of (not to mention sanction supporting) approaches to administra-tive decision-making that seek to be disinterested, unbiased and fair; there is less agreement on the right way to make intervention decisions in day-to-day practice.

Evidence and reasonable decision-making

A helpful way to think about this point is to think about the legal and admin-istrative side of social work practice. It is very clear to see how, in these areas, there are guidelines, legal criteria and categories or rules of entitlement that limit your freedom. The NHS and Community Care Act 1990, for instance, says you have to assess someone who appears to be in need of community care, and the Act also tells you what community care services are. It also tells you that, amongst other things, once you have made your assessment, you then have to decide whether or not any of the needs identified should be met by the local authority. All this is set out in law, guidance and local procedures. This illustrates the idea of the room you have and the limits set on your free-dom for decision-making – and, although there are limits, there is still room within the rules to exercise discretion.

Running alongside formal rules setting the limits of your freedom, there are also assumptions about how you should make decisions and use evidence to put the rules into effect. These requirements can be summarised under the rubric of 'natural justice'. They are rules based on legal tradition and some statute law which recognise that decisions about who gets services, or whether steps are taken to protect a child or vulnerable adult, involve the exercise of public authority. These decisions significantly affect citizens; it is important that they are made in a fair and unbiased manner, and that they are given care-ful and thoughtful consideration. There is an expectation, for instance, that when making a decision officials look at all relevant factors, but exclude evidence that is not relevant to the matter at hand; and that a response will be within the bounds of reasonableness and will be in proportion to the problem (Brayne and Carr, 2010).

These requirements are about avoiding maladministration. This is not just about applying the law or a procedure correctly, but also doing it in a fair and just manner. An example would be that, in allocating services, you need to have a full picture of a person's need before you can come to a judgement; popping your head around the door and taking a look would not be sufficient. Similarly, a decision about a person's need for help with getting in and out of bed should not be based on whether you think they are a nice (or unpleasant) person. This is not relevant and should not enter your consideration. Fairness is also about being open about the decisions you are taking, when those decisions affect people's lives, so that you can check the facts and get all sides of the story. For instance, if you are undertaking an assessment of need your liking for the person (or not) should not be a consideration. Your focus should be their needs – not your prejudice. You should also be careful to weigh the strengths and weaknesses of the actual facts, rather than force them into pre-existing stereotypes (Brayne and Carr, 2010).

You need to be consistent – treat similar cases in similar ways, but also be aware of differences that may call for different treatment. These and other principles combine to govern the way in which you can use the discretion in relation to the legal-administrative aspects of your work.

Evidence-based decision-making

As we saw earlier in the chapter, evidence is an important part of administrative decision-making. Here, it is helpful to be aware of a potential confusion that can occur in discussing evidence and decision-making. People often see evidence in this way as having the facts to support a decision. In evidence-based decision-making, the idea of 'evidence' tends to be used in a more restricted way to refer to research evidence about what works. Other knowledge has a place in the decision-making process, but research evidence has a particular prominence. The principles underpinning the use of legal and administrative discretion are designed to promote disinterested and rigorous decision-making to reduce the chance of bias or prejudice. Similar concerns about the need to reduce bias in professional decision-making have been evident since the 1990s in the development of evidence-based practice. Evidence-based practice has been concerned about the biased thinking that can undermine effective professional judgement.

At the individual level, there is a large body of evidence from psychology and behavioural science contrasting the ideals of rational behaviour with the faulty way in which humans reason (e.g. Taylor, 2013). According to this research, we are inherently biased in the way we approach decisions, relying on assumptions, habits, stereotypes and short-cuts in thinking about what to do:

> We are vulnerable to a variety of cognitive biases that may lead us astray such as confirmation biases, wishful thinking, and hindsight bias. We search for data that confirm our views. We weigh data in support of preferred views more heavily than we weigh data against them. We overestimate our competencies and are subject to wishful thinking. (Gambrill, 2011: 29)

At the level of the profession as a whole, advocates of evidence-based social work are concerned about the way they believe social work gives too much credence to the authority of famous names, popular ideas, traditions and consensus as the bases for making decisions in practice (Gambrill, 2011;

Sheldon, 2001). Evidence-based decision-making seeks to bring in evidence from a range of sources to reflect what it sees as a range of legitimate sources of evidence for professional decision-making. However, it sees science as the fundamental criterion of sound decision-making – and gives particular emphasis to the role of evidence, in the sense of clinically relevant research, as a foundational guide to practice (Gambrill, 2011).

Central to evidence-based practice's perspective is a commitment to Karl Popper's approach to the nature of scientific enquiry. This can be seen in the criticism of the authority-led, particularly theory-led, approaches to social work (Gambrill, 2011; Sheldon, 2001). The evidence-based approach is critical of approaches such as psychoanalysis which are based on the authority of texts and authors (e.g. 'Freud said …') rather than scientific evidence. Drawing on Popper, advocates argue that Freudianism is not scientific but is a pseudo-science. Science, according to Popper (2002), is not about having a theory and finding evidence that proves it right. Rather, science is sceptical, and it is characterised by its commitment to test and challenge ideas through experience. If an idea survives it is useful, until someone manages to disprove it; if it is disproved, then it is back to the drawing board. Science, for Popper, is not the accumulation of evidence in the absence of theory, but is the continuing questioning and challenging of theory by observation:

> This method assumes a more and more scientific character the more freely and consciously we are prepared to risk a trial, and the more critically we are looking out for the mistakes we always make. And this formula covers not only the method of experiment, but also the relationship between theory and experiment. All theories are trials; they are tentative hypotheses, tried out to see whether they work; and all experimental confirmation is nothing but the result of tests undertaken in a critical spirit in an attempt to find out where our theories err. (Popper, 1944: 131)

This approach to reliable knowledge has been influential in social work, beyond a narrow, evidence-based practice paradigm, and it can be seen in policy and practice injunctions to retain a 'respectful uncertainty' and a 'healthy scepticism' about your first impressions of situations and working hypothesis about what might be 'going-on' (Lord Laming, 2003; Munro, 2011).

While Popper distinguishes 'scientific' and 'non-scientific' knowledge, he does not consider non-scientific knowledge to be meaningless – it may contain interesting ideas that could lead eventually to more robust knowledge. In this respect, it is valuable to draw a distinction between Popper's view and 'positivism'. Positivism is the idea that scientific knowledge is built up by the accumulation of facts about the world, with theory then capturing some basic truth about the world about us. Popper (2002) was sceptical about treating knowledge as the accumulation of facts. As you accumulate facts, you might get the idea of how one thing tends to follow from another – this is your interpretation, your theory. You may have always seen swans flying in from the east to over-winter in Britain. From these observations you say, with authority, that swans are white birds; and next week, when you go to the zoo, the swans you will see will be white. But previous observations can never guarantee what is going to happen next. When you go to the zoo most of the swans you see are white but there are some black swans, too. You will need to rethink your assumption that swans are always white birds. Furthermore, when you see regularities, this is your interpretation of what you have seen, a working idea, and for this reason you should always retain some scepticism towards it.

The process of evidence-based decision-making

As discussed in earlier chapters of this book, evidence-based decision-making is usually presented as a five-stage process following on from completion of the assessment (Gambrill, 2011; McCracken and Marsh, 2008). The aim of the practitioner is to intervene as effectively as possible in people's lives. The assessment identifies the 'presenting problem'. The first stage of the process is to consider whether you already know how best to help, or whether you need additional information about the best course of action (McCracken and Marsh, 2008: 303). If you decide you do not know enough, you need to identify your 'clinical priorities' and use these to develop clear and focused questions to search for information for the most effective intervention.

Having formulated the questions, the next step is to search for the answers to fill the gaps in your knowledge. From an evidence-based perspective, this means looking for evidence from 'valid and clinically relevant research ... especially from [client-centred] clinical research' (Strauss et al., quoted in Gambrill, 2011: 32). Alongside the aim of looking for the best evidence is the practical imperative to be efficient – using knowledge of the strengths and weaknesses of different databases, and the best database to answer particular questions (see Chapter 2, for a fuller discussion of how best to do this). This is a practical imperative to balance rigour with an eye to the efficient use of time and resources (Gambrill, 2011: 32).

As a result of the search, you will have gathered together research evidence. The third step is to evaluate the research in terms of its methodological quality and practical use: 'This step includes two equally important questions for clinical decision-making: Did my search yield high-quality information? If so, does it apply to my client?' (McCracken and Marsh, 2008: 305). See Chapter 3, for some tips about critical appraisal of research.

After having weighed the evidence, the fourth stage of the process is to incorporate what you have found to be sound and useful into your practice:

> deciding whether evidence found (if any) applies to the decision at hand (e.g. is the client similar to those studied? Is there access to services described?) and considering client values and preferences in making decisions as well as other application concerns. (Gambrill, 2011: 32)

The final stage of the decision-making process is evaluation. This seems to involve two tasks. Gambrill (2011: 32), for instance, emphasises evaluating the decision-making process itself (the four stages outlined above), while McCracken and Marsh (2008: 307) focus on the intervention and its outcome from the point of view of the practitioner, service user and practitioner's employing organisation.

At one level, the process is unexceptional – who could disagree with the need to fill gaps in your knowledge, and to be organised and efficient in going about searching for the information to fill the gaps? In this regard, the early stages look like a literature review, balanced by a practical acknowledgement that you can only do your best in the time and with the resources available.

Perhaps the most discussed aspects of this process are the notions that some forms of research evidence are better than others, and the emphasis on a clinician characterisation of the relationship between practitioners and users. The idea is that there is a hierarchy of evidence by which you can rank the quality of intervention research and the paucity of (and limitation on producing) the sort of evidence best described as good-quality. This aspect of evidence-based decision-making has been widely discussed and I do not propose to look at it in any detail here. For a summary, see Evans and Hardy (2010: ch. 2), or Chapter 1 in this volume.

A strength of evidence-based decision-making is the way in which it seeks to involve (rather than pathologise) the preferences and views of service users. However, this commitment is very much located within an idea of clinical expertise, in that decision-making is understood as an expert process in which the service user is cast as the consumer of expert knowledge. Service users should be informed about the best course of action, and their views and concerns are discussed and put into the balance when deciding how/whether to proceed. But they are treated very much as an audience for expert knowledge.

Evidence-based decision-making seeks to incorporate a range of factors in the decision-making process. The practitioner's own skills and knowledge are taken into account, as are the facts of the situation and how these two identify gaps in knowledge. Economic concerns are also present, in that the process of looking for information cannot be endless but must take account of resources. Furthermore, service users' views are important in deciding what to do and how to do it. The emphasis, though, is on the compelling nature of intervention research, as judged against a hierarchy of evidence to inform and guide decisions about how to intervene.

However, there are two aspects of evidence-based decisions that are puzzling – the absence of consideration of the role of theory, and assumptions about the nature of ethics. I will look at each of these issues in the final sections of this chapter.

Theory and evidence-based decision-making

Evidence-based decision-making characterises itself as challenging unthinking approaches to decision-making. It is sceptical (in the best sense) decision-making. Advocates of evidence-based decision-making often present their approach as a challenge to practice that takes for granted certain theories and uses these in an uncritical way to make decisions about interventions. They characterise current practice in terms of a range of false paradigms (Gambrill,

2011: 27). The other side of this argument is that the aim is to replace these paradigms with a new paradigm for social work based on scientific approaches to the nature and role of evidence in decision-making (Gambrill, 2011; Sheldon, 2001; Sheldon and Macdonald, 2008).

Here, it is useful to reflect on Kuhn's (1970) account of the nature of paradigms. The shift from one paradigm to another is not about a move from a worse to a better understanding of the world; rather, it is about a shift in focus from one set of problems, and what is seen as a good way to research and understand them, to another. Paradigm shifts reflect changing social concerns, rather than the inexorable, onward and upward progress of knowledge. Furthermore, paradigms are systems of control and authority. They tend to promote ways of understanding the world that comply with the favoured paradigm, seek to dismiss and explain away challenges to the authority of the paradigm, and marginalise other approaches to concerns and perspectives. Paradigms close down debates and naturalise ways of understanding and investigating the world, and this is all the more powerful because it is taken for granted.

Khun was a historian of science, and his account of paradigms reflects what he found to be the practices of scientists and the broader scientific community to which they belonged. As we saw earlier in this chapter, Popper's concerns are quite different. He was concerned with the nature of claims to scientific knowledge. He distinguished science from pseudoscience on the basis that science tests ideas to destruction; as long as they survive they are useful, but we always have to remember that they are not universal truths. The key process in science for Popper is falsification, identifying ideas and testing them against the evidence. In this respect, he was critical of 'positivist' ideas of knowledge that emphasised the accumulation of evidence towards a claim to general truths.

Here, I want to consider two points that follow from this for understanding the role of evidence in decision-making. First, being clear about the ideas you hold and the theories you assume in your practice is central to understanding the role of evidence in decision-making; and, second, evidence has a central role in challenging these assumptions and theories underpinning practice.

PRACTICE REFLECTION 5.2

Appraisal of first reactions and expectations

Think of a new piece of work you have taken on recently. Write down what you remember about your first reactions to the referral. Now look over this description and make a note of the ideas that you feel underpinned your reaction. When you started work, was there anything that you did not expect? Thinking now about these ideas and assumptions in your practice, what are their limitations as well as their strengths? Are they helpful? Do they help or restrict you in seeing the situation in the round?

Theory, ideas and assumptions are central and basic in scientific understanding:

> Out of uninterpreted sense-experiences science cannot be distilled, no matter how industriously we gather and sort them. Bold ideas, unjustified anticipations, and speculative thought, are our only means for interpreting nature. (Popper, 2002: 280)

But consideration of theory is surprisingly low key in the evidence-based approach to decision-making in social work. However, even in the short summary of evidence-based decision-making above, it is clear that theories of practice – (tentative) ideas about the nature of problems and what could help – come into play at key points. For instance, at the very beginning of the process McCracken and Marsh (2008) highlight a fundamental decision the practitioner must take – whether they already know how best to help and whether they need additional information about the best course of action. This reflection of one's own knowledge and ideas about how best to help – your theory of practice – is important. This is more, though, than just 'background information' (McCracken and Marsh, 2008: 303); it is the ideas and theories by which you understand 'development' and the relationship between things such as individual cognition and cultural context. Reflection needs to be more probing and critical to uncover the taken-for-granted ideas underpinning theories of practice (Fook and Gardner, 2007) so that they can then be examined: what is taken for granted as significant? Is there any evidence that challenges my approach? Is there evidence that may require revision of any practice ideas?

McCracken and Marsh (2008) also point out that, at the fourth stage of the decision-making process – integrating evidence into practice, you should acknowledge that any evidence is unlikely to provide a clear and simple answer to the question you are trying to answer. 'The practitioner must also decide whether the intervention can be used as described in the literature or in a practice guideline or whether it needs to be adapted to one's client or practice environment and if so how' (McCracken and Marsh, 2008: 306). Here, the issues are not only questions of population difference, outcome differences and delivery personnel, but also the theoretical assumptions in the research such as ideas of how people learn and change behaviour.

Why, for instance, might the fact that the research was undertaken with different populations be relevant – or not? Why might the fact that different professionals or organisations delivering an intervention be significant – or not? To combine these studies, or to translate findings from one context to another, you need to know what theoretical perspective they employ, what are their assumptions about what makes people tick, what ideas they are testing – unless you already know what makes people tick, that is! The answer in relation to evidence-based decision-making seems to be the latter option – advocates of the approach simply accept that there are 'empirically validated theories of human behaviour, such as social learning theory. The principles of social learning theory ... are universal in their application' (Macdonald, 2001: 23). However, this leaves the classic account of evidence-based decision-making in social work with the problem that, while it is advocated on the basis of Popperian scepticism about absolute and empirically validated knowledge, its practice seems to rely on an unPopperian faith in 'empirically validated theories of human behaviour' (Macdonald, 2001: 23).

The role of evidence in evidence-based decision-making resembles 'normal science' in Kuhn's use of the term. However, a more scientific approach (in Popper's sense) would be to think of evidence in terms of a way to test and challenge theoretical assumptions. In relation to decision-making, this would involve taking some time to make explicit the ideas and theories underpinning assessment and decisions, and then formulating questions to seek evidence to test and challenge these theories. There have, of course, to be questions of what constitutes sufficient evidence to falsify the ideas and theories on which you rely, but the basic point is that testing and challenging your own ideas is central to rigorous critical thinking in practice. What we think we know works is not 'the truth'; it is best thought of as tentative knowledge; it is a starting point, one we should not simply assume is right or just seek to confirm. It is important to fill in gaps, but it is also important to test and challenge those areas of our thinking we take for granted. In short, a crucial aspect of evidence in decision-making is seeking out information that challenges our assumptions, and which questions what we think is the case.

Decision-making authority and ethics

The last observation I would like to make here is about the moral injunction to engage in evidence-based decision-making. Gambrill, for instance, is emphatic that evidence-based decision-making is one's professional duty:

> EBP emphasize the close connection between evidentiary and ethical issues and describe a unique five-step process, related tools, and systemic requirements designed to help practitioners to honor this connection in everyday practice.... Ethical obligations emphasized in original sources include the obligation to help clients and avoid harming them and the obligation to involve them as informed participants. Transparency (honesty) regarding what is done to what effect (e.g. the evidentiary status of services) is a hallmark. (Gambrill, 2011: 31, 33)

What is intriguing here is that ethics seems to be treated as a system of requirements that professionals must follow; a set of law-like injunctions, rather than principles and aspirations. But this mistakenly equates the goals and commitments of professional membership with the basic rules that are enforced through regulation and registration. In this respect, evidence-based decision-making seems to be rejecting thoughtful deliberation in favour of convention and authority. This is what Weinberg describes as:

> The canonical approach ... that prescribes the correct conduct a practitioner should undertake with clients ... it is assumed that by applying the code in a prescriptive, linear fashion, in combination with good decision making and a method for tracking harms, a worker will be able to avoid ethical breaches. (Weinberg, 2010: 34)

Weinberg points out that the problem with this approach is that it tends to collapse ethics into narrow principles prescribing the right solution in which conflicts and tensions are played down and concerns for broader structural issues of poverty, inequality and oppression are seen as 'idiosyncratic', 'outside the lens of ethics' and 'political'. Ethics becomes the application of general rules in clinical encounters that can – and, for some, should – be separated off from questions of social justice, commitments and relationships. This approach to ethics, though, does not engage the experience of ethics in practice, which encompasses dilemmas, conflicts, and intuitions and feelings, as well as principles.

Ethical decision-making is complex. Williams, for instance, contrasts authority-based approaches – what he calls 'the peculiar institution' of morality (Williams, 1993: 174) – with ethics. Morality, he argues, entails the imposition of unyielding, law-like rules, recognising only obligations as ethically significant, ignoring other reasons for ethical action and obscuring the tensions and feeling tied up in making a decision about the right course of action. In place of morality, Williams argues for ethical decision-making that is grounded in the engagement with evidence and experience, not merely principles.

Williams' idea of ethics has a place for reason, but stripped of the theological reverence it was ascribed in traditional morality, and brought down to earth as one of a number of considerations in ethical decision-making. He provides an example of the character of the contrast between the unyielding absolutism of moral injunction and his more grounded ethical thinking (Smart and Williams, 1973). He asks us to imagine a situation: Jim stumbles on a hostage situation and the hostage-taker offers Jim the choice of one hostage to be killed. If Jim refuses to choose one, the hostage-taker will kill twenty at random. In practice, you will often be faced with choosing between options set by policy, resources or managers. Jim's dilemma is extreme but do you find yourself in practice having to decide between unattractive alternatives?

There may be any number of ways to do something – or even, in the most dreadful circumstances, there may be a way to act that will do something to mitigate the dreadfulness of the situation. In Jim's circumstances, though, a moral code such as utilitarianism would give him no option but to choose what it would characterise as the lesser of two evils and choose one person to kill and so save nineteen others. But, Williams points out that, as such 'reasonable solutions' are often thought of as beyond the pale, we cannot bring ourselves to do these things: 'Entertaining certain alternatives, regarding them indeed as alternative, is itself something that he regards as dishonorable or

---

CASE SCENARIO 5.1

Mary and Tom

Imagine a situation where you have assessed Mary and feel that, without immediate help, her situation will seriously deteriorate. You take this to your manager, who points out that Mary's current need/risk is below the threshold of intervention and there is insufficient money available for preventative work. 'But', the manager suggests, 'what about closing Tom's case? I know you'd planned to do a couple more weeks' work with him, but if you close his case now you'd be free to do some work with Mary'. What do you do? What does it feel like to make this sort of decision?

absurd' (Smart and Williams, 1973: 92). Rather than simply dismissing our intuitions and commitments with our reason, we struggle – it should be more of a two-way flow; the evidence of our intuitions should sometimes curtail our more fantastic rational calculations. Important unalienable projects should establish the boundary of the thinkable – they express a deep commitment, a meaning and purpose for the agent, which if he is forced to relinquish is an assault on his integrity. 'It is to alienate him in a real sense from his actions and the source of his actions in his own convictions ... this is to neglect the extent to which his actions and his decisions have to be seen as the actions and decisions which flow from the projects and attitudes with which he is most closely identified' (Smart and Williams, 1973: 116–17). Jim may feel he considered the utilitarian argument, but this judgement would not be taken in isolation from his sense of identity and his commitments: 'to reach a grounded decision in such a case should not be regarded as a matter of just discounting one's reactions, impulses and deeply held projects in the face of a pattern of utilities, nor yet merely adding them in – but in the first place to understand them' (Smart and Williams, 1973: 118).

Conclusion

In this chapter, I have looked at evidence, decision-making and discretion in relation to the ways in which social workers engage in a range of different tasks in their work. While they have some freedom within these tasks to make decisions, the extent of this freedom varies according to the nature of particular tasks. Decision-making in relation to legal and administrative tasks tends to be more circumscribed by formal rules than professional judgements about the nature of need and risk, and how to respond. Furthermore, decision-making in these different areas draws on different assumptions about evidence and the nature of decision-making. The idea of evidence in relation to legal and administrative work, for instance, gives particular emphasis to the facts of the matter at hand, how these relate to legal and organisational rules, and background consideration about the nature of unbiased and fair decision-making; for example, consider all the relevant facts but exclude those facts that are not relevant. Professional judgements about 'need' and 'risk' and how to intervene tend to be less circumscribed. In this area of practice, evidence-based practice ideas about the role of research evidence in decision-making have become increasingly influential. And, while this sort of professional decision-making is much less constrained by formal rules than legal and administrative decision-making, it still operates within a set of assumptions about the nature of evidence and the process of decision-making.

Evidence-based decision-making is critical of 'unscientific' approaches within social work. However, when the practice of evidence-based decision-making is compared with the account of scientific thinking presented by Popper, questions emerge about the limited consideration of the role of theory in understanding, assessing and using research evidence. Furthermore, while the evidence-based approach emphasises independent thinking, it tends to characterise professional ethics as authority-based – simply rules to be applied.

However, an alternative view of ethics, which would seem to sit more comfortably with independent thinking, is Williams' approach, which recognises a wide range of forms of evidence – including intuitions and beliefs – that need to be considered in ethical decision-making.

In looking at different aspects of social work practice, it is important to recognise that, while it is possible to distinguish these different areas analytically, in practice decision-making often involves juggling a mixture of different tasks in the same piece of work. Decision-making almost inevitably involves simultaneously balancing different concerns, different modes of decision-making and different ideas of evidence. Particular approaches to decision-making have their strengths and limitations and, in some circumstances, the nature of the decision you have to make may emphasise particular approaches and play down others. However, more often than not, evidence in social work decision-making takes a range of forms including 'the facts of the case', 'research evidence' and intuitions. Furthermore, this evidence does not speak for itself (Popper, 2002); its significance lies in the questions we ask of it and how we seek to use it. To understand any evidence you have at hand, you have also to recognise the ideas, assumptions and theories that may have informed the research studies you use to make sense of things, and to guide your practice.

FURTHER READING

Evans, T. and Hardy, M. (2010) *Evidence and Knowledge for Practice* (Cambridge: Polity). Chapter 2 examines the evidence-based practice approach in social work, including debates about issues such as the idea of a hierarchy of research evidence informing practice decision-making.

Fook, J. and Gardner, F. (2007) *Practising Critical Reflection: A Resource Handbook* (Maidenhead: Open University Press). Fook and Gardner present reflection as a critical strategy for making explicit theories of practice. They also offer practical approaches to critical reflection in practice settings.

McCracken, S. and Marsh, J. (2008) 'Practitioner Expertise in Evidence-Based Practice Decision Making', *Research on Social Work Practice*, 18(4): 301–10. McCracken and Marsh provide a clear, practical and grounded account of evidence-based decision-making and the role of practitioner expertise within an evidence-based practice framework.

Weinberg, M. (2010) 'The Social Construction of Social Work Ethics: Politicizing and Broadening the Lens', *Journal of Progressive Human Services*, 21(1): 32–44. Weinberg presents an approach to ethics as a process of thoughtful engagement with the dilemmas and day-to-day complexities of practice.

CHAPTER 6

Using Research Evidence in Practice: A View from the Ground

Victoria Hart

Evidence in practice? The what, why and how

Using evidence improves practice. As a social worker in a busy frontline team, it is important to be able to look at how we can incorporate research evidence into day-to-day work and explore how this is possible even when a caseload is bulging at the seams and time is short. In this chapter, I explore the practicalities of incorporating research evidence into a work style and approach, sometimes in spite of an environment which may not be conducive to it.

As well as sharing some of the tools and systems I have used both personally and within the teams I have worked in, I will look at some of the ways research evidence has been shared across health and social care professions. Social work, in some ways, has a great deal of learning which it can take from allied health professions and it is important that we identify shared ways of learning. I will also explore how social work students can both play a crucial part in bringing current research into a practice placement opportunity and also display an awareness of the place of evidence-based practice to build solid foundations for successful and effective practice.

The reality of social work practice 'in the field' can be vastly different to the way it is perceived in academia and it is important that professionals in practice do not become detached from the process of building an evidence base for the profession as a whole. The pressure of the job can make time very scarce and there is a danger that time for personal and professional growth will be trimmed at the expense of pursuing organisational targets. As social work professionals, we need to take responsibility for our own learning and training, and to display the clear links between up-to-date, responsible, knowledgeable and responsive practitioners and those organisational targets which will be better met with a better-skilled workforce.

The reality of social work practice can be rushed and pressured. There are, though, reasons to hope. Building strong foundations of evidence-based practice can have an almost immediate impact on us as practitioners and students, as well as, more importantly, the quality of the services which we provide. As Aveyard and Sharp argue:

> Evidence based practice is practice that is supported by a clear, up-to-date rationale taking into account the patient/client's preferences and using your own judgement. If we practice an evidence-based approach then we are set to give the best possible care. (Aveyard and Sharp, 2013: 4)

While there may not be many opportunities for practitioners actively to undertake original research, it is vital that we are aware of current research in the fields that are directly relevant to us, as well as more general work being undertaken in the field. If we are not in a position of seniority that would allow us to change policy, we can, in whatever position we find ourselves, challenge policies with knowledge. We can also look at ways of changing our interactions and make small changes which may be of some significance to those with whom we are working and which help us to achieve the best possible outcomes for them.

In this chapter, I shall first look at how evidence is currently used in practice through others' perspectives on this topic, as well as reflecting on my experiences. I will then look at some of the ways we can access immediately useful evidence and research, particularly as access to journals cannot always be assumed.

I will then look at why it is important to build research evidence into daily practice while reflecting on the responsibilities we have individually to ensure that our practice is up-to-date and as useful as possible. As social work practitioners, we remain responsible for ensuring that our own development and learning is up-to-date with practice developments, so it is vital that we do not become complacent in spite of pressure of work. I will look at some of the challenges that exist and the reasons why it is not always possible to develop competence in evidence-based practice, before looking at some of the practical ways these barriers can be challenged and broken down.

In the final part of the chapter, I will approach the more practical details. I will explore how we can use supervision, team work and critical reflection to develop a research- and evidence-friendly environment, and to create or strengthen evidence-literate practitioners and students.

Do social work practitioners use evidence in practice?

Many text books considering the use of evidence in social work practice refer to how well a social work practitioner or student might be engaged in understanding and using research in their day-to-day role. This should be something that happens as matter of course, but is this really happening in social work settings at the present time? Clearly, a great deal will depend on the setting and work environment itself, the culture of particular teams, and the attitudes of managers and directors within those organisations. But it is important to remember that individual practitioners share some of the responsibility for making this happen.

Applying research in practice

To what extent are you able to use research to inform your day-to-day practice? What are the main barriers and challenges you face in doing so?

Some authors suggest that a lack of ability of practitioners to undertake research betrays a lack of interest in using research. For example, Corby argues that:

> Research probably occupies the minds of more social work lecturers (and now students) much more than it does those of most practitioners. It would be reasonable to think that many social workers, faced with trying to meet the needs of disadvantaged and sometimes challenging service users, might be sceptical about the usefulness of research in helping them tackle these problems. (Corby, 2006: 158)

Alongside his assumption about the lack of engagement of social workers with research findings, he cites a study undertaken by Sheldon and Chilvers (2002) which found that social workers did not tend to keep up-to-date with research. Over a decade later, we are perhaps fortunate to have many more ways to access research information than would have been the case when Sheldon and Chilvers collected their data, but it is important to question the extent to which practitioners are able to do this now.

Dominelli is more emphatic and critical saying:

> The current social work labour force lacks the requisite research knowledge and skills and is poorly equipped either to undertake or use research in a critical reflexive manner ... this reality constitutes a compelling reason to encourage social work educators, practitioners and students to take an active role in promoting social work research. (Dominelli, 2009: 251)

In Dominelli's view, undertaking and using research are inextricably connected and practitioners' failure to engage in either produces the same outcome of a poorly-equipped social work workforce. Uncritically bringing together the very different activities of undertaking and using research indicates some of the difficulties in the blanket statement approach favoured by both these academics.

Corby and Dominelli are harshly critical of the ability of social work practitioners (ironically, the same people they helped to train) to use the skills of critical reflection to interpret research. This is a standpoint that serves to increase divides between academic social work and social work practitioners, and is not helpful for the profession.

The only way to challenge these assertions is to ensure that practitioners and academics work more closely together and build bridges, rather than create divides. It is crucial that, as practitioners, we exceed the particularly low expectations that have been set for us by some social work academics. It is possible that these opinions that social workers are ill-equipped to interpret and use research could be an indication of the way that evidence-based practice is taught on social work courses and in post-qualifying social work programmes. However, it is better to challenge negative attitudes by demonstrating that it is possible, relevant and important to understand and use research in practice. Whether as a newly qualified social worker, or a highly experienced social work practitioner of many decades, the skills of interpreting research can be learnt and applied in practice.

Much of the current literature about research and evidence-based practice in social work explores research methods and how research can be conducted in practice. In reality, very few social work practitioners have an opportunity to conduct their own research. That may, and should, change in the future but, at the time of writing, local authority-based social work in the UK does not readily encourage practitioner-based research.

By looking more closely at how we use and interpret the research that already exists, and the reasons why it is necessary to do so, I hope to reach a point by the end of this chapter where it is possible to challenge some of the assumptions made by Dominelli and Corby (p. 93).

Owning social work

For as long as there is a perception (which may well be based in reality) that practising social workers have little time for, or interest in, using research evidence in their practice, the focus, growth and knowledge base of the social work profession will move away from those engaged in frontline practice and move towards social work educators. It is crucial for the profession that the locus of expertise does not remain fixed within one area.

The word 'expertise' itself can confer power in terms of where it is located, so it has to be very carefully claimed. Dominelli (2009), by establishing researchers as experts in social work, shifts the balance towards academia in claiming the knowledge base for social work. She explains that the introduction of a greater evidence base for social work practice will build its status as a profession. This is a solid assumption. It is vital, though, that the expertise of social work practitioners and the status of social work 'experts' does not reside exclusively within academic institutions. The best way the profession can grow, as a whole, and the only way it should do, is by drawing in evidence-based expertise from a wide range of sources. A broad evidence base needs to exist, one established by educators, researchers, practitioners and students, and disseminated in a broad and open manner, so that people who use social work services can experience improved outcomes.

Expertise in the subject, practice, analysis and development of social work needs to be shared between service users, social work practitioners, social work educators, social work researchers and social work students who all have extremely valuable narratives to contribute. However, only when expertise is shared will the best results for practice be achieved, which should be our ultimate goal.

While there is a small, but significant, group of people who are committed to and engaged in practitioner research, it pales in comparison with practitioners in other fields who are engaged in both clinical work and research work;

for example, in clinical psychology or medicine. The structures which exist in the National Health Service in the UK to support practitioner research should be duplicated in local authorities and other social work organisations. But there is a long way to go to achieve this.

So, in the absence of extensive social work practitioner research, I shall look at ways in which we can make small changes, even in some of the most diffi-cult and stressful working environments, to the way we use and interpret social work research in our day-to-day practice.

Where is the research?

We may search for research findings in specialist databases (see Chapter 2), or in particular journal articles and research papers. While this will be a rich source of information, it is important that we look more broadly, particularly as access to journals can be difficult and costly when one is not aligned with a particular educational institution. Building libraries, particularly without the support of an employer, can be expensive, and there may be limited access to academic papers. Some papers are written for other social work academics, rather than to be of immediate use in practice. Aveyard and Sharp gave exam-ples of publications that interpret and use both direct and indirect research:

- government or professional organisations' policy, reports, guidance or stan-dards – Care pathways or protocols;
- results from audits;
- reports from international, national or local organisations;
- information from trusted websites;
- patient/client information leaflets;
- information leaflets/letters from manufacturers regarding products;
- textbooks. (Aveyard and Sharp, 2009: 45)

To supplement this list, which is primarily aimed at health care professionals, I would add government white and green papers, local authority and commu-nity policy documents, and information which often has research embedded in it.

> PRACTICE REFLECTION 6.2
> **Keeping up-to-date with research findings**
> Which databases, journals or sources of research evidence can you access via your employer or professional association? It is important to request access to these to ensure you have the opportunity to stay up-to-date with new research findings.

Using research to drive change

In the agency where I previously worked, we were involved in a consultation on proposed changes to the service. Because I had read a recent research paper which I had obtained from an internet forum, I was able to collate with my colleagues a more robust response to this proposal, which would have had a significant impact on service users with whom we worked. By doing this, and building the paper into our response, we were able to demonstrate an interest in our own personal and professional development and also present a cogent challenge to some of the plans for the service. Although the outcome of the consultation did not change as a result of this, it allowed us, as a group of staff and particularly as social workers, to demonstrate our interest in building responses that related to evidence, rather than emotion. It also indicated in a very real sense the usefulness of research studies to colleagues in the team when they saw they could be used to challenge the rationale of decisions made by the organisation.

Finding information

Fortunately, we have access to many more tools than would have been the case even as recently as 2010 and the wealth of accessible information is growing daily. The boom in social media tools such as blogs, Twitter, Facebook and online forums which link to resources, as well as more information being published online, have created a wealth of freely accessible information. While there are some websites such as the College of Social Work (www.tcsw.org.uk), Research in Practice (www.rip.org.uk), Research in Practice for Adults (www.ripfa.org.uk) and Community Care Inform (www.ccinform.co.uk) which may require a subscription to access additional resources, there are substantial resources available without cost.

Often, literature searches as described in Chapter 2 can be a good starting point for discussions in team meetings or within supervision. For example, Research in Practice for Adults publishes a freely available series of pamphlets in a series called 'OutLine' which summarise a particular issue and present literature reviews. For example, 'OutLine 12: What forms of support are effective for family carers of people with dementia (2008)' is a paper which can be read quickly and brought into a team meeting for discussion about how some of the research in this field could be brought into current local authority practice.

As well as finding research online, we now have more opportunities to disseminate, share, and review the quality of research evidence not only with both colleagues and managers, but also with those who are involved in conducting or commissioning the research. While reflexive journals can be useful, there is also scope to establish an online space to invite comments, either within closed communities or publicly, to share the learning as it happens. There are ever-increasing online resources which share up-to-date research in accessible formats and allow comment for conversations to develop around them. There are also substantial resources in other disciplines which can be particularly useful. For example, the Cochrane Library (www.cochranelibrary.com), which primarily focuses on health care research at a very high level, has useful evidence for social work in health and mental health.

As discussed in Chapter 2, it is possible that we want to find evidence in relation to a particular issue, or locate the answer to one question, rather than looking generally at a topic. Aveyard and Sharp (2013) suggest using the acronym PICOT to help identify and determine whether a particular piece of research will be of use. The acronym has a slightly different interpretation depending on whether the piece of research used either qualitative or quantitative methods.

- P is for population (the group of people who the study is about – it might be older people, children in care, or social work students, for example);
- I is for intervention or issue (the phenomena or practice which the study is investigating);
- C is for comparison or context (an intervention or service used to compare the intervention with, or it could be an explanation of the context of the study);
- O is for outcome (what the intervention aimed to achieve or, in qualitative studies, experiences or attitudes, for example);
- T is for time (a length of time is relevant for some studies).

Either explicitly or implicitly, these are useful to consider when searching for any piece of research from any source.

Can we 'do' research?

As stated previously, there are some opportunities for practitioner research but these are very much an exception, rather than the rule. Increasingly, though, opportunities are growing for practitioners to feedback and input into research projects, even if there are few opportunities to lead them. While these opportunities may be transient, there may be a growing awareness of the need for research to be useful. In order to identify what might be useful directly in practice, and in the development of policy within local authorities and organisations which employ social workers, it is increasingly important to engage practitioners in research projects.

As a part of their initial training, students usually carry out a dissertation project which might link with their work on placement. When I have provided a placement for social work students in my agency, I have sometimes asked them to undertake short research tasks while on placement in addition to their university work. This might be to locate and feedback information about a particular client group, or the impact of a certain theoretical approach on practice, for example.

As practitioners or students, we can also carry out small pieces of research independently, although time becomes a crucial factor. 'Research' does not have to be an all-encompassing major task that leads to assessment or publication. 'Research' exists in many places and it is important not to become reliant on a single source. It is crucial to take the responsibility to distinguish, particularly when time is limited, between useful and less than useful information when presenting it back to a team or manager (the critical appraisal tips in Chapter 3 can help with this).

Corby argued that 'linking research and practice in social work has never been straightforward because ... the goals of researchers and social workers often do not coincide' (2006: 5). Fortunately, these increasing opportunities open up the possibility for more solid links to be built between those who commission research, those who carry it out and those who work in frontline social work teams. The hope is that more service users will also be supported to participate in, undertake and disseminate research in the social work field.

Moving to co-production

One area where social workers can take a lead is in the encouragement of people who use the services we provide to become involved in research projects and discussions. Social work values include putting co-production and advocacy as central to our practice. Including those most affected by the services we provide in research and evidence gathering can be a key point to this. This may be done in a practical sense by working with or creating user focus groups in the area we work in and encouraging discussions about what subjects would be useful to pursue. It may, and probably should, lead to areas we had not necessarily considered. Just as the priorities between social work academics and social work practitioners can change due to the differences in perspective, so the priorities between practitioners and users, or carers of those who use services, can differ. It is important that the voices of those who are ultimately the ones whose lives are most significantly affected by social work practice should be at the heart of decisions about the evidence sources and, if there is any scope for original research, they should be actively involved and engaged in the process. Even when original research is not possible, due to lack of interest or funds from employing organisations, having time and space to share literature searches can only improve practice. It is important, though, that this channel is a two-way process and that professionals and practitioners do not 'instil' information in people who use the services. Rather, it should be an opportunity to learn from each other about information sources and evidence.

Good channels of communication between those who commission, undertake and use research are vital to the development of an increasingly useful evidence base for the profession and to ensure that there are fewer instances of repeated research studies which tell us the same thing over and over again.

How can we use research in practice?

Corby (2006) described three models which explain how research-mindedness can be built into social work practice. He called them the 'research-practitioner' model, the 'embedded research' model and the 'organisational excellence' model.

The 'research-practitioner' model places the responsibility for bringing new research into practice solely on an individual practitioner. In contrast, the 'embedded research' model, he explains, does not need to involve the practitioner at all, as it would be undertaken by policy advisers within the agencies that employ social workers. There is an assumption in this model that research evidence from the relevant field would inform the agency's policies and procedures. Finally, the 'organisational excellence' model would operate somewhere between the two, where the agency's procedures and policies would be based on research evidence and its practitioners would take an active part in engaging with relevant research so that the organisation as a whole becomes research-minded.

Corby provided a case study where social workers within a local authority team were given space actively to pursue practitioner research. However, as they were not given protected time away from their substantive posts, casework and emergency work took priority over research work. While the model seemed positive, in practice it was not successful, as the pressures of practice did not give those involved time to engage fully with the research. So, if employers want actively to encourage social work practitioners to engage in research, it is important that this is supported by both time and space, rather than a half-hearted attempt to do the 'right thing'.

Time which is spent on research participation and engagement needs to be valued by employers as contributing positively to service provision and benefiting both the practitioner and the service as a whole.

Although Corby accepts it is not the ideal approach, I will look primarily at the 'research-practitioner' model because, despite his scepticism, it may be the only approach available to many social workers. While we can hope that more work will be done in relation to active practitioner research, the only thing we can be actively responsible for is our own development and learning.

Personal and professional responsibility

It is important to remember that a personal undertaking is made, as part of registration as a social worker, to ensure that practice is up-to-date and that robust continuing professional development is undertaken. This can take many guises but it can include the search for, and use of, research evidence.

As discussed in Chapter 1, registered social workers are legally and professionally accountable for their practice, providing a strong rationale for being committed to using research to inform your practice. For example, the standards of proficiency established by the Health and Care Professionals Council (HCPC) (2011) for social workers in England specify that all registered social workers should:

12.3 Be able to engage in evidence-informed practice, evaluate practice systematically and participate in audit procedures. (HCPC, 2011: 12)

In addition, they should:

14.6 Be able to recognize the value of research and analysis and be able to evaluate such evidence to inform their own practice. (HCPC, 2011: 13)

These are individual and personal responsibilities to which all registered social work practitioners in England have to adhere. Similarly, Scottish social workers, under the Scottish Social Services Council, are expected to be:

> 6.8 Undertaking relevant training to maintain and improve your knowledge and skills and contributing to the learning and development of others. (Scottish Social Services Council, 2009: 34)

Even if the culture of the organisation in which someone works is not supportive and does not provide an environment which is conducive to professional development, these are the individual responsibilities to which social work practitioners must adhere. Registered social workers are not absolved from the responsibility of ensuring that all the standards of their regulatory body are upheld and respected. Students, likewise, are accountable to their universities. While it is absolutely vital that support is given, there has to be a level of personal responsibility and endeavour which has to be self-guided and self-motivated.

Most social work in the UK takes place in large public sector organisations, usually within local authorities or health services. But it is by no means the only setting in which social work takes place and it is important to understand the needs of social work in a variety of settings and sectors.

While social work training remains largely generic, social work jobs tend to be much more specific. There are different streams and strands of professional development depending on whether one works primarily with children, adults or within mental health services. Post-qualification training can therefore be narrower in scope, as it will tend to happen around a specific sector. In order to ensure that we are rounded as social work professionals, though, returning to those generic routes can be vital. Learning about other areas of social work beyond the ones in which we are employed may be something that is not automatically offered through work settings alone.

For example, I have worked in a mental health service where my post-qualification training pathway was very much focused on current mental health practice and legislation. However, families do not naturally divide into 'children/adults/mental health' with the same clarity as services which are provided for these groups of people. I have found it important to have a good understanding of child development and the research which relates to the impact on children, as well as adults, when a parent has a period of mental ill health. While the limit of my 'training' in relation to children is around basic child protection procedures, I have found it important to seek out and identify current policy, practice, research and legislation to ensure my knowledge base is secure and safe. As a practitioner working with adults, I have found it important to know when to refer issues with children on and, while recognising my own professional role has been limited in terms of services that I can deliver, I have needed to have an awareness of the needs of all family members.

Similarly, working in a multi-disciplinary team I have found it very important to be able to extend beyond social work research and draw on the valuable learning which is available in nursing, medical and allied health professional evidence, journals and information sources.

In order to practice effectively, honestly and in an ethically robust manner, it is vital that we are able to explain with clarity the reasons for the particular decisions we make. We must also be able to undertake and interpret our assessments effectively using the knowledge base that we have. Even if we cannot always make the changes we would like to be able to, due to the power differentials or the positions that we hold within an organisational structure, it is important to ensure our research knowledge remains up-to-date so we can explain the background and reasoning for the actions which we take.

What prevents us accessing research in practice?

There are a number of reasons – some already alluded to above – which prevent a social work practitioner or student actively making use of new research in their practice. Aveyard and Sharp (2013) identify some of the blocks which exist and explain why the reality of implementing evidence-based practice may be different from text book models which exhort practitioners to embrace it in order to improve practice and outcomes for service users.

They note that there is likely to be not only a lack of time, but also a number of priorities competing for the attention of the frontline practitioner. This is both on personal and professional levels, as different circumstances may lead to an individual having less time to use outside work to study or read. There also may be skill deficits in terms of practitioners knowing how to locate, interpret and evaluate the literature in a useful way. While more social work qualifying programmes are including this in their curriculum, there are still many practitioners who may have difficulty in finding useful information and studies. Access to relevant information is also a stumbling block as journals and books can be costly. Access to libraries which contain peer-reviewed social work journals and the finances to pay for access to online journal articles may be limited. Further, time can be wasted reading research which is repetitive or irrelevant, which may deter the reader from searching for more potentially useful studies.

Organisational attitudes towards research and study have a significant impact on the ability of an individual or team to spend paid time identifying and reading relevant research and policy papers. The need to complete particular tasks at work will override the time which may be spent by staff reflecting on the way current practice is being carried out in the context of new research findings.

As budgets are being cut throughout the public sector in the UK, time and other resources invested in staff development are under increasing threat unless tangible benefits are seen. However, the potential benefits of research literacy are generally less measureable. There is a move towards quantifying social work practice outcomes, but ethereal qualities such as 'being up-to-date with research' are difficult to measure, or do not produce immediately discernible results.

Hewitt-Taylor (2011) identifies a similar list of reasons why it is difficult to use research evidence in practice. She emphasises the importance of individual authority within a team, which can create and sustain a positive learning and working environment. She also argues that opposition to presenting new ideas can be expressed not only overtly through direct challenge within a team, but also by covert undermining of new ideas which may be brought into a team. Team dynamics and support, or lack of support, can be crucial in influencing the ability of a practitioner or student to remain engaged with learning 'on the job'.

Corby, meanwhile, also identifies barriers and says that:

> practitioners are just too busy because of intensive workloads, the bureaucratic demands of various new procedures and the crisis nature of much of their work. The argument is that social workers simply have no time to pursue the sorts of activities that would lead to more direct research-informed practice. Of course being too busy could be seen as an excuse ... it could be that social workers simply do not see the value of research-based approaches. (Corby, 2006: 162)

Authors in this field appear to identify similar barriers, with time and organisational culture being the main threats to applying research in practice. While there is only a finite amount of time and, although it can be difficult for an individual practitioner to manage or change organisational culture single-handedly, it is possible to tackle some of these challenges. We can ensure that we build our own knowledge base as practitioners and put research-based approaches at the heart of all the work that we do.

How can we overcome the barriers?

It can be easier to define the problems with using research in practice than to find the solutions. Also, what works for one person may not work for another. However, I will explain some of the ways I have found to access and use research evidence in my day-to-day work in a very busy frontline team, which has helped to ensure that my practice remains up-to-date.

Time is limited but there is a need to carve out time within the day to ensure that information can be read and internalised. This may be reading over lunch or defining an hour in a week which can be protected in order to ensure that this happens. It may also need to happen outside a work setting, if a working environment does not permit it. Either way, it is important that there is time for reading and reflecting on what has been read and what can be learnt.

Keeping an evidence log

It can be useful to keep a diary of information that is found and the relevant sources (similar to the suggestions made in Chapter 2 about locating research evidence). Using some of the free resources detailed above (pp. 95–6), literature reviews, policy documents and/or specific research papers can be accessed, depending on what sources of information are available to you at work or home. I have found jotting down the key learning points to be a useful way both of coming back to the information at a later date, and of recording what has been done in terms of continuing professional development.

The diary may be kept in the form of a blog online which could allow for comments and broader sharing of information with others, or it could be a paper-based private resource. At the very least, though, it is useful to share what you have found within your team.

Sharing information locally

I have worked in teams which have a monthly learning meeting, often over a lunch hour, to discuss papers or learning that has been undertaken independently by team members. This is a useful way to develop a learning culture from the ground up within a team, if there are enough people who feel it would be useful and it is supported by a manager. Another model which could be used is that of the journal club, where a particular research paper is chosen and then discussed among peers, as in a book club, in order to appraise and share particularly relevant information.

Ensuring that research evidence is used in a practical way is also a good way of building a positive reputation for you within an organisation, whether as a student on a first placement or a confident practitioner of many years standing. It can be done through introducing relevant research evidence into consultations which take place locally, for example. If there is a consultation about a change in the way a service is delivered, it may be possible to respond with a particular piece of research which speaks of the challenges or benefits of the proposed change. For example, there are a number of studies about the use of direct payments with older people. If this is a policy which is being developed further within the local authority, this body of research could be searched to identify how other local authorities have overcome some of the barriers or blockages to providing direct payments and offer solutions to the policy team leading the service changes.

As a part of my job I did some work on trying to develop a pilot project for older people with functional mental health problems to access individual service funds. This is a way of using personal budgets with provider organisations to ensure that people have more flexibility and choice around their packages of care, if they are not able or do not wish to manage the budget, or become an employer directly. As there was little information in this area, I researched the use of individual service funds for people with learning disabilities, an area in which it has been much more commonly used. I found some information about how pilots in other areas had worked which could be used to transfer the process to the client group with which I worked. The reliance on, and use of, pre-existing research gave the project and my paper credibility and moved it to the next stage of implementation. However, the project came to an end when it was determined that it would be too expensive to pursue; however, it enabled me to push for greater involvement and creativity in developing personal budgets in different ways for older people and people with fluctuating mental health needs.

Using supervision

Supervision is an ideal time to discuss research evidence which you have found. While much of supervision can be very task focused, particularly for more experienced social work practitioners, there should be time devoted to personal and professional development and learning. As supervision is owned by both the supervisor and the supervisee, and the agenda should be jointly established, there is an opportunity to reflect on research within the space provided. In a practical sense, this may not always be welcomed by a manager when there is a limit on time, but it is important to establish the need for learning within supervision and to try to broaden the focus beyond discussion of casework alone.

Building links with universities

Even if there are no formal networks available, and this will vary between local authorities and universities, making connections with academic social work departments is something that can be done proactively by practitioners to indicate an awareness and desire to grow as professionals. Sometimes, there are formal structures in place, as universities have practice education arrangements with particular local authorities and other social work employers. If you are a practice educator, you are likely to have key contacts within academic social work departments. If you are not a practice educator or your employer is not in a partnership with a university social work department, it can be worth trying to establish contacts and networks independently. They would rarely be refused. Offering to speak to social work students can establish an initial contact which could be reciprocated by inviting academics to come into team meetings or organisations and to talk about the relevance of their research work to practice. While contacts can start informally, they can grow into networks. We now have greater ways to create connections whether through social media or more traditional exchanges, and it is a useful resource on both parts. As practitioners, it is important that we do not lose sight of the value we have to bring to social work students and so we can ask for some input in the other direction when we are trying to find time to analyse any local relevant evidence. There may even be the possibility to engage actively in research as a result of the links which are made.

Creating learning spaces

It may be possible to establish groups within an employing agency who are interested in discussing and updating knowledge, even if a particular team is research-resistant. Cross-team forums can help ensure that these conversations take place more broadly. Some organisations may place more emphasis on learning than others but, even when the space is not specifically created in terms of funding for practice research, or even allowing time to discuss broader issues such as the place for research and use of evidence in every day work, there is a case for forcing the issue. As it is a professional requirement to keep up-to-date with research, you could demand space within team meetings and supervision to move discussions beyond casework and managerial issues, and that evidence bases for practice delivery are explored and discussed at more length.

Increasingly, there are more opportunities to find space for discussions about new research online and in secure spaces, if it is not possible in a face-to-face environment, or during working hours. While it is important to try to encourage a research-friendly focus within all teams, it will not always be possible if a team or manager is resistant. While in an ideal world this would be welcomed, it is important to acknowledge that a research-friendly environment does not always exist for social work practitioners.

PRACTICE REFLECTION 6.3

Using research in practice

What do you think about these suggestions? Do you think they will help you to overcome the barriers you face in using research in your practice? What other suggestions do you have?

Moving forward

Despite the scepticism of some social work academics in the ability or willingness of social work practitioners to engage with research, it is essential that practitioners are provided with access to research, and the resources to engage with it, for social work to become more respected as a profession.

Unfortunately, the idealised vision of research-informed practice is not one that exists in reality except, perhaps, in localised areas. The reality is that frontline social work practice is fast-paced and unlikely to involve proactive managers who encourage time to be spent on research and in the promotion of new ways of working based on research evidence provided to them by practitioners, rather than what they are told to implement by senior managers. As social workers and social work students, we have a professional responsibility to ensure that our practice knowledge is current and is based on the best available research evidence.

Some steps can be taken by every practitioner and student, even if the larger barriers to implementing research findings in practice are more difficult to tackle. By referring to the evidence base at work, in reports, in team meetings and in reflective diaries, in whatever format is chosen, the profession as a whole grows.

Ideally, we would see more practitioner research, and there are increasing opportunities for social workers to contribute to research. In the meantime, though, it is important to demonstrate that you can be a responsible, responsive and knowledgeable practitioner, even in some of the most difficult circumstances.

CASE SCENARIO 6.1

Jane

You have been asked to work with Jane, an 85-year-old woman who has vascular dementia and no family support or informal networks, and who has constantly refused care that has been offered to her. You have been told she has Diogenes Syndrome and that the condition of her property is posing a potential environmental risk to her and those living nearby.

PRACTICE REFLECTION 6.4

Applying research evidence and experience

Read Case scenario 6.1 and consider these questions:

1. How can research evidence be used to inform the decisions you make about her needs and the action you can take?
2. You have found a way to provide support for Jane, having explored some of the alternatives available and reached some decisions. How can you help others in your local authority and in local third-sector organisations and universities learn from your experience?
3. How can you involve Jane in the learning and use her views to inform future research?

FURTHER READING

Aveyard, H. and Sharp, P. (2013) *A Beginner's Guide to Evidence-Based Practice in Health and Social Care*, 2nd edn (Maidenhead: Open University Press). Although aimed more squarely at those working in health care settings, this book provides some good practical examples and pointers to using research on a day-to-day basis while working in a public-facing role. It covers ways to appraise the quality of research evidence and non-research evidence, which is sometimes one of the greatest challenges as we move towards having access to more material

SOME USEFUL WEBSITES

http://ifp.nyu.edu/ Information for Practice. A US-based website from a New York-based academic, Gary Holden, who collates sources relating to social work including open access articles, journals and news from around the world.

http://www.ripfa.org.uk/ (for social care with adults) and http://www.rip.org.uk/ (for social care with children and families). While there are paid parts to these websites, they also have free resources including regular downloadable digests of latest information and updates on research. They are very useful to dip into, although the author has almost exclusively used the adult version.

http://www.scie.org.uk/. This is a constant source of useful information including papers that reflect and use evidence to promote good practice in many areas of social care. The resources are free and easily accessible.

http://www.thementalelf.net/ The Mental Elf. This is a website that collates and summarises research papers that specifically look at a wide range of mental health issues. The site is particularly useful and is clearly written to make research papers accessible and usable.

See also:

The Cochrane Library (http://www.thecochranelibrary.com): health-based research and literature reviews

Community Care Inform (http://www.ccinform.co.uk/): paid research site for children's social work

College of Social Work (http://www.collegeofsocialwork.org/home/)

Joseph Rowntree Foundation (http://www.jrf.org.uk/): think tank that focuses on social policy

The Kings Fund (http://www.kingsfund.org.uk/): think tank that focuses on health and social policy

Applying Research Evidence in Different Social Work Contexts

Introduction to Part II

Part II of this book applies the general principles discussed in Part I to specific domains of social work practice. Each chapter follows a similar pattern and includes:

- an overview of research relevant to the specific practice field;
- a case scenario which a social worker may typically encounter within the specific practice field; and
- a discussion of how research evidence could inform a social worker's assessment, decision-making and intervention in the context of the case scenario.

It is not possible to include every practice context in which a social worker may find themselves. However, Chapters 7 to 14 cover the main social work practice domains. Each is written by experienced social work academics and researchers with considerable expertise in their respective fields:

Chapter 7: Karen Broadhurst and Andrew Pithouse explore the research evidence which is used to inform safeguarding children.

Chapter 8: Robin Sen discusses the research evidence used to inform working with looked-after children.

Chapter 9:   Steven Walker focuses on the research evidence used in working with young people with additional needs.

Chapter 10: Wulf Livingston and Sarah Galvani engage with the research evidence which informs working with people who misuse substances.

Chapter 11: Nick Gould is joined by social work practitioner and Approved Mental Health Professional Tom Lochhead to discuss the research evidence which is used to inform working with people with mental health problems.

Chapter 12: Hannah Morgan focuses on the research evidence used in working with disabled people.

Chapter 13: David Smith discusses research evidence used to inform working with offenders.

Chapter 14: Jill Manthorpe explores the research evidence which informs working with older adults.

You are encouraged to select practice domains of interest to you and focus on the chapters which relate to these. Though, of course, you are welcome to read as much or as little as you like!

Finally, Martin Webber reflects on the core themes of the book in Chapter 15 and looks to the future of bringing the domains of social work practice and research closer together.

CHAPTER 7

Safeguarding Children

Karen Broadhurst and Andrew Pithouse

Introduction

Since the mid-1990s, we have witnessed a significant expansion in research designed to inform policy and practice in the field of social work with children and families. From population studies that seek to measure need (Axford, 2010), to studies that focus on specific processes and outcomes arising from new policy initiatives (Neil *et al.*, 2010), there has been an unprecedented increase in the generation of knowledge reflecting a broader national and international trend towards evidence-based practice in public services. Research knowledge can be clustered around the following topics that are central to the work of safeguarding children: 'child development', 'family ecology', 'early intervention and prevention', 'child maltreatment', 'attachment', and 'substitute care and adoption'. Drawing from across the disciplines of psychology, sociology, law and medicine, an interdisciplinary knowledge base now informs policy and practice development. The growth in research has been paralleled by an increase in both the range and number of institutional and web-based portals that bring research in accessible formats direct to the practitioner. In this context, it is imperative that the research-minded practitioner is able to understand the antecedents of current trends, and to sift and filter high-quality material from the mass of information available and appropriately apply research to practice.

To understand the range of influences and the changing nature of social work research, this chapter revisits key moments in the recent history of the profession, draws out core learning and signposts readers to classic works, as well as contemporary material that can be explored further. Our account of the knowledge base that underpins contemporary child and family social work is inevitably selective and our discussion starts with the continuing influence of postwar psychosocial science, with its emphasis on clinical observation. This is briefly considered and contrasted with the later rise of a 'what works' paradigm that has spawned a raft of evaluation or intervention studies since the mid-1990s. Shortfalls in the extant knowledge base are highlighted, in particular the limited number of longitudinal studies that afford valuable insights into the longer-term outcomes of interventions. Thereafter, we consider the application of research to practice. Picking up on themes outlined in the earlier discussion, a case scenario is introduced that provides readers with a practical illustration of how practitioners might navigate the sensitive world of child safeguarding and apply research to practice.

Key moments: psychosocial science and clinical observation

The theoretical developments in the postwar years are particularly salient for current practices of child and family social work, given the ground-breaking work that was undertaken during this period and which underscored the importance of stability and continuity in care-giving relationships. Influenced by the growing credibility of psychosocial science in the 1950s and 1960s, Bowlby's classic works on attachment drew the mother–child relationship clearly into view, theorising the impact of early childhood separation on account of 'maternal deprivation' (Bowlby, 1969; 1973). This work was further developed by Mary Ainsworth et al. (1978), who began to map attachment styles and offered a categorical framework of 'secure', 'ambivalent' and 'avoidant' attachments.

Running in parallel, a tradition of psychosocial casework emphasised the therapeutic power of the practitioner–client relationship as the vehicle for addressing deficits in interpersonal relationships and promoting change. The credibility lent to psychosocial science in the postwar years directed academics and practitioners to focus on early experience, personality development and the individual's 'adjustment' to his/her environment. Clinician observations were essential to the production of social work's knowledge base, with leading texts developing explanatory frameworks from detailed reflection on casework or direct observation. For example, if we examine Biestek's classic text, *The Casework Relationship* (1957), the use of case notes and observations was central to the development of his theoretical principles.

While it is important to situate social work in the postwar years in a context of 'home and hearth' (i.e. an orientation to supporting traditional gendered household relationships), concepts and ideas have been refashioned through subsequent research such that the legacy of this period continues. Indeed, knowledge of attachment theory is pivotal to the child and family social worker's repertoire of expertise, and underpins contemporary approaches to family preservation and permanence planning (Howe, 1995; Howe et al., 1999). In this context, kinship care and adoption remain the gold standards in respect of alternative family care. Where children must remain in long-term foster care, emphasis is placed on how these forms of care can provide a secure emotional base (Maluccio et al., 1986; Schofield and Beek, 2005; Selwyn, 2010). Inspired by early casework, there is also a substantive body of work that espouses a relationship-based approach to practice, again translated into contemporary models based on a 'common factors' approach (Cameron and Keenan, 2010).

Where there is a notable departure from the tradition of postwar psychosocial science is in a shift away from the clinician or caseworker's observation as the foundation for knowledge building, towards what is seen as a more systematic approach to research. For example, contemporary analyses of attachment relationships tend to employ a range of validated tools to assess attachment patterns and styles. Variants of the adult attachment questionnaire are used in both research and practice to progress understandings of parent–child relationships and to make assessments about parental potential for change within child protection (Mikulincer and Shaver, 2007). Thus, research has tended to focus on refining tools and subjecting them to further validation, although arguably retaining much of the foundational learning of postwar years.

The Client Speaks: service user perspectives, family ecology and the rise of identity politics

Postwar psychosocial casework professed something of an *expert diagnostic* position. However, towards the end of the late 1970s a challenge to this standpoint emerged from a number of different camps that called for a fundamental re-think of the knowledge-making process. The work of Mayer and Timms, *The Client Speaks* (1970), was ground-breaking in bringing the service user into view and challenging those developing services to foreground a service user perspective. This work was followed by a raft of studies that sought to democratise the practitioner–service user relationship, giving 'voice' to those who had traditionally held only limited influence in policy arenas. It is now commonplace for research to seek to include the perspectives of service users, with studies documenting topics such as the child's experience of domestic violence (Buckley *et al.*, 2007; Cleaver *et al.*, 2007). Understanding family violence through the lens of the child has enabled an understanding to be gained of the vulnerability of young children in respect of their limited coping skills, and has drawn attention to the importance of protective informal networks (Stanley *et al.*, 2012).

During the late 1970s, questions about the relationship between socio-economic disadvantage and service involvement took centre stage, challenging both research and practice that focused exclusively on individual history and intra-familial relationships at the expense of wider context. Garbarino (1981) called for an ecological approach to understanding child maltreatment. A leading study by Bebbington and Miles (1989) identified a clear relationship between socio-economic disadvantage and reception of children into care. An ecological approach underpins contemporary national guidance, as can be seen in the statutory instrument *Working Together to Safeguard Children* (Department for Education, 2013b), which aims to co-ordinate the actions of a multi-agency workforce. An ecological approach directs the practitioner to consider housing, neighbourhood and the broader systemic context of family life, with the relationship between child poverty and problems of parenting now firmly established. Although socio-economic disadvantage is not deemed strictly *causal* of parenting and family difficulties, it is now very clear that children's life chances are significantly influenced by family resources in their multiple guises (Marmot, 2010).

The late 1970s and 1980s also saw the rise of a feminist-informed challenge to the gendered nature of welfare practice. As household family formation began to shift significantly, patriarchal assumptions within child and family practice were exposed (Scourfield, 2003). Proliferation of what are termed 'identity politics' also saw the views of minority groups given far greater profile. Ethnocentric values associated with family functioning were challenged as a volume of literature called for more cultural competence in social work practice and research. Although the 1970s and early 1980s have been described as 'turbulent times' (Pierson, 2011), this period paved the way for a participatory turn in social research that has been seen as broadly positive. The influence of this period has continued to ensure that researchers resist treating participants as passive subjects and seek co-production of knowledge and shared learning.

Demise of the bureau professional and rise of a 'what works' agenda for research and practice

The 1980s are generally considered to mark a significant point of departure in respect of the demise of the postwar welfare state and loss of confidence in the bureau professional. Unfavourable economic conditions during the early 1980s saw a New Right government making a profound shift within public services through the introduction of a business ethos, designed to increase efficiency and hold professionals to account in respect of evidencing the impact of their activities (Harris, 2003). In a drive to cut back and target public sector spending, new directions for social research emerged that were decidedly *policy*-driven, bound up with calculating service demand, impact and outcome. This has been described as the start of an 'instrumental turn' in both policy and practice (Butler and Drakeford, 2005). In the work of safeguarding children, standardised or 'evidence-based' programmes began to emerge that could demonstrate proven effectiveness. This trend was consolidated under New Labour from 1997 and an endless pursuit of 'what works' continued, with successive administrations favouring helping 'products', such as the parenting skills programme that could be implemented *sui generis* (Broadhurst, 2009). Attempts at the standardisation of practice through proceduralisation and work-flow systems began in the 1980s and have continued as a consistent organisational trend, although a backlash has been witnessed in the form of the Munro Review (Munro, 2011). Following Munro, it is now firmly established that the complexity of family need requires a responsive, durable and multi-faceted relationship-based approach; reductive programmes that are overly behaviourally focused and short term have often failed to deliver the desired outcomes.

New Labour and early intervention

There is no doubt that, during the New Labour administrations, investment in children was considered a key political priority. In particular, New Labour invested heavily in early intervention based on a belief that the quality of child care and education in the early years was pivotal in respect of a child's subsequent life chances. The flagship programme Sure Start was launched, with Children's Centres initially targeting disadvantaged communities. An equally complex and ambitious evaluation was commissioned to run alongside this project, with the aim of achieving systematic measures of improvements in children's development and well-being (National Evaluation of Sure Start, 2005). However, the evaluation seemed to leave many questions unanswered, and of significant concern was that the aspirations of the scheme were not met easily, if at all, in respect of some 'hard to reach populations' (Clarke, 2006). A belief in early intervention continues, as evidenced in the Allen Review (Allen, 2011). However, we are arguably witnessing something of a new moment in respect of policies of early intervention, as neuroscientific research gains traction in policy circles. An explicit emphasis on intervention in the *early years* has found cross-party political support and is legitimated through concerns about the impact of neglect on infant brain development. However, running counter to this are important messages from robust reviews of the research evidence that, as yet, an applied biological perspective cannot yield conclusive evidence about the biological embedding of child maltreatment (McCrory *et al.*, 2012). In terms of effective early intervention, it is critical that studies of parents' perspectives about what they consider to be the most valuable forms of family support are not obscured by the latest scientific fashions. As Penn and Gough (2002) noted in an article entitled 'The price of a loaf of bread', parents consistently cite child care respite and financial assistance as the most helpful forms of assistance. Critics have argued that early intervention programmes in the UK have failed to achieve their potential because they are too closely tied into political agendas such as workfare, rather than aligned to research findings concerning parents' priorities (Grover and Mason, 2013).

Social work research, child abuse tragedies and the media

A discussion of research in respect of safeguarding children would be incomplete without considering risk and the unabated media coverage of child abuse tragedies. Again, looking back in time, the media coverage of the deaths of Maria Colwell (Committee of Inquiry into the Care and Supervision Provided in Relation to Maria Colwell, 1974) and Jasmine Beckford (Brent Borough Council and Brent Health Authority, 1985) were the first of many tragedies to be given high-profile attention and which fundamentally impacted on child and family safeguarding practice and research. The case of Jasmine Beckford, in particular, ushered in a raft of child protection procedures and joint working arrangements, which were to bring about fundamental change to the conditions of safeguarding practice. While public enquiries might bring some sense of justice and closure for the public, for practitioners engaged in the work of safeguarding children successive scandals served to heighten the sense of risk attached to their work. Regarding research on safeguarding, the impact of media coverage has been to stimulate a body of research that is specifically focused on the safety of child protection systems and the causes of human error (Broadhurst *et al.*, 2010a; Broadhurst *et al.*, 2010b; Munro, 1999).

In addition, with the advent of the Serious Case Review, local authority materials have created a wealth of new data for research analysts. The work of Brandon *et al.* (2009) has provided a consistent set of messages about the kinds of failures in frontline practice that result in children slipping through the net of preventive services. The messages are that practitioners fail to share information; they are not good at seeing and communicating with children, or identifying the point at which child neglect becomes unacceptable or dangerous. Social workers' difficulties in understanding household composition, and working effectively with men in families, have also been a consistent theme in this body of work.

Such is the consistency of these messages that research has, more recently, shifted to consider their implementation, rather than simply rehearsing the pitfalls of practice that occur and recur (Sidebotham *et al.*, 2010). There is also a clear thrust towards understanding the systemic context in which practitioner errors happen in order to reduce the often misguided tendency to blame individuals. Risk is ubiquitous in child safeguarding work – and produces a very particular context for child welfare research and practice, which can mean that practice is dominated by a narrowly focused, forensically orientated concern with child harm or neglect. Thus, the current research interest in what makes complex protection systems effective may prove a useful counter to this (Munro, 2011).

Progress and shortfalls in the extant knowledge base

There is no doubt that the wealth of research approaches described selectively above has delivered a substantive body of knowledge to inform child safeguarding practice. In particular, consistent findings in respect of children's needs for secure and consistent care-giving have stood the test of time. While the risk focused literature may have inadvertently fuelled a defensive climate for child and family social work practice, this literature has also spawned a range of tools for identifying and assessing matters such as domestic violence, child developmental harm and the impact of parental mental health (Tunnard, 2004). A raft of participatory studies has certainly brought the views of parents and children far more into prominence, but has often indicated a mismatch between how practitioners and service users frame and understand the interventions offered.

Social workers are arguably the operational embodiment of social policies and, by extension, social work research is also closely aligned. The tendency for research, since the mid-1990s at least, to have become rather dominated by short-term policy-focused objectives at least has, arguably, served to limit the scope of social work research leaving some distinct shortfalls in the knowledge base. In particular, longitudinal studies are few in number. This form of study is a particular challenge for the human services, but their absence may also reflect short-termism in funding linked to policy objectives. The problem is that the outcomes of certain practice interventions may not be detectable for many years, but an absence of longitudinal studies renders equivocal any assumptions of attribution. Ironically, while randomised controlled trials (RCTs) are currently in vogue, there are actually few such large-scale enquiries in social work, which may be indicative of the practical and ethical difficulties in setting up such studies. The problem is that social work practice can be difficult to reduce to its constituent elements (Broadhurst and Mason, 2012) – actions do not always give rise to neat measurable changes. However, qualities of care that are difficult to quantify may be at risk in result-oriented and evidence-based child welfare services. Commentators have talked of a short-term pragmatism in research, with government tending to fund research to support policy objectives (Butler and Drakeford, 2005). A distinction can be drawn between research that seeks to illuminate process and outcome, and that which aims to develop explanatory or theoretical frameworks. Arguably, the push towards 'what works' has tended to mean that research funding is available more for evaluation research than further 'blue sky' exploratory work.

The challenge for the professional tasked to safeguard children is to be able to identify, synthesise and appraise research findings, and then apply these in working with individual children and their families in a way that is sensitive to the specifics of the case. Here, the practitioner is challenged to resist oppositional tendencies within schools of thought (that this or that methodological approach is weak). Rather, the task is to identify rigorous studies whatever their methodological orientation. Some of the most instructive work is that which illuminates the subjective experience of service users. Equally, influential epidemiological studies of the background of children entering care that have stood the test of time illustrate the value of a range of approaches (Bebbington and Miles, 1989).

In summary, we seem to be at a point in UK social work whereby there is an even greater emphasis on evidence-based programmes. The current coalition government has, in the context of austerity and constraints on public spending, asserted the primacy of proven technologies of intervention. For example, the latest policy guidance on early intervention in child and family problems comes in the form of the Allen Review (Allen, 2011), where much unreflective faith is placed on a somewhat simplistic taxonomy of methods for conducting research, with the RCT emerging as the clear 'winner'. While there is undoubted value in some studies that adopt a controlled/experimental model, it is not the case that this must be the first choice for any robust research design. Such studies run into problems when dealing with complex matters such as family life due to familiar problems of isolating and abstracting cause and effect. When we work with families to preserve relationships and safeguard children, improvement may not always follow a clear and measurable upward trajectory – rather, the unexpected challenges of family life are more likely, in research terms, to create oscillations that call forth more nuanced methods to capture change and its multiple causes.

PRACTICE REFLECTION 7.1

Longitudinal research

Why might longitudinal studies be hard to set up? What is the value of this kind of research design? How can longitudinal research inform safeguarding?

To help you think about these questions, go back to Chapter 1 and read about cohort studies.

Safeguarding and research: the case of the Common Assessment Framework

An interesting example of a new innovation in practice that became subject to careful evaluation involving practitioners and service users is the Common Assessment Framework (CAF).

Its primary aim is to help deliver better outcomes for children through a shared e.system of assessment and planning that enables information-sharing and promotes, by means of an identified lead professional, earlier intervention. CAFs tend to have in common a conceptual base drawn from the *Framework for the Assessment of Children in Need and their Families* (Department of Health, 2000). These meticulous methods to assess children across a range of domains and dimensions have been adapted and (substantially) reduced in different versions of the CAF. There is no uniform or universal CAF, but most frameworks emphasise prompt identification and delivery of preventive services in order to improve children and young peoples' quality of life and reduce the likelihood of more serious problems. In doing so, the CAF aims to enhance safeguarding and well-being.

The CAF has its genesis in ground-breaking research by Ward and Peel (2003), who introduced an intentionally detailed, highly schematic and pedagogically driven model of assessment. This proto-type was replicated to some extent and tested by Pithouse *et al.* (2004) (see also Pithouse, 2006), who deployed mixed methods action research in which practitioners (social work, education, police, health, voluntary sector) and service users helped design and test an assessment schema linked to different age-bands of children and thresholds of concern. It was geared to key domains around child development, parenting capacities and environmental themes. Its evaluation suggested better inter-agency information collection and sharing and some reduction in inappropriate referrals. Other CAF research found multi-agency working to be improved and that the CAF prompted a more holistic understanding of the child's needs (see Brandon *et al.*, 2009). The shortcomings of the CAF have not gone unnoticed, such as concerns about lack of user involvement in assessment practice, the focus by some workers on 'problems', rather than strengths and needs, and concerns over CAF as a mode of surveillance, rather than prevention. The many shades of CAF also inhibit any consistent application across children's services (see also Broadhurst and Pithouse, 2009; Gilligan and Manby, 2008; White *et al.*, 2009). The development of the CAF (and of new information technologies in safeguarding more generally) provides an instructive case study into the way research provides essential insights into the strengths and weaknesses of e-based innovations in social work and, in doing so, has decisively shaped policy and practice in the UK.

Applying research to child safeguarding practice

We now turn to the matter of practice and how we might apply a more research-minded approach to the sorts of challenges that social workers often face when safeguarding children. Before introducing an example from practice, first, we set out our position on research and its potential application in everyday work. It should be clear by now that we do not see social workers as 'practitioner-scientists', engaged in the purist application of a hierarchy of knowledge, privileging the evidence derived from experimental studies over other sources of valid knowledge, such as qualitative research or single case studies. Indeed, much training and practice in social work mirrors key elements of the research act in qualitative studies – confidentiality, empathic listening, being clear about aims and responsibilities, ethical orientation, disciplined enquiry and reflection, and good analytical skills. The effective researcher, like the good worker, avoids the search for verification of hunches and, instead, uses working hypotheses in order tentatively to test whether the 'data' fits our 'theory' about what is going on (see Farmer and Owen, 1995). We challenge our preferred explanations in order to avoid a natural tendency to seek confirmation of our initial bias or to resist the pressure of 'group think' in meetings (see Milner and O'Byrne, 2009). What is certain in our day-to-day work is the uncertain world of human interaction and here the notion of a working hypothesis helps us structure our thinking and analysis, and resist the attraction of received wisdoms. In doing this, the explorative genius of qualitative methods is well-suited to the indeterminacy of social work and, particularly, the occupational world of child safeguarding where forensic approaches to gathering clues, analysing evidence, estimating risk and designing an intervention require clear analytic and reflective skills, including a capacity to evaluate practice.

Assuming some prior exploration and hypothesis-testing, we may have identified the need for some intervention and wish to apply a methodology to understand its appropriateness for the case in hand. This calls for a search of the research literature to locate supporting evidence; but the question then is what should guide us in this endeavour? We argue for a pragmatic approach to research evidence which recognises the value of pre-existing high-quality quantitative and qualitative research that describes proven interventions. The primary test here is: Are these studies of a reasonable standard and are they *relevant* to the context? In our thinking about this we are much persuaded by Dodd and Epstein (2011: 19) who assert the importance of flexibility in worker orientation to research tools and evidence, and commend the virtues of compatibility and applicability of research to the problem at hand; the motivation being the benefits this will bring to the client, the service and the practitioner.

So, how might practitioners utilise research in their response to a child safeguarding concern? This deceptively simple question has no easy answer, particularly when we have known for some time (see Epstein, 1987; McLaughlin, 2007: 151) that social workers for various reasons (time, crisis work, multi-stranded problems of families) display some scepticism about the value of applying research in their pressured daily practice and, often, rely on experience-based methods of conceptualising and acting in response to cases. Yet, there have been clear expectations within occupational standards that UK social workers become research-minded (Munro, 2011). Similarly, since the 1990s, as we stated in the introduction to this chapter, we have seen an ever-expanding body of knowledge in social work about what might be effective interventions promoted by a growing number of research translation bodies in social work (e.g. Research in Practice, Centre for Excellence in Children's Outcomes). The sheer scale of national and international sources may seem bewildering and impossible to navigate to all but the most experienced researchers. But in seeking to apply research to practice, we might impose some basic order on the seemingly infinite materials that are potentially relevant. Assuming some research literacy on the part of the worker (not all workers will have this, or be as 'good' as some of their peers) and an organisational culture that endorses a research-minded approach to practice – by no means a given – we suggest that the worker approaches the research literature in a step-by-step process as discussed in Chapters 2 and 3 to answer a practice-based research question.

Case scenario

The following child safeguarding referral has been fictionalised from different cases known to the authors in order to create an example that might resonate with frontline workers.

The Rogers family has been long known to their local authority; this has not been a 'live' case for several months but one seen as requiring preventive support which is provided through a health visitor scheme that offers additional health care to young mothers and their infants.

CASE SCENARIO 7.1

The Rogers family

Julie Rogers was in care for some years and left foster care at 16 with little in the way of stable family connections. She is white British, now aged 24, the mother of three children (a boy aged eight, a three-year-old girl and another girl of six months). The two older children are of mixed heritage by different fathers. The family live in a two-bedroom social housing flat which is cramped and where there is little room for the children to play. The neighbourhood is an outer-city area of some deprivation and few local amenities. Her partner Anthony, aged 33, often absent, is of eastern European background, is the father of the youngest child and has convictions for petty theft. There have been previous referrals because of domestic violence. A new referral has come in from the health visitor after finding the youngest child being looked after by the oldest, together with concerns about home conditions and neglect regarding the three children.

We now draw on our earlier discussion but, particularly, the important work of Holland (2011: 169) in tackling this referral in a research-minded way through two key stages. As a social worker new to the family, as a qualitative researcher might, (see McCracken, 1988) at stage 1 we would develop some initial 'culture check' about our own assumptions or preconceived views which might affect our observation of what is 'going on' in the family, and which we need to acknowledge and restrain. Thus, the worker might start by asking her or himself:

■ What do I know about families in the UK today where children and parents may be from different ethnic backgrounds and what is the source of this knowledge?
■ What do I know about people from new accession states in the EU, such as Romania and Bulgaria, and what is the source of this knowledge?
■ What do I know about care-leavers and their lives in the community?
■ How will I and my agency be seen by the family?
■ What are my main techniques, knowledge(s) and values for assessing risks in this family?
■ What information gaps, assumptions and prejudices are likely to apply?

In addressing these questions, there is, for example, a sizeable research literature on care-leavers and the challenges they face. Likewise, there is a large body of work on domestic violence, child poverty and new family structures in late modernity. As ever, the issue is the time and skills needed to search and audit multiple sources. It is also the case that sources may provide little more than general pointers to assist assessment and reflection. It is highly unlikely that there is some matching piece of research that will reveal all that is needed to be known about the neglect of children with mixed heritage in adverse material circumstances looked after by a mother who was in care, has limited parenting skills and whose current partner is from a much discriminated European minority. But broadly relevant research will stimulate interpretations that may not have been previously considered.

Having considered the reflective insights and likely actions arising from this audit of relevant sources, the worker might then move to stage 2, where she develops some working hypotheses based on various strands of knowledge and suppositions to be tested by her initial assessment.

Hypothesis 1: The eight-year-old child left to look after the infant did not represent much of a risk, the child is sensible, often helps the mother, who was only away from home for less than 10 minutes in going to the corner shop for essential ingredients for lunch.
(This was the mother's version of events according to the health visitor (HV).)

Hypothesis 2: The infant and middle child are regularly left in the inappropriate care of the eldest while mother goes out with her partner, or visits nearby friends.
(This was the HV's version.)

Hypothesis 3: All three children are at risk of neglect, or being neglected, because of mother's poor parenting skills, unsatisfactory home conditions, and previous incidence of domestic violence by Anthony.
(This is the version that would arise from a surface reading of the case file.)

Hypothesis 4: Home conditions are more disorganised and chaotic rather than materially 'poor'. The mother loves her children and they her. Mother is overwhelmed and not very capable, has learning and literacy problems. Anthony has struggled to find legitimate employment but has been in low-paid shift work for last nine months and there have been no new domestic violence reports for over a year.

(This was the worker's version, whereby case events are framed to allow an alternative testable interpretation of what is going on.)

It may be that none of the above hypotheses, singularly or combined, can capture current events and that 'what is going on' may be different altogether. However, the evident differences of these working hypotheses do assist in keeping an open mind in approaching the family and can help avoid an overly concrete interpretation of what is happening based on inevitably partial information from referral and historical case notes.

In approaching the family, the worker expects some hostility and anticipates a role that recognises strengths while not oblivious to the dangers of optimism about the abilities of some neglectful or abusing families to change (see Haringey Local Safeguarding Children Board, 2009). In working with families, there are several validated interventions that can be applied should they correspond to the problems at hand (family therapy, cognitive behavioural approaches, attachment therapy, task-centred practice, ecological approaches and so forth). In this case, it may be that the multiple adversities faced by the family require a theory and method that connects at different levels. The priorities and processes of the intervention(s) would need to be established with the family. In selecting the theory and method of intervention, the social worker needs to apply some judgement about the evidence to support their choice. In so doing, the worker could usefully apply the 10-question appraisal checklist offered by McLaughlin (2012), or other frameworks as discussed in Chapter 3, in their reading of the relevant research.

Returning to the case scenario, let us assume that the social worker co-works with the health visitor. The health visitor confirms that immunisations are up to date but developmental milestones are causing some concern; the older child, in particular, is not doing well at school because he is being called on to help his mother too much. Anthony has been difficult to engage and claims shift work is the reason he is rarely available to meet the social worker. As is often the case, the social worker is faced with unknowns and uncertainties in looking to the future. Patterns of risks and strengths do not reveal what actually happened, neither do they reliably predict the mother's capacity to cope looking ahead, or her partner's willingness to engage. In trying to find a way forward, the worker has used her reading of research to deploy an ecological approach that will: (a) engage with parenting skills (mainly the mother's, in the short term); (b) support the children's emotional and physical development; (c) generate a safe home environment; (d) deal with mother–partner relationships; (e) update welfare benefits; (f) provide school support; (g) investigate a housing upgrade. An ecological approach requires a systemic approach to intervention that attends to the range of potential resources that might provide holistic support to this family and strengthen 'protective factors'.

Evaluating the impact of any intervention is critical to effective practice. This requires that the practitioner is attuned to the objectives of his/her actions and intended outcomes in particular cases. Here, we stress the particularity of cases and tailored responses which require excellent observational and analytic skills, rather than simple reliance on a manual or procedure. Tools that encourage practitioners to map child and family strengths, such as the resilience matrix designed by Daniel *et al.* (2010) or the Graded Carer profile (Srivastava *et al.*, 2003) can certainly aid the inexperienced practitioner – provided they are used thoughtfully, rather than as a substitute for professional judgement. That workers must establish meaningful relationships with family members – not only to understand children's social and emotional worlds, but also motivate change in parents – is a consistent finding in the research literature (Horwarth, 2013). Hence, family members need to participate in and share their perceptions about what works at all stages of intervention and evaluation, as this is key to capacity-building within families.

There are very clear parallels between evaluation research and everyday evaluation in practice. Here, we draw on six principles for evaluation research (see Shaw, 2012b: 377–9), which the reader will readily appreciate is directly applicable to the reflective cycle of practice discussed above. Summarised, these comprise:

- concentrated critical reflection in the way we describe practice and people in relation to some intended outcomes;
- try to understand one's own taken for granted orientations to the issue at hand and seek to challenge or falsify simple or convenient truths;
- be open to the sometime unpalatable or uncomfortable views of service users and their worlds from which such perspectives may emanate;
- utilise reflectively the evident overlaps between the basic research skills in qualitative research and social work practice;

- seek to broaden the impact of the results of evaluation in practice beyond the solo worker and individual case via team or network engagement;
- prioritise and sustain participatory evaluation with users and carers and understand their world.

This approach to family support and child safeguarding draws on available research outputs (what research says) as well as applied research processes (how to think and work with families in a research-minded way – hypotheses and reflection and analysis). The 'real world' messiness of human interaction cannot be restrained, or made wholly transparent. But, by using prior research and using research skills in a reflective way that compares, contrasts and critiques the available information in collaboration with participants, the worker can impose some essential analytic rigour within their safeguarding practices. In this case, what we know is that family functioning can be greatly improved by enhancing protective factors, which can then significantly improve developmental outcomes for children.

The practitioner-researcher, in drawing on an ecological approach (Bronfenbrenner, 1979; Pardeck, 1988), needs to identify the sub-systems that surround the family (extended family, community, other services, economy) and their likely impact (Kerson, 2004). In the case in question, the ecological mapping is likely to implicate a mix of interventions that have different stakeholders, timelines and outcomes, and cannot somehow be integrated into a single evaluable event. Consequently, the worker might adopt a flexible strengths approach (Holland, 2011) informed by safeguarding priorities whereby evaluation of progress is a mix of methods, skills and sensitivities to determine whether initiatives are actually helping the family. Much depends on clarity of needs, intervention objectives and intended benefits that both worker(s) and family agree (Dodd and Epstein, 2011: 42). Thus, with regard to the case study, we could envisage a worker deciding to try and assist, first, in practical ways to promote trust and generate early impact. Hence, some preliminary focus on checking welfare benefits may produce useful results and, likewise, some visible advocacy over housing may demonstrate worker commitment to the issues that families see as most pressing. Such efforts are more easily calibrated in terms of transparent outcome to the parents, as is for example using a tested 'checklist' approach to working with families to help them make their home environment safe for children. The children's emotional, cognitive and physical needs are clearly a matter for careful joint-working with the family and its interface with health and education services. This is likely to entail specialist and routine appraisal of development which can inform multi-disciplinary intervention that will impact on family well-being and can be evaluated. The skilled worker could also use validated tools to promote and appraise parenting skills in ways that empower and build on strengths. From these initiatives – which may include proven techniques, as well as novel empirically unsupported activities based on practice wisdom and professional judgement – it should be possible to generate a mosaic of data and analytic insights that allows some modest descriptive evaluation of progress over fixed points.

Conclusion

There are those that insist that only the credibility of rigorous measurement tools to evaluate interventions can resist the accusation that social work is somehow pre-scientific and, in some instances, dangerous quackery. Such heated but often sterile debates can be noted elsewhere (Stoesz, 2010) and, in our view, fail to connect with the 'real world' problems of children, families, communities and the professionals that support them, the complexity of which makes the idea of searching out some experimentally proven 'silver bullet' technique illusory at best. The often multiple and chronic difficulties of people in culturally diverse and poor or challenging environments require a much more systemic approach in which practice wisdom and experience combine with the insights of a research-minded approach. The pitfalls of relying too heavily on matching some presenting problem to an evidence-based product is that this fails to understand the nature of practice which reaches an emergent, rather than an a priori, understanding of family difficulties. The effective practitioner must be wary of being drawn into wrong-thinking that practice is simply common sense but, equally, that family work is a technical matter constituting little more than the judicious application of evidence-based programmes. Both ends of the spectrum can be described as epistemological boot camps (Staller, 2013) that undermine critical engagement with a wealth of research evidence and astute, process-focused social work practice.

FURTHER READING

Dodd, S.-J. and Epstein, I. (2011) *Practice-Based Research in Social Work: A Guide for Reluctant Researchers* (London: Routledge). The authors provide a clear and compelling exposition of the relevance of basic research methods to good practice. The accessibility and applicability of the text makes this a really useful book for the research hesitant.

McLaughlin, H. (2012) *Understanding Social Work Research*, 2nd edn (London: Sage). This introduction to the research enterprise in social work allows a more thematic treatment of general issues and key concepts: philosophy of social research, research ethics, user involvement, anti-oppressive practice, inter-disciplinary approaches and application to practice. It is geared to practitioners and students, and is a key source for reflexive thinking about research in practice.

Munro, E. (2011) *The Munro Review of Child Protection: Final Report. A Child-Centred System* (London: Department for Education). This final report from the national review of child protection, stimulated by the high-profile death of Baby Peter, clearly highlights the negative impact of excessive procedure and standardisation on professional practice.

Shaw, I. (2012) *Practice and Research* (Farnham: Ashgate). Shaw offers a landmark compendium of methodological wisdoms, guidance on applied research and evaluation techniques, and a wealth of insights into the complex relationships between practice and research.

Webb, S. (2001) 'Some considerations on the validity of evidence-based practice in social work', *British Journal of Social Work*, 31(1): 57–79. This seminal article provides a critical overview of assumptions that can underpin approaches to evidence-based practice.

CHAPTER 8

Working with Looked-After Children

Robin Sen

Looked-after children: the context

In 2012, there were around 91,000 children in the care system in the UK. (In this chapter, 'child' or 'children' is used to refer to those aged 0–18. Where there is specific discussion of those aged 12 and over, the terms 'young person' or 'young people' are used.) Following a number of years of decline, the number of children in the care system rose between 2008 and 2012 (see NSPCC, 2013). The latest available statistics for England show 62 per cent of children entered care due to abuse or neglect (Glenndenning, 2012), though some research studies (Quinton and Rutter, 1988; Wade *et al.*, 2011) have found higher proportions of looked-after children may have had such experiences. Other principal reasons for children entering out-of-home place-ments are: 'family dysfunction' (where parenting capacity is deemed chroni-cally inadequate) 14%, 'family in acute stress' (where a temporary crisis renders parenting capacity temporarily diminished by external circumstances) 9%, 'absent parenting' 5%, parental illness or disability 4%, child disability 3% and socially unacceptable behaviour by the child 2% (see Glenndenning, 2012). A large proportion of those entering care come from families already known to social work teams (Cleaver, 2000), while young people of twelve and older are more likely to have entered care due to their own behaviour or family breakdown, and are more likely to exhibit emotional and behavioural difficulties (Sinclair, 2005).

Although the largest proportion of children who return to parental care still do so within the first six months of becoming looked-after (Biehal, 2006), practitioners should be aware that the proportion of children entering the care system due to abuse or neglect has increased substantially since the 1990s and, partly as a consequence, children are spending longer periods within the care system than previously (Biehal, 2006; Sinclair *et al.*, 2007). This focuses attention on the need for practitioners to organise tailored indi-vidual packages of support to help children address the impact of such abuse or neglect. Effective provision is likely to include a tailored but holistic programme of educational support, therapeutic or psychological support, carers who can manage difficult behaviour while maintaining a child's self-esteem, and sensitive assessment of the child's needs and wishes around birth family contact (Gilligan, 2000; Sen and Broadhurst, 2011; Sinclair *et al.*, 2007).

In the most complex birth families, multiple factors – such as parental substance misuse, domestic violence, mental health difficulties, child neglect and poverty overlap – create a highly challenging context for good parenting (Cleaver *et al.*, 2007). Research highlights that social workers should be intervening earlier to place children in care where parents are clearly not meeting young children's needs (Selwyn *et al.*, 2006; Ward *et al.*, 2012), albeit the importance of effective parenting support has also been emphasised (Quinton, 2004). Ward *et al.* (2012) stress that knowledge of child development is crucial to making informed assessments. Regardless of the primary reason for entry into care, the vast majority of looked-after children will have had experiences of poor and insecure housing, difficult family settings and poverty (Sinclair, 2005). Living in poverty in deprived localities is far from synonymous with poor parenting, but parenting well in such circumstances is substantially harder (Utting, 1995).

Longer-term outcomes for children who have been in the care system are poor compared with peers in terms of educational attainment, employment, mental ill health, involvement in the criminal justice system and homelessness (Wilson *et al.*, 2004). However, Wilson also warns that simple comparisons with the general population are misleading as the origin of many of the difficulties care-leavers experience will pre-date their entry into the care system. Practitioners should be aware that emerging evidence suggests that children remaining in parental care on 'home supervision' with social work support are also vulnerable to experiencing poor outcomes (Gadda, 2012) and they may fare worse in terms of educational attainment (McClung and Gayle, 2010). While there is room for improvement in the care system, evidence shows it tends to improve the well-being of children entering it (Forrester, 2008); the majority of children in care are content to be there (Sinclair, 2005); and those children who enter the care system and then return home tend to fare worse than those who remain in care (Quinton and Rutter, 1988; Sinclair *et al.*, 2005b; Wade *et al.*, 2011). There is a clear implication that leaving children in parental care which is clearly not meeting their needs will lead to poorer outcomes for them.

PRACTICE REFLECTION 8.1

Child abuse and neglect

Figures now indicate that a higher proportion of children are entering the care system due to abuse or neglect. Why do you think this is? Are the characteristics of children entering the care system fundamentally different than in previous times; if so, why should this be? Or do you think that increasing awareness of abuse and neglect, together with changes in the way these are recorded, is more significant?

Placement options

There are three broad placement options for a child entering care: foster care, kinship care and residential care. Although other factors such as a child's age and placement availability will influence placement decisions, it is important to be aware that research suggests different placement types are associated with different outcomes in terms of, for example, placement stability and psychological well-being. In most cases, placements will initially be temporary while the possibility of a return to parental care – 'rehabilitation' or 'reunification' – is assessed. Where it has been decided that a long-term placement outside parental care is required, the same three placement options plus adoption are possibilities.

Rehabilitation/reunification

Returning children to parental care is principally a consideration while children are in 'short-term' placements, but children can return from nominally 'permanent' substitute care. Recent evidence is worrying on the outcomes of reunification in terms of placement breakdown rates, the likelihood that children are re-abused and broader outcome measures. Lutman and Farmer's (2013) five-year follow-up of returned children found that just over half of returns did not last and that child well-being for those who were stable at home was worse than for those who were in settled placements outside of parental care. Also, 59 per cent of children experienced maltreatment within two years of return. Farmer and Wijedasa (2013) and Sinclair et al. (2005a) both found re-abuse rates of just under 50 per cent for returning children. Farmer and Wijedasa (2013) also found that re-abuse rates were still higher in cases of parental substance misuse, while Sinclair et al. (2005a) found that children in long-term care who had returned home at any point fared worse in terms of school performance and behavioural difficulties.

It cannot be said that all children who return and experience poor outcomes should have remained in care: a lack of clear planning, the failure to build gradually towards full rehabilitation, the gaps in service provision for parents with substance misuse issues and the absence of intensive post-return support are identified as key gaps within practice which need to be addressed for reunification to work better (Lutman and Farmer, 2013; Wade et al., 2011). Nonetheless, practitioners should be aware that the need for better assessment of whether rehabilitation is the right option for children is highlighted. Notably, where parents display a strongly positive disposition towards contact, and evidence a motivation for reunification through addressing concerns which led children into care in the first place, children's return it is more likely to succeed (Biehal, 2006; Cleaver, 2000; Wade et al., 2011).

Adoption

Where a child is unable to return to parental care, adoption is an attractive option in terms of the legal, emotional and psychological security it can provide a child. National and international evidence suggest that, while adoption does not allow children who have experienced adversity to catch up on all measures of behaviour and well-being, it can be more effective in promoting healthy attachments than other placement options (Selwyn *et al.*, 2006; Sinclair *et al.*, 2007; Van Ijzendoorn and Juffer, 2006). However, long-term fostering can be equally effective in terms of other measures, such as placement stability and behavioural change where children of similar age and characteristics are compared (Sinclair, 2005). Evidence suggests that the younger a child is when adopted the better the likely outcomes, with the best developmental catch-up achieved where children are placed under 12 months of age (Van Ijzendoorn and Juffer, 2006). However, research on resilience suggests that positive later life experiences can overcome early adversity and emphasises that the early years are important because they precede the later years, not because of a 'critical period effect' (Rutter, 2007: 199).

Two UK studies (Rushton and Dance, 2003; Selwyn *et al.*, 2006) showed the adoption of 'older young' children (aged 3–11) can work well, but each study also found there were at least some difficulties in over half of the adoptive placements, suggesting the need for ongoing effective post-adoption support. Adoption becomes increasingly unlikely as the child's age at entry and length of time in care increases (Selwyn *et al.*, 2006) and, in practice, it is rarely used for children who are over five when they first enter care (Sinclair *et al.*, 2007).

In considering adoption therefore, practitioners should be aware that it is an attractive option in terms of outcomes, but successful outcomes are less pronounced as a child's age at adoption increases. This does not mean adoption should be ruled out for older children but, rather, that attention should be focused on identifying whether adoption is a viable option for a child in care as soon as possible. Delays in placing children for adoption should be minimised, where possible, without compromising the identification of suitable adopters or the assessment of rehabilitation as a possibility.

Fostering

Fostering is the most common placement option for children in the UK. There is evidence that both short-term and long-term foster care improves child well-being (Forrester, 2008) and some evidence that the majority of children in it wish to stay there (Sinclair *et al.*, 2005b). Long-term foster care is a far more likely destination for older children in long-term care, both because of a lack of adopters for older children and because of many older children's lack of willingness to be adopted (Sinclair, 2005). There are some concerns, though, regarding the number of placement moves that children can have within foster care (Sinclair *et al.*, 2007; Wilson *et al.*, 2004). While foster care does not perform noticeably worse than other placement options in terms of placement disruption, breakdown rates for teenagers in foster care can be as high as 50 per cent, with those with emotional and behavioural difficulties more likely to experience disruption (Sinclair, 2005). There are also concerns around adequacy of provision: one fostering organisation has estimated that there is a shortage of 10,000 foster carers in the UK (Tearse, 2010). There is a particular shortage of specialist foster placements which are able to meet the complex and challenging needs of those children for whom disruption is most likely (Sinclair, 2005). Practitioners should be aware that fostering placements provide an effective and flexible placement option for both short-term and permanent care. Outcomes for children in foster placements taken as a whole are worse than for those adopted, but those in foster care constitute a far wider range of children. When comparisons are made of children of similar age and characteristics, long-term fostering can achieve similar outcomes to adoption, albeit that it lacks the 'permanence' of adoption (Sinclair et al., 2007).

Kinship care

Where extended family members are willing to care for children, kinship care provides an alternative to unrelated substitute care; this can offer greater continuity of relationships and networks for children (Aldgate and McIntosh, 2006). Evidence suggests that outcomes in kinship care are not markedly different from unrelated foster care (Farmer and Moyers, 2008; Hunt et al., 2008). Farmer and Moyers' (2008) comparative study of foster care and kinship care placements did not find significantly different levels of placement disruption. Kinship carers were also found to persevere more despite difficulties in placement, but disruption rates for children over 10 were greater in kinship placements than foster care. Sinclair et al., (2007) paradoxically found kinship placements were of poorer quality but had better outcomes, and recommend that the use of kinship care could be increased; Ward et al. (2012) are more cautious about it as a placement option in high-risk cases on the basis of their study of very young children.

Family group conferences (FGCs) have been suggested as one worthwhile mechanism for harnessing family networks and exploring possible kinship care options when children are about to enter care, or are already in care (Holland et al., 2005; Hunt et al., 2008), although there is some evidence that kinship carers themselves have mixed views on their value (Hunt et al., 2008).

Overall, these somewhat divergent research findings support the view that kinship care is a viable placement option, and can be highly effective in terms of both short-term and longer term care. However, it is not without its own difficulties and a common finding is that practitioners need to undertake better assessment of potential kinship placements, and provide better financial and practical support to them.

Residential child care

Residential child care in the UK is now principally used for young people over 12, where their high level of needs, behaviour, preference against family-based care or previous placement breakdowns make foster or kinship care untenable (Kendrick, 2008). Despite the fact that it tends to care for children with higher levels of need, there is still evidence that the residential sector improves child well-being (Forrester, 2008), and there is some evidence that young people in residential care may themselves prefer it to foster care (Kendrick, 2008). However, there is less evidence of its effectiveness in improving child welfare than other placement choices (Forrester, 2008).

Sinclair *et al.* (2005a; 2005b; 2007) found that children in long-term foster care and adoptive placements exhibited fewer emotional and behavioural difficulties than those in residential child care, while international evidence shows that developmental catch-up is significantly poorer for young children placed in institutional care (Van Ijzendoorn and Juffer, 2006). The label of 'institutional care' does, though, group together a wide range of different residential provision. Comparing the outcomes of residential care with other placement options in the UK is also difficult because it serves some of the children with the highest level of need (Kendrick, 2008). However, due to the limited evidence of its effectiveness, alongside its relative expense, residential care is now seldom a first-choice placement, especially for those under 12. For children with marked emotional and behavioural difficulties – those involved in significant offending or risk taking behaviour, those who refuse a family placement, or those who have experienced multiple placement breakdowns – it may, though, be the only viable placement option.

Birth family relationships in care and adoption

Since the 1989 Children Act, there has been a legislative presumption in favour of looked-after children's contact with birth family members and significant others, although this contact must be practicable and consistent with a child's welfare. There are now significantly greater levels of contact than prior to the 1989 Act (Cleaver, 2000; Sinclair, 2005). Contact can provide children with reassurance about family members' welfare and support existing relationships. Looked-after children usually want contact with their birth families and can be highly distressed by a lack of it (Sen and Broadhurst, 2011). However, research over the last 15 years has increasingly emphasised that not all contact is likely to lead to positive outcomes for children: where there has been prior maltreatment, frequent and unsupervised contact increases the risk of placement breakdown and re-abuse (Sinclair *et al.*, 2005a; Sinclair *et al.*, 2005b). Contact alone is insufficient for there to be a return to parental care, far less a successful one (Biehal, 2006). In managing contact, focus is therefore put on the need for practitioners to think through the purpose of contact, its context and safety, as well as giving due weight to a child's and birth family's wishes (Sen and Broadhurst, 2011).

When a child is adopted, courts should consider contact with the birth family; however, there is no assumption that there should be contact. The most usual form of post-adoption contact is 'letterbox' contact of low frequency; however, there have been increasing moves towards some direct contact with birth families (Neil and Howe, 2004). The emerging research suggests such contact can work positively for all concerned, albeit the evidence is currently based on children who were placed for adoption when young, without significant pre-existing relationships with birth family members. Practitioners should be aware that such contact may be a less positive proposition where it involves the adoption of older children, or children whose birth family history means contact is more likely to be problematic (Neil and Howe, 2004).

Sibling co-placement

There is some evidence that placing siblings in the same placement can be a protective factor, offering better continuity of relationships and mutual support (Kosonen, 1996). The impact of co-placement for siblings is less clear: Holland *et al.* (2005) found some, but not strong, evidence that sibling co-placement increased placement stability and, where sibling relationships are difficult, it can destabilise placements (Sinclair, 2005). The individual needs of siblings sometimes dictate that separate placements are required (Rushton *et al.*, 2001). However, this does not fully explain why a high proportion of siblings – up to two thirds – are not placed together (Kosonen, 1996; Sinclair *et al.*, 2005b). Separation is more likely when there are significant age differences, large sibling groups and entry into care occurs at different points in time (Kosonen, 1996; Shlonsky *et al.*, 2003). Where siblings are separated, the vast majority of siblings want contact (Office for Standards in Education Children's Services and Skills, 2009) and this is not prioritised as it should be (Kosonen, 1996; Sinclair, 2005). The research evidence supports the legislative presumption in favour of sibling co-placement, but also suggests the need for assessment of whether a child's needs can be met in the same placement as their other siblings. Where separation is deemed necessary, clear consideration and documentation of plans for maintaining links between siblings should be undertaken.

Working with children in care

The concept of resilience developed from evidence of young people's ability to overcome marked adversity occurring in earlier childhood (Rutter, 1981). Previously, research into attachment had emphasised that early child experience has a marked impact on later development: neurological development is affected by experiences of nurturing from the very first days after birth onwards (Howe, 2005). Notably, children will ordinarily start to form discriminating attachments to their primary carer(s) from around seven months (Schaffer and Rudolph, 1990). In social work, resilience theory has been principally applied to consider the protective and enabling factors in a looked-after child's life which can support them to overcome obstacles to optimal developmental progress despite previous experiences of adversity (Gilligan, 1997).

Some of these factors relate to qualities 'within' the placement itself, some 'outside' it but impacting on it. Sinclair *et al.* (2007) found that the single most important factor in promoting well-being for looked-after children was the quality of their placement. Equally, Gilligan (2000) has illustrated how a stimulating school environment can support emotional, health, social and educational development; out-of-school activities can foster self-esteem, social skills, positive social networks and improved health, as well as the development of specific knowledge and skills.

Research identifies key characteristics of placements which are supportive of looked-after children's development as providing:

- at least one person the child can trust, in whom they can confide, and who provides acceptance and emotional warmth;
- the capacity to manage difficult behaviour in a way which imposes clear boundaries for the child while maintaining their self-esteem;
- support for the child to explore and understand their identity, including their birth relations and history prior to entering care;
- tailored programmes of therapeutic support where the child has mental health support needs (see pp. 143–55);
- support for the child in their educational setting, including an individu-alised plan of additional educational support where necessary;
- support for the child to develop interests and skills (Gilligan, 2000; Sinclair *et al.*, 2007; Triseliotis, 1983; Wilson *et al.*, 2004).

Listening to children's views is often emphasised from the standpoint of chil-dren's rights. However, there is evidence that children's meaningful participa-tion in decisions about their care supports their development and makes decision-making more effective – children actively involved in choices of place-ment may enjoy greater placement stability, for example (Thomas, 2009). There are challenging practice dilemmas to be negotiated where a looked-after child's wishes are in tension with professional assessment of what is in their best interests – such as around contact, or a return to parental care. There is some, albeit limited, evidence that children in care value being consulted even when the final decision made is one with which they disagree (Children in Scotland, 2005). Where a decision is made against a child's expressed wishes, research highlights the importance of practitioners carefully explaining why that decision was taken (Thomas, 2009).

> ### PRACTICE REFLECTION 8.2
> **Children: the importance of listening**
> The importance of listening to children's views about their care has been established for a number of years. However, research suggests many looked-after children feel that, at points in their lives, their views were not heard or taken seriously. Why do you think this might be? What might be done to avoid it in future?

Social workers should be aware that the prevalence of mental health issues amongst the looked-after child population is up to five times that of the general child population (Meltzer *et al.*, 2003). Tailored therapeutic work is required where such needs are identified, with research showing that such work needs to include carers and, where appropriate, parents in order to be effective (Davies and Ward, 2011; Rushton and Minnis, 2008). Some evidence- based tools may help within this process: The Strengths and Difficulties Questionnaire is validated to help identify emotional and behavioural difficulties in children (Goodman, 1997), while some interventions with an evidence base in the USA have started to be employed in the UK. Multi-Systemic Therapy for Child Abuse and Neglect (MST-CAN) can be used for children in short-term placements, while Multi-Treatment Foster Care for Pre-schoolers (MTFC-P) is employed with younger children moving to permanent placement (Davies and Ward, 2011), although evidence of their effectiveness in UK settings is yet to be established. Finding good-quality therapeutic input for children in care is not easy due its scarcity. Selwyn *et al.* (2006) discovered that only 7 per cent of looked-after children had received therapeutic help despite many more needing it. This suggests the importance of practitioners identifying needs for specialist input as early as possible, trying to find appropriate resources to meet it and, where they are not available, emphasising cases of unmet need to highlight the need for service development.

Leaving care

Where young people are supported to prepare to leave care, there is evidence that they are more likely to move on from care successfully (Stein, 2012). Young people can feel forced to leave their placements at an earlier age than they want: it has been suggested that foster placements should generally go beyond the age of 18 and be available as a resource for young people to return to once they have left their placement (Sinclair *et al.*, 2005b; Stein, 2012). In a number of other Western European countries, young people stay in care until their early 20s (Stein, 2012). Tailored programmes of support for young people leaving care need to be established considering accommodation and tenancy management, future training and education plans, and support to help a young person manage their health needs (Stein, 2012). It is also important that there is recognition of the relationships young people have already built up as there is some evidence that over-zealous preparation of young people for independent living can unhelpfully distance young people from long-term carers (Selwyn *et al.*, 2006; Sinclair *et al.*, 2007).

Using research evidence to inform practice

Case scenario 8.1 involves the Connell/Turner family, where the three children in the family are placed in care. Decisions about their care will be explored at two points in time: when they have just been placed in care, and eight months later, when a long-term decision about their future care is made. Box 8.1 illustrates how research helped inform key decisions in the case.

Parental refusal to engage meaningfully with services where there are serious child protection concerns is a common factor where children have gone on to experience serious harm (Brandon *et al.*, 2008). Additionally, research confirms that serious parental substance misuse severely compromises parenting capacity (Cleaver *et al.*, 2007). The social worker working with the Connell/Turner family was mindful of research on neglect, which underlines

CASE SCENARIO 8.1

The Connell/Turner family

Caitlin Connell (12), Kieran Connell (7) and Rhianna Turner (9 months) were placed in local authority care via an Interim Care Order. Leanne Connell (30) is the mother of all three children and, her partner, Pete Turner (25) is the father of Rhianna and step-father to Caitlin and Kieran. Kevin Hurst (30) is the father of Caitlin and Kieran. There has not been any sustained contact between Kevin and the family since Leanne and Kevin ended their relationship in 2007.

The social work team had been working with the Connell/Turner family for two years following initial concerns about Caitlin and Kieran's very low school attendance, and dishevelled and dirty appearance when at school. It was established that Leanne and Pete were addicted to heroin, and also using amphetamines. Following engagement with addiction and social work services, they had stabilised on methadone programmes and the family situation initially improved significantly during Leanne's pregnancy with Rhianna. However, during the six months leading to November 2012 concerns increased. Caitlin and Kieran's school attendance dropped to less than 30 per cent. When at school, while Caitlin was well-presented, her behaviour was often disruptive and aggressive. Kieran was invariably poorly-clothed, withdrawn and sometimes also tearful in class. After initial positive engagement with the intensive support health visitor, both the social worker and health visitor were unable to gain regular access to the children within the family home despite many planned and unplanned visits. Rhianna had also missed a number of immunisation appointments and developmental checks. The parents denied they were again misusing illicit substances but, when they were seen, their physical presentation, together with the mounting child care concerns, suggested otherwise.

the importance of assessing whether a child is making appropriate development progress, and intervening when they are not (Ward *et al.*, 2012). On the last occasion the social worker had seen Rhianna prior to the children's accommodation, she was in a soiled nappy and the parents were unresponsive to her crying. While a detailed developmental assessment was not possible, the social worker had concerns that Rhianna's fine motor skills did not appear to have developed to those of a nine-month-old child and that Rhianna also displayed no signs of distress when her parents were not physically present in the room with her, as might be expected of an infant of her age who is developing a healthy attachment to her primary carers (Schaffer and Rudolph, 1990). The parents were required to attend an emergency GP appointment for Rhianna later that day to assess her well-being due to these concerns. However, the parents were not in when the social worker called back to take them to the appointment and they did not attend by themselves.

Placements

Before the children came into care, aware that research has shown that kinship care can provide a viable placement option with greater continuity of family relationships (Hunt *et al.*, 2008), the social worker had arranged a family group conference to explore care options available with the extended family network. She had also tried to contact Kevin and his parents at their last known addresses, but without success. The conference was, however, extremely difficult with Leanne and Pete's families blaming the other parent for the deterioration in the children's care. It was clear that a viable kinship placement was not available.

Recognising the potential benefits of sibling co-placement (Kosonen, 1996), the social worker pushed to find a placement for all three children together. In doing so, she was careful to provide a clear assessment of the different care needs of each of the three children, given that effectively matching children with carers is an important factor in successful foster placements (Sinclair, 2005).

Permanence decisions

A decision was taken to seek permanent placements outside parental care for all three children: an adoptive placement for Rhianna, long-term fostering for Kieran and a residential placement for Caitlin. In assessing the possibility of the children returning to their parents' care, the social worker was aware of research showing high breakdown rates for children returning home, and high rates of re-abuse, particularly where there is parental substance misuse (Farmer and Wijedasa, 2013; Lutman and Farmer, 2013; Wade *et al.*, 2011). However, she also knew that research underlines the need for individualised assessment of the possibility of rehabilitation, considering:

- the children's needs and the parents' ability to meet these needs if they were returned;
- evidence of whether the parents have made clear progress on the issues which brought the children into care;
- the nature and quality of relationships between the parents and the children, and the views and motivation of all parties towards rehabilitation. (Biehal, 2006; Sen and Broadhurst, 2011; Wade *et al.*, 2011)

The children's needs

Rhianna made good developmental progress in her foster placement and her general health improved. Her fine motor skills were assessed as being age appropriate and she was talking, although the health visitor noticed that she was not stringing words together as might be expected at her age (see Sheridan, 2000) and referred her to a child development centre to monitor her progress.

Kieran settled within his foster placement, making strong relationships with both his carers. He was prone to emotional outbursts in both the placement and at school which necessitated authoritative and patient responses from his carers and teachers. He was behind his peers academically and had a tailored programme of educational support within school. Kieran's educational psychologist and social worker were aware not only of the importance of Kieran getting appropriate support for his educational development, but also that a child doing well in school promotes their resilience (Gilligan, 1997) and placement stability (Sinclair, 2005).

Caitlin had experienced a number of difficulties. There had been two foster placement breakdowns as her carers felt unable to manage her behaviour and her third foster placement was also at risk of disruption. Her behaviour towards her foster carers had been consistently challenging, particularly towards female carers. Caitlin's social worker believed this was connected to her fierce loyalty to her mother. On occasion, Caitlin also self-harmed by cutting herself on her stomach and wrists. A referral to child and adolescent mental health services was made by the social worker, recognising the importance of tailored therapeutic input in such circumstances (Davies and Ward, 2011; Selwyn et al., 2006).

Family relationships

The social worker put a plan for regular supervised contact in place, aware of the value that families place on contact, the social worker's key role in facilitating contact plans and that contact was necessary for there to be a realistic prospect of rehabilitation (Sen and Broadhurst, 2011). Supervised contact presents parents with a pressurised context in which to have their parenting assessed but the social worker knew it would also provide some valuable insights into family relationships and the parents' underlying motivation to regain full time care of their children (Cleaver, 2000). The information from contact was mixed: during the first three months, the parents attended every contact and there were clear indications of the positive relationships within the family. However, following a visit where Leanne attended under the influence of drugs there had been a marked deterioration, with a number of missed contacts without explanation. This caused significant distress to Caitlin and Kieran. In later contacts which did occur, there was a marked pattern of Leanne focusing all her attention on Caitlin, and Pete focusing on Rhianna, causing Kieran to become very distressed. The social worker was aware that childhood experiences of rejection can have long-lasting consequences into adult life (Howe, 2005).

Parental circumstances

The parents' situation had remained unstable. Both were re-referred to addiction services and initially engaged very well for the first two months but their attendance then became sporadic. Drug analysis tests later showed they were using opiates again. Research (Cleaver et al., 2007; Farmer and Wijedasa, 2013) shows such circumstances provide a very unfavourable context in which to parent well. The social worker met with the parents on a number of occasions to discuss concerns about their previous care of the children and to support them to make positive changes. The parents acknowledged there were ongoing difficulties but stated they were desperate to have their children returned. Given the parents' early progress, the court agreed to extend care proceedings beyond six months to see whether they could manage to address their substance misuse, on the proviso that the local authority also started to identify substitute placements for the children. Unfortunately, the parents' engagement with addiction services remained sporadic in the subsequent two months. The parents' genuine love for their children was not in doubt, but the social worker knew that research (Biehal, 2006; Wade *et al.*, 2011) showed that without significant positive changes in the parents' circumstances, particularly around the issues leading to the children's placement in care in the first place, successful rehabilitation was unlikely.

The children's views

Rhianna was too young to express a view therefore it was clear that a decision should be taken based around assessment of what was in her long-term best interests. The social worker undertook a series of exercises with Kieran about where and with whom he felt safe and happy, recognising the importance of getting his views as appropriate to his age (Thomas, 2009). Kieran frequently mentioned his carers and siblings in these exercises, but rarely mentioned Leanne. Pete was hardly mentioned at all. In the previous five months, Kieran also frequently wet the bed on the night before family contact was due to take place. The social worker noted in her assessment that Kieran has settled well in his placement and that this presentation suggested some anxiety about a return to his parents' care. Caitlin expressed an unequivocal wish to return to her parents, and consistently refused to discuss the possibility of a long-term placement. The social worker was aware that children's views about their care are highly important (Thomas, 2009) but that research highlights their views should not be decisive where there are clear child welfare concerns (Davies and Ward, 2011). The social worker discussed with Caitlin why it was not thought in her best interests to return to her parents on a number of occasions, recognising the importance of explaining to a child why a decision has been taken against their expressed wishes (Thomas, 2009). Caitlin, however, still fiercely opposed the decision.

Long-term placement choices

In making a permanence decision at this stage, the social work team prioritised moving Rhianna to an adoptive placement as soon as possible, having already started to search for a suitable match. In doing so, they were aware of research suggesting that adoption earlier in a child's life is generally more successful, allowing the best chance of developmental catch-up (Rushton *et al.*, 2001; Van Ijzendoorn and Juffer, 2006).

Kieran was settled in his foster placement, the quality of care provided to him was good, and his foster carers agreed that Kieran could stay with them until adulthood, and potentially beyond. Aware that adoption offers greater legal and emotional security (Rushton *et al.*, 2001), the social worker explored options for the adoption of Kieran alongside Rhianna and also had discussions with the foster carers about adopting Kieran. However, placement services could not identify prospective adopters who might take Rhianna and Kieran together, and Kieran's foster carers were reluctant to give up the social work support a fostering arrangement provides. The social worker was aware that Kieran's age, as well as his birth family links, meant adoption was an unlikely option and that the quality of care within the foster placement would itself be supportive of positive outcomes for him (Sinclair *et al.*, 2007). Therefore it was decided that Kieran should stay in his placement, with the possibility of special guardianship to be explored.

Caitlin's age, previous placement breakdowns, challenging behaviour and negative attitude towards a permanent substitute placement meant another foster placement breakdown was significantly more likely (Sinclair, 2005). The social worker was aware there is less clear evidence that residential child care improves child well-being (Forrester, 2008) but that young people can themselves prefer residential care (Kendrick, 2008) – particularly where they have strong family loyalties. Given this, and taking account of some of the key characteristics of successful placements (Gilligan, 1997; Sinclair *et al.*, 2007), it was decided initially to find a specialised residential placement for Caitlin where she would receive intensive support from residential care staff while receiving specialised psychological therapy to help her with the emotional and behavioural difficulties she was experiencing. The importance of care staff being actively involved in the programme of psychological input (Rushton and Minnis, 2008) was emphasised within Caitlin's care plan, as was the importance of a tailored educational programme to help Caitlin catch up academically (Sinclair *et al.*, 2005b).

PRACTICE REFLECTION 8.3

Competing needs and wishes

What competing needs and wishes might be at play for each child in the Connell/Turner family when considering permanent placement options for them? Which of these competing needs and wishes might be met within the plans set out above for their future placements? Which might not be met?

Though some years away, the social worker was aware that a planned programme of leaving care and aftercare support would be needed for Kieran and Caitlin when they reached that stage. This would need to be delivered in a way which did not undermine positive existing relationships in their placements (Dixon and Stein, 2002; Selwyn *et al.*, 2006).

In making these choices, the social worker team was aware that some difficult compromises had to be struck in applying research evidence to the complexities of the children's situations. Splitting up the sibling group meant maintaining close sibling relationships would become very hard (Kosonen, 1996). However, the sibling group had already become separated through Caitlin's first foster placement breakdown and there was no placement which could effectively meet all their differing long-term needs. Noting the impor-

BOX 8.1 KEY DECISIONS MADE IN CASE SCENARIO 8.1 AND THE INFLUENCE OF RESEARCH

Decision	Research influencing decision
Placing the children in substitute care	▪ Established need to place children in substitute care when parents are consistently failing to meet their developmental needs (Ward et al., 2012) ▪ Identification of consistent absence of parental engagement with support services as an indicator of potential future harm to children (Brandon et al., 2008) ▪ Established negative impact of severe parental substance misuse on parenting capacity (Cleaver et al., 2007)
Assessment of the possibility of rehabilitation to parental care	▪ Awareness of high breakdown rates and rates of re-abuse where children return home, particularly in cases of parental substance misuse. Need for thorough assessment of the possibility of rehabilitation as a result (Lutman and Farmer, 2013; Wade et al., 2011). ▪ Assessment of rehabilitation should focus on parental ability to meet children's needs if returned (Cleaver, 2000); evidence of progress on the concerns that led to the children's accommodation (Biehal, 2006; Wade et al., 2011); the quality of relationships between children and parents, and the motivation of all parties towards rehabilitation (Biehal, 2006; Cleaver, 2000).
Meeting the children's needs in placement	▪ Evidence of the importance of education not only as a means to academic development for looked-after children, but also due to its positive impact on placement stability, self-esteem, and development of skills and interests (Gilligan, 2000; Sinclair et al., 2005b). ▪ Evidence that the quality of care provided is one of the most important variables affecting outcomes for children in the care system (Sinclair et al., 2007). ▪ The importance of identifying the need for specialist psychological or therapeutic support and providing it where it is needed (Davies and Ward, 2011; Selwyn et al., 2006).
Long-term placement choices for the children	▪ Evidence that a young person's sense of stability, placement stability and developmental outcomes are most positive within adoption (Sinclair et al., 2007; Van Ijzendoorn and Juffer, 2006). However, this needs to be considered alongside research findings that the possibility of poorer outcomes increases with a child's age (Rushton et al., 2001; Selwyn et al., 2006). ▪ Evidence that foster care is a wide-ranging and flexible placement option that can successfully meet most children's needs in a range of situations and circumstances (Sinclair et al., 2005a). However, this needs to be considered alongside research findings that, while foster care can provide long-term stability for children, it does not do so as frequently as it might, particularly where children have challenging behaviour and have experienced multiple previous placement breakdowns (Sinclair, 2005). ▪ Evidence that residential care improves child well-being (Forrester, 2008) despite principally caring for older children, many of whom have higher levels of pre-existing need, and for whom other family-based placements would not be available (Kendrick, 2008). However, this needs to be considered alongside research findings that outcomes for children in residential care tend to be worse than for children in family-based settings (Sinclair et al., 2005a; Sinclair et al., 2005b; Van Ijzendoorn and Juffer, 2006).

tance that most separated siblings place on maintaining links (Office for Standards in Education Children's Services and Skills, 2009), plans for sibling contact were put in place. Plans for contact between the children and Leanne and Pete were also revised, recognising that the frequency of direct contact would likely reduce for Kieran and contact would most likely be indirect for Rhianna once adopted (Neil and Howe, 2004; Sen and Broadhurst, 2011). In revising these plans, the social worker knew the children's individual wishes, the parents' and carers' responses, the impact of contact on each child and the implications of the different placement pathways and the need for flexibility would all be influential.

FURTHER READING

Davies, C. and Ward, H. (2011) *Safeguarding Children Across Services: Messages from Research on Identifying and Responding to Child Maltreatment* (London: Jessica Kingsley). This provides the latest digest of government-commissioned studies on children's services in England. Several of the studies were not specifically about looked-after children; however, the book contains a range of findings of which practitioners working with looked-after children should be aware.

Kendrick A. (2008) (ed.) *Residential Child Care: Prospects and Challenges* (London: Jessica Kingsley). This presents a range of important theory and research on a sector that has received relatively scant research focus in the UK in recent years.

Schofield, G. and Simmonds, J. (2009) (eds) *The Child Placement Handbook. Research, Policy and Practice* (London: BAAF). This assimilates a wealth of evidence on a wide range of issues related to looked-after children. Each chapter is written by leading researchers and writers in their field.

CHAPTER 9

Working with Young People with Additional Needs

Steven Walker

Introduction

This chapter will provide an overview of the evidence in the field of social work with young people with additional needs. It will illustrate how reliable research evidence can be used in social work practice using a hypothetical case study, which illuminates the conceptual points made. This will enable readers to engage critically with debates about how research evidence informs this complex area of social work practice. The chapter contains a macro perspective of Child and Adolescent Mental Health Services (CAMHS) to show where social work engages with a service increasingly dominated by medical and psychological management and interventions, provides definitions of commonly used terms, outlines the political, social and economic context of service provision and, finally, offers the latest empirical and clinical research studies for readers to absorb and reflect on as they seek to apply this knowledge to their practice contexts.

Contextual factors

Evidence of the rising numbers and specific characteristics of child and adolescent mental health problems has been thoroughly documented since the mid-1990s, prompting widespread professional, public and private concern (Dimigen *et al.*, 1999; Green *et al.*, 2005; Kurtz *et al.*, 1995; Mental Health Foundation, 1999; Office for National Statistics, 2007; Rutter, 1995; Rutter and Smith, 1995). Social workers are at the heart of this phenomenon, working in the frontline where children, families, parent/carers, schools and communities are experiencing the destructive consequences. Recent studies from several different countries agree fairly closely that the prevalence of mental health problems in children up to the age of 18 years is 10 per cent, with higher rates among groups that suffer a number of risk factors, such as those who live in deprived inner city environments (World Health Organization, 2010).

It is estimated that, in Britain, one in five children and young people mani-fest mild emotional or behavioural difficulties, or the early stage of significant problems that do not require long- term specialist intervention. However, only a small proportion of these children actually present to services for help, mani-festing difficulties in a variety of contexts where the cause of the problem is not adequately addressed. Many social work staff lack confidence in assessing and intervening, even when they suspect a mental health component to the difficulties being presented (Mental Health Foundation, 1999).

The latest data from the charity Young Minds reveals that:

- 1 in 10 children and young people aged 5–16 suffer from a diagnosable mental health disorder – that is, around three children in every class at school;
- between 1 in 12 and 1 in 15 children and young people deliberately self-harm, and around 25,000 are admitted to hospital every year due to the severity of their injuries;
- more than half of all adults with mental health problems were diagnosed in childhood with less than half treated properly at the time;
- nearly 80,000 children and young people suffer from severe depression;
- over 8,000 children aged under 10 years old suffer from severe depression;
- 60 per cent of children in care have a mental health disorder – these are some of the most vulnerable people in our society;
- 95 per cent of imprisoned young offenders have a mental health disorder; many of them are struggling with more than one disorder;
- the rate of suicide in young ex-soldiers is three times that in the equivalent civilian population. (Young Minds, 2010)

High rates of mental health problems among young people have many causes. The decline of traditional family life and globalisation are just two features of modern life which underpin these rates. Additionally, armed conflict has increased the number of asylum seekers with economic and social dislocation, a known correlate of mental health problems (Walker, 2011). However, in spite of high rates of mental health problems among young people, access to CAMHS is restricted to those with the greatest need.

Child and adolescent mental health services

The last major review into CAMHS in 2008 concluded that there were 22,000 children unable to access specialist CAMHS due to long waiting times. The proportion of young people waiting more than 26 weeks ranged from 3.5 per cent to 18 per cent (Walker, 2011). In particular, the review highlighted the lack of provision for children with learning disabilities or developmental prob-lems. Seminal research (Kurtz *et al.*, 1995) came to similar conclusions as the latest independent review, which starkly illustrates the lack of progress in this important area.

Data on CAMHS effectiveness released in 2010 comparing self-reported total scores at local authority level for 2008 and 2009 showed that, out of 87 local areas, 48 did not change and 13 experienced a decline (Department for Children Schools and Families, 2010). Part of the aim of this chapter is to ask how this could be the case and what social work can do to improve things for a child similar to one born in 1995 when that research was published; a child who, at age five, showed disturbed behaviour at primary school; at eight years of age, the early signs of depression; at 11 started self-harming and now, aged 18, has been admitted to an in-patient psychiatric unit with a serious mental health problem which will have consequences for the rest of their lives.

There is no coherent national strategy for CAMHS, primarily because it falls between the Department of Health and the Department for Education, who each consistently fail to comply with the practice of the much-lauded government strategy of 'joined-up thinking'. Children's mental health needs have to compete with other demands in child protection, other children's services, and especially the health care system, and the GP-led Clinical Commissioning Groups who are newly responsible for commissioning services but are struggling to manage their role. Multi-agency partnerships are meant to be the modus operandi of CAMHS but there are problems because of the different expectations from each partner agency of what CAMHS outcomes should be. This, then, leads to the question about what research base is being used, developed and implemented to provide valid data on which to base decisions about what, where and how to provide services to meet what is acknowledged to be an increasing need (Walker, 2011).

Part of the problem with the organisation of CAMHS is whether to conceive it as a comprehensive or specialist service – in other words, a preventive or a reactive provision. A preventive focus requires a planned training and educational programme for primary care, social work, and health and education staff. Reactive provision is against universalist principles, is likely to be more costly in the long run and cannot contribute to health promotion.

The increasing trend towards including children and young people as active, rather than passive, recipients of health and social care research means that the task of developing robust methods for obtaining children and young people's perceptions is important. Enabling them to collaborate in the design of research studies and to be consulted fully about the areas they consider important to research can only enrich these studies. The impact such research has in terms of the immediate effect on the child or young person, and also on later service and practitioner development, are areas requiring attention from social work researchers involved in this area of work. This particularly highlights the need for continued vigilance and effort by social workers in the area of children's rights.

Children are also not a homogeneous group. The age ranges from childhood to adolescence incorporate several developmental stages which suggest attention should be paid to the design of developmentally appropriate methods of intervention. It is important in this context to continue the task of finding out what works best for which children in what circumstances, and to link this with why some children fail to develop mental health problems even in highly disadvantaged situations, while some in the wealthiest and higher social class self-harm and commit suicide.

In 2008, the Secretary of State for Children, Schools and Families said that children and young people's emotional well-being was everybody's business – meaning it was not the sole responsibility of specialist Tier 3 child and family consultation services or the medical psychiatric professionals (Walker, 2011). In the same way that social workers have argued for decades that child protection is not their sole responsibility, so social workers can now accept that they, too, have considerable responsibilities in the area of child and adolescent mental health. So, the question is: What social work research is there that can be of some use in the CAMHS context and how can this be adapted, modified and then applied?

PRACTICE REFLECTION 9.1

Supporting children and young people with additional needs

From your reading in this chapter, reflect on the different professionals and agencies that might work with children and young people with additional needs. Consider whether, and how, the communication between these professionals and agencies could be improved.

Definitions of terms

The concept of the young person with additional needs is both new and, at the same time, quite old. This is because terminology in social work and other professional domains is always developing in step with, ahead of, (and sometimes behind) real world changes in the circumstances of young people. Contemporary evidence illustrates this most vividly and, as our perceptions of young people are shaped by our developing knowledge and research evidence, new formulations of how to describe and understand the needs of modern young people invariably change. Euphemisms such as 'challenging behaviour' or 'special needs' are ploughing similar ground. Was it ever thus?

In terms of this chapter, 'additional needs' is defined as the specific area of CAMHS which itself incorporates a diversity of practice and a wide variety of different agency domains, such as youth offending, learning disability, fostering and adoption, drug and alcohol abuse, special educational needs, domestic violence, emotional and behavioural difficulties, S47 assessment, safeguarding and child protection. In addition, the presenting issues could range from parent–infant bonding, post natal depression, attachment disorders, attention-deficit hyperactivity disorder (ADHD), depression, anxiety, autism and Asperger's syndrome, cyber bullying, school phobia, post-traumatic stress disorder (PTSD), child abuse and neglect, self-harm, child sexual abuse and suicide.

Research evidence

The evidence base relating to children with additional needs is strongly dominated by health and especially psychiatry, so immediately social workers are challenged to examine an evidence base which, with some notable exceptions, focuses on medical, behavioural and epidemiological factors, written in the language of the bio-medical model rather than a more familiar psychosocial paradigm. The Social Care Institute for Excellence (SCIE) is the main repository for the social work evidence base (e.g. Brodie *et al.*, 2011; Parrott *et al.*, 2008; Social Care Institute for Excellence, 2005).

The western health-dominated and psychiatric model of mental illness tends to ignore the religious or spiritual aspects of the culture in which it is based. However, Eastern, African and Native American cultures tend to integrate them (Fernando, 2010). Spirituality and religion have only recently featured in the mainstream social work literature, yet they can be critical components of a family's well-being, offering a source of strength and hope in trying circumstances (Furness and Gilligan, 2010). Social work research in this area is still in its infancy. Social workers need to address this dimension as part of the constellation of factors affecting children and adolescents, avoiding stereotyping, and bearing in mind the positive and sometimes negative impact spiritual or religious beliefs might have on their well-being (Gray *et al.*, 2010; Wong and Vinsky, 2009).

Early intervention

Early intervention, and the policies associated with it, is the touchstone of progressive social work practice. Yet, it is impossible to verify or provide concrete evidence of its effectiveness due to the number of social, psychological and ecological variables, and the lack of empirical longitudinal studies. It does always seem to make sense at the intuitive and instinctual level, though. The evidence base which informs practice at the early intervention or preventive stage of social work practice is derived from multiple sources. There is no research model that has been devised to encapsulate the factors that impede a child's development, or identify linear causation to pinpoint a stage when a child can clearly be defined as having additional needs. Often, symptoms can appear suddenly, or slowly grow in strength and frequency. They are most often identified in primary health care contexts but, even here, many health professionals are reluctant to offer a clear diagnosis or prognosis because children can change very quickly where natural resilience, genetic predisposition or environmental factors can mitigate developmental problems.

Parents often intuitively know when something is not right with their child before a health professional can ascertain definitive symptoms. At worst, this means some parents enduring a frustrating delay in receiving support, which is always better started sooner rather than later. At best, this can be a false alarm or, conversely, indicative of Munchausen's Syndrome by Proxy (a syndrome characterised by carers deliberately inducing health problems in the people for whom they care). Various initiatives aimed at children and their families living in disadvantaged areas in the UK are evidence of the practical implementation of the implicit preventive aspects of this early intervention policy, which was based on evidence of success from the US Head Start scheme (Gross *et al.*, 1995). Gross *et al.*'s study demonstrated long-term reductions in antisocial activity, marital problems, child abuse, adult mental health difficulties, and unemployment in later life in a group of children who received the intervention in contrast to a group of children who did not receive the intervention.

The Sure Start initiative was the British equivalent and the signature family support policy of the early twenty-first century (Walker, 2012). Recent research to evaluate its impact has produced positive findings (Hutchings *et al.*, 1998). However, a systematic review of family group conferences linked to Sure Start shows that, to succeed as a family support intervention, they need to be part of a range of helping services and the start of a continuum of support, rather than a crisis intervention into a complex and established chronic situation (Shlonsky, 2010).

Family support

Measuring or quantifying the impact of preventive family support work is complex and achieving systematic results is expensive. Therefore, there is little in the way of evidence of long-term effectiveness in Britain, or the rest of Europe. However, while outcome measures from various government projects are intangible (Robbins, 1998), there are signs small-scale social action projects could show changes in relationships between parents and professionals, as well as demonstrate how to work in partnership and engage positively with parents, all of which contribute to better family support and user-focused approaches for children with additional needs (Lloyd, 1999; Miller and Prinz, 1990).

The expansion of parent education or training programmes in the face of exponential demand for help from parents to deal with a range of child and adolescent difficulties – from toddler tantrums to self-harm, suicide, and drug and alcohol addiction – has meant this form of intervention is popular and expected to be offered as part of a repertoire of contemporary family support measures. Studies of parent education programmes, while limited in number, show they can be an effective way of supporting families by improving behaviour in pre-adolescent children (Lloyd, 1999; Miller and Prinz, 1990). They highlight the impact of group-based behaviourally oriented programmes in producing the biggest subsequent changes in children's behaviour and are perceived by parents as non-stigmatising. Programmes where both parents are involved and which include individual work with children are more likely to result in long-term changes.

Parent education

While enjoying a growth in popularity in Britain and other European countries, parent education programmes are generally not subject to rigorous evaluation (Donnellan, 2003; Nybell *et al.*, 2009). In a number of studies, 50 per cent of parents continued to experience difficulties. Further, it is not clear to what extent changes are due to the format or method of intervention, group support or practitioner skill. High attrition rates from some programmes are attributed to practitioner variables, such as their level of qualification and experience, and qualities such as warmth, enthusiasm, or flexibility (Barlow, 1998). It may also be that some programmes are inappropriate for parents lacking motivation, especially when they are compelled to attend under the pressure of child protection concerns and legal orders.

Few British studies have used randomised controlled trials which, as stated in Chapter 1 and elsewhere in this book, are considered to be the most robust method of evaluating intervention effectiveness in health and social care. Social work has tended to rely on qualitative or mixed methods research models mirroring the history of psychosocial practice and the desire to reflect service users' perceptions and articulate their voices. The most readily available evidence for social work practitioners takes the form of narrative-led, case study descriptive content at one end of the spectrum through to mathematically dense, statistical quantitative data often using small cohorts with poor wider applicability at the other. This inhibits identification of the most beneficial elements of a programme and, because most provision is geared to rectifying problems in disadvantaged groups, available research evidence reflects this bias.

Those that have been conducted, nevertheless, have yielded important qualitative data from stakeholders' perspectives (Ghate and Daniels, 1997; Morrow, 1998). It has been argued that managerialist preference for evaluating work on the basis of the three Es (efficiency, effectiveness, and economy), which reflects service managers' agenda for quantitative outcome measures, fails to reflect the whole picture (Leonard, 1997; Walker, 2001). Others argue these data need to be supplemented with the three Ps (partnership, pluralism, and process), which better reflect professional social work principles seeking to incorporate service users' perspectives (Beresford, 2001; Dominelli, 2004; Powell and Lovelock, 1992). And there is the famous saying: What can be counted is not always important, whereas what is important cannot always be counted.

Further studies paying attention to normative models of parenting in the community counter this bias by identifying skills leading to successful parenting and focus on what went right, rather than what went wrong. For example, when Winnicott (1965) famously suggested that 'there is no such thing as a baby', he was simply drawing attention to the concept that it is not enough to consider a baby (or, in this case, a child with additional needs) as a separate entity from the family and main carer. So, research evidence to inform social work practice in this specialist area has to be conducted at the community, family, parent and individual levels, in order to achieve an isomorphic fit with the foundation assessment tool of the Common Assessment Form (CAF) (Department for Education, 2013a). Webb (2001) takes this concept further when he argues that the appetite for research evidence may have paradoxical consequences, drawing social workers into designing a narrow, prescriptive range of practices which imposes a planned order in the delivery of social work, and ending up with losses in efficiency and higher costs.

Transition from youth to adult services

Transition from youth to adult services is a vexed issue within CAMHS, as it can be difficult to achieve a smooth journey between two very different practice cultures. Transitions are unfortunately sometimes characterised by young people becoming lost in the system, or disappearing between two rigid bureaucracies and their eligibility criteria. Recently, the large numbers of young people being inappropriately contained on adult wards in hospitals has been exposed (Young Minds, 2010).

Transition has received a considerable amount of attention from researchers for several years. A range of important studies and reviews of the research literature have taken place (Brodie *et al.*, 2011). One of the most recent primary studies, the TRACK study, took place in London and the West Midlands. It aimed to identify the organisational factors that either help or impede effective transitions between CAMHS and adult mental health services (AMHS), and to make recommendations about the organisation and delivery of services that promote good continuity of care. A range of methods was used, including document analysis, case studies and qualitative interviews with young people and professionals. It is of concern that, of 155 potential referrals, only 90 were made and about 50 finally accepted into AMHS.

PRACTICE REFLECTION 9.2

Transitions in practice

More research is needed in transitions. Consider how research in post-transition outcomes and service use for different groups of young people (including those not moving to AMHS), and the effectiveness of practices and different service models to improve transition, could be conducted and applied to your practice.

Evaluating practice interventions

Evaluating practice interventions is notoriously difficult. Previous government initiatives have tried to address this problem, and a national programme of research was commissioned to evaluate responses from local authorities and health trusts trying to meet the challenge of finding better ways of responding to the needs of troubled young people (Department of Health, 1997). The key aspiration was that innovative responses should create preventive, early intervention inter-agency working, and more effective inter-professional cooperation, thereby resulting in better outcomes for troubled children within their own communities. The findings from this research, however, were that evaluations were difficult to quantify and generalise from the specific characteristics of different forms of service delivery and research methodologies being employed (Walker, 2011).

Linking specific interventions with agreed outcomes is also problematic due to the network of variables potentially impacting on a child or young person's development. One important issue to emerge from the evidence base is the way children acquire different *at risk* labels – such as 'looked-after', 'excluded', or 'young offender' – and the variety of perceptions of their needs from the care system, education system, or youth justice system. Each professional system has its own language and methodology with which to describe the same child, invariably resulting in friction between agencies and misconceptions about how to work together and integrate interventions. In this climate, the mental health needs of such children can be neglected.

There is, however, good evidence for effective interventions for most of the common problems presenting to CAMHS (Fonagy *et al.*, 2002; Wolpert *et al.*, 2006). A list of evidence-based interventions includes: cognitive behavioural therapies (CBT), behaviour therapy, parent training, medication, family therapy, interpersonal therapy (IPT), social skills training, multi-systemic therapy (MST), treatment foster care, and, to a lesser degree, individual psychodynamic therapies (Walker, 2011). The striking feature of these studies is that the predominant factor, regardless of theoretical orientation, is the quality of the personal relationship between practitioner and service user. This evidence reinforces those social work practitioners and academics who strongly advocate a return to relationship-based practice (Ruch *et al.*, 2010).

The other striking feature is how little young people are involved in the design, implementation and evaluation of research evidence in CAMHS. It is also important to take account of the natural history and environmental context of children's problems in relation to their developmental stage, and acknowledge that there are no standardised ways of measuring childhood functioning. Many of the classic measures are based on white Eurocentric models that are not nowadays consistent with culturally competent practice. What is consistent in all the major studies is the general absence and rarity of service user evaluation of, and involvement in, the design of child and family research. The implication is that by enlarging the focus of effectiveness measures it is possible to see children not merely as having problems, but also as having positive and constructive elements in their family lives, and to build on these and amplify them wherever possible. They also have much to tell us about how *they* feel about research into their lives and how research methodologies can become more child-centred.

This view is echoed in recommendations based on thorough research into interventions targeted at the child, teacher and parent which demonstrate that the combined effect produces the most sustained reduction in conflict problems, both at home and at school, and in peer relationships (Walker, 2011). Recognising and building on the children's own perspectives provides new opportunities for social work with young people, guided by possibilities of which adults are not aware, or to which they fail to pay sufficient attention. Thus, it is possible to adhere to the Children Act tenets of the paramountcy of the child's welfare while employing a theoretical research paradigm that permits an effective analysis of the child's emotional, psychological and environmental family context.

Children's perspectives have rarely been explored in relation to the help they receive towards their emotional and mental well-being (Walker, 2003). The prevalence and upward trends of mental health problems in childhood, together with findings that young people with such difficulties are reluctant to make use of specialist services, or quickly cease contact, is worrying (Office for National Statistics, 2007). This indicates the importance of developing appropriate sources of help that are experienced as useful and relevant, and therefore going to be used effectively.

In order to do that, methods of consulting with children and young people to gather research evidence need to be developed that are appropriate, effective and methodologically robust. The CAMHS literature has tended to neglect individual experience, and the voice of the child is almost unheard in most evaluative studies. Here, social workers have the opportunity to refine research models to include a child's perspective. There is a growing literature on the subject of the rights of children and young people to influence decisions about their own health and health care (Fraser *et al.*, 2004). However, this remains an area of contention for some professionals who believe that the notion that children can think, comment and participate in a meaningful way in evaluations of the help they receive is, at best, misguided or, at worst, undermining of parental and/or professional responsibility.

Applying the evidence

The primary aim of intervention in Case scenario 9.1 is to assist the decision-making process about Anton's future, and gain an understanding of the mental health needs of all the children. Assessing Sharon's parenting and her own need for support is a priority. Research consistently shows that a holistic, systemic perspective is required to incorporate the whole picture, rather than compartmentalising – and, thus, scapegoating – individuals (Walker, 2011).

Anti-racist and anti-discriminatory theory should be a cardinal element in any work with this family. Research with children of parents from different ethnic backgrounds and blended cultures show they are particularly vulnerable to personal and institutional racism and prejudice. For example, Robinson (2013) clearly provides compelling evidence of this endemic problem. The family dynamics in the case scenario indicate that this needs to be a major focus of discussion and exploration.

The assessment should include what impact the child protection system has had on the family and acknowledge that their functioning will be affected in that context. A wider focus will include the current role of the grandparents and children's fathers, and what support they might be prepared to offer in future. Murphy (2004) provided good evidence of the dangers of focusing too narrowly on parenting deficits, rather than potentially supporting people in the family system – especially during the child protection process, which can be experienced as judgemental and persecutory.

A combination of various models for different aspects of the intervention process might be appropriate, as would using other professionals in contact with the family, to contribute their perspective and skills. For example, a psychodynamic model could help explore with Sharon the effects of past experiences on her current parenting capacity. Attachment theory would be a primary model to employ in exploring the various attachment typologies within the family and individual children. A task-centred model could assist in

CASE SCENARIO 9.1

Anton, Sharina and Byron

Anton (6) has been accommodated for two months at the request of Sharon, his mother, following bruising to his right leg and right upper arm. She lost her temper after Anton had a tantrum and allegedly held him, hit him and shook him strongly. Sharina (3½), Anton's half-sister, lives with her maternal grandmother. Previously perceived as a happy child developing normally, her behaviour now seems to be regressing. Nursery staff report infantile behaviour and language, with long spells of thumb-sucking during the day. Byron (12), a full brother to Anton, has previously shown aggressive behaviour towards other children at school. He is recorded as punching, kicking and the attempted strangling of younger children. He recently started stealing money from Sharon and lighting matches around the flat. Byron has poor school attendance and recently complained about hearing voices inside his head.

Sharon (26) is currently in a relationship with Sharina's father. Anton and Byron have the same father but he is not involved with them in any way. Sharon is expecting her fourth child in five months. She finds it hard to cope and is asking for help. She has poor health and a past history of post-natal depression, and also childhood physical and sexual abuse. She has required the support of a community mental health team in the past and has criminal convictions for possession and dealing drugs. Sharon has worked as a prostitute to increase her income, particularly when extra money is needed to buy birthday or Christmas presents for the children. Sharon was in state care herself between the ages of 5 and 8, and is isolated from family and friends. Multi-agency review meetings have taken place, triggered by mental health, primary care or social work staff concerned about the safety and well-being of her children. Sharon does not welcome social work support, in particular because her overwhelming feeling is that they are persecuting her and simply preparing to take her children away from her. She had a traumatic time in state care and alleges that she was molested by a male member of staff in her residential home.

Sharon's partner, Malik (30), comes from a large Bangladeshi family in East London. His parents are elderly and he has three brothers and two sisters. He is the youngest sibling. He has experienced several years of periods of unemployment and then part-time low-paid work in the clothing industry in Tower Hamlets. He has also worked for cash as a waiter at a curry house in the evenings, which results in him sometimes working 15-hour days.

His family generally disapproves of his relationship with Sharon. His parents are most hostile. They do not speak English and are either unwilling or refuse to talk directly to Sharon. However, his sisters are more supportive and are willing to help Sharon when she lapses into periods of depression and exhaustion. Sharon's parents also disapprove of the relationship between her and Malik. Her father is particularly unpleasant about the relationship. He is a racist and refuses to speak directly with Sharon, saying she has brought shame on their family. Her mother tries to be supportive but cannot hide her feelings about Malik and his ethnic background; however, she admits to adoring her granddaughter Sharina.

mapping out the steps necessary for Anton's return. Individual counselling or play therapy with the other children could help enable them to manage their feelings, while a systems theory model could enable all the important aspects of the family's context to be included. The research evidence in each of these domains can be harnessed to fine tune the conventional and limited elements of the CAF, for example, so that effective, evidence-informed interventions can be formulated in the context of multi-disciplinary practice.

Conclusion

Social workers in CAMHS draw on research from cognate health disciplines and the social sciences to inform their work. Research on social models and interventions in CAMHS is slow to emerge, but there is potential for social workers to influence the development of this. In particular, we can champion the voices of young people with additional needs in research about them and for them.

Working in CAMHS requires a careful blending of social work theory and research to engage with young people with additional needs and their families in order to improve their care experiences and outcomes. As with other areas of social work discussed in Part II of this book, it is not simply a case of applying evidence about effective interventions to practice. Professional judgement, expertise and practice wisdom is required to integrate insights from research to assessments, decisions and interventions in CAMHS.

FURTHER READING

Fonagy, P., Target, M., Cottrell, D., Phillips, J. and Kurtz, Z. (2002) *What Works for Whom? A Critical Review of Treatments for Children and Adolescents* (New York and London: Guilford). A seminal text that brings together rigorous examination of the evidence base in a comprehensive and authoritative compendium.

Malek, M. and Joughin, C. (eds) (2004) *Mental Health Services for Minority Ethnic Children and Adolescents* (London: Jessica Kingsley). A very good collection of evidence-based recommendations for improving service delivery as part of a multidisciplinary project based at the Royal College of Psychiatrists' Research Unit.

Timimi, S. and Maitra, B. (eds) (2006) *Critical Voices in Child and Adolescent Mental Health* (London: Free Association). Excellent reading for the progressive worker who seeks solid evidence of institutionalised racism in psychiatry and a refreshing alternative to orthodox thinking in CAMHS.

Walker, S. (2011) *The Social Workers Guide to Child and Adolescent Mental Health* (London: Jessica Kingsley). Extends points raised in this chapter, providing more depth and breadth, especially in specific areas of interest to different practitioners.

Walker, S. and Beckett, C. (2011) *Social Work Assessment and Intervention*, 2nd edn (Lyme Regis: Russell House Publishing). A highly-acclaimed and popular book illustrating the seamless link between assessment and intervention, and the perpetual synchronicity between the two.

USEFUL WEBSITES

FOCUS (http://www.rcpsych.ac.uk/cru/focus/index.htm): provides resources relevant to promoting effective practice in child and adolescent mental health, including guides on searching and critical appraisal tools.

Web of Addictions (http://www.well.com/user/woa): aims to provide accurate information about alcohol and other drug addictions.

Kids Link (http://sargon.mmu.ac.uk/welcome.htm): aims to provide information, relevant links and support for parents of children with special needs.

Eating Disorders Shared Awareness (EDSA) (http://www.eating-disorder.com): includes information on definitions, causes, treatment with links and online support.

Dyslexia (http://www.dyslexia.com): contains online bookstore and library plus links, training information and a discussion board.

Autism (http://www.autism.org): aimed at parents, carers and health care professionals, this site provides information related to or about autism and related disorders.

Social Care Institute for Excellence (SCIE) (www.scie.org.uk): provides access to the electronic Library of Social Care (eLSC) that includes CareData, a searchable database of social care abstracts.

Social Policy Research Unit, University of York (www.york.ac.uk/inst/spru/pubs/researchwks. htm): provides details of studies conducted in the related fields of social security, social care and health care with many studies concerned with disabilities.

Research in Practice (www.rip.org.uk): a Department of Health/Association of Directors of Social Services funded organisation set up to promote evidence-based practice in social care; searchable evidence including summaries (brief appraisals) of key reviews.

CHAPTER 10

Working with People who Experience Alcohol and Other Drug Problems

Wulf Livingston and Sarah Galvani

Introduction

Alcohol and other drug use (hereafter referred to as 'substance misuse') is a significant factor in determining the well-being, health and social care of many social work service users. Substance use and the problems related to it span many specialist areas of adults' and children's social work practice. Some social workers choose to specialise in substance use; the majority do not. Social workers, through their roles, knowledge and skills, are tasked with responding to the situations and concerns that arise in people's lives as a result of their substance use. This response includes identifying, assessing and intervening with substance use. There is increasing evidence for the success of substance use interventions and their appropriateness for use by non-substance specialist frontline staff.

Until the turn of the twentieth century, literature – and, more specifically, research focusing on social work with alcohol and other drugs – was relatively sparse. There were three key social work texts which summarised twentieth-century developments (Barber, 1995; Collins, 1990; Harrison, 1996). In addition, there was some influential research – which primarily concentrated on social workers' confidence, preparedness and supportive educational experiences – in undertaking work with substance use (Harrison, 1992; Lightfoot and Orford, 1986). More recently, substance use and its impact on families, children and young people, in particular, has risen up the political agenda (Advisory Council on the Misuse of Drugs, 2003; Her Majesty's Government, 2008; 2010; Lord Laming, 2009). There has also been a broadening of the research which identifies the use of substances by adult service user groups and adds depth and strength to earlier concerns about the lack of preparation social workers receive for working with substance use (Galvani and Forrester, 2011). This has coincided with a number of new summary texts for social work on substance use policy and practice (Collins and Keene, 2000; Galvani 2012; Goodman, 2007; Keene, 2010; Paylor *et al.*, 2012).These developments have been accompanied by the publication of practice guidance and resources targeting frontline social workers working with specific service user groups (Forrester and Harwin, 2011; Galvani and Livingston, 2012a; 2012b; Livingston and Galvani, 2012; McCarthy and Galvani, 2012). Furthermore, there has always been an extensive volume of literature and research in the alcohol and drug domain, which is highly relevant to social work practice.

This chapter will provide a summary of the key messages from this research literature, using a case scenario to highlight how some of the evidence supports specific interventions relevant to social workers.

Messages from research

Social workers work regularly, if not daily, with people with substance problems and there are various effective interventions for use within social work practice.

Clients with substance problems

There is plenty of research that seeks to establish the volume, patterns and changes of overall general population use of alcohol and other drugs (Davies *et al.*, 2012; Department of Health, 2007; Robinson and Harris, 2011). As this is frequently survey data, care must be taken in its interpretation, as it reflects under-reporting and subjectivity (Galvani 2012).

Data from the annual General Lifestyle Survey (Dunstan, 2012) show that 36 per cent of men and 28 per cent of women in the UK reported alcohol consumption above recommended levels on at least one day in the previous seven, with a substantial number (19 per cent of men, 13 per cent of women) drinking 'heavily' on more than one of the previous seven days. Given these are national prevalence data, they translate into significant numbers of people in the UK drinking at levels deemed to pose medium- or high-level risks to their health. In relation to other drugs, the most recent statistics of illicit drug use in the general population show that 36.5 per cent of people aged 16–59 years reported ever having taken an illicit substance, with 8.9 per cent reporting use within the past year (Home Office, 2012). The most widely used drug remains cannabis. It is worth noting that drug data are collected differently from alcohol data. Drug use statistics relate to *any use*, rather than risky use, as reported above in the alcohol data.

The prevalence of such levels of substance use among large elements of the population translates into a range of individual, familial and societal problems (Department of Health, 2007), including negative impacts on the individual's wider networks of family and friends, work and community. In addition to these national prevalence data, there is some good evidence to support heightened levels of use and consequences among particular social work client groups (Galvani 2012; Paylor *et al.*, 2012). Some of the evidence for substance use among key social work groups is highlighted in Box 10.1.

BOX 10.1 EVIDENCE ON SUBSTANCE MISUSE IN DIFFERENT SERVICE USER GROUPS

Service User and Carer Group	Prevalence	Consequences	Sources
Children and families	■ Significant factor in social work caseloads, particularly where there are child protection concerns. ■ General population estimates suggest 22% of all children aged under 16 live with parent who drink hazardously and 8% with a parent who has used other drugs in the past year.	■ Parental substance use can cause a complex range of harms for children, particularly if problematic. ■ Substance problems can affect the parenting of the non-using parent, too. ■ Research identifies a range of negative physical, psychological and social impacts from parental substance use. ■ This, in turn, can result in behavioural change, educational problems and increased risks of suffering and perpetrating abuse. ■ Unborn children can also be damaged by maternal substance use.	■ Advisory Council on Misuse of Drugs (2003); Forrester and Harwin (2011); ■ Kroll and Taylor (2003); (Manning et al., 2009); ■ Templeton et al. (2006).
Mental health	■ Evidence consistently suggests that approximately half of the people attending substance use or mental health services experience these as co-existing issues.	■ Substance use can exacerbate mental distress although some people will use substances because they feel this helps their symptoms. ■ It is possible that substance use can trigger psychological and psychiatric distress. ■ It can be difficult to intervene if the substance use effects mimic mental distress symptoms.	■ Bartels et al. (2006); ■ Manning et al. (2002); ■ Moselhy (2009); ■ Needham (2007).

Young people

- The number of young people using alcohol and other drugs is falling overall. However, the UK still has high rates of substance use among young people, particularly cannabis use. Also, prevalence is higher among groups of young people who experience high levels of parental conflict; where parents condone substance use; among young people who are excluded from school; and among those who have lived in institutional care.

- Many young people experiment with alcohol and other drugs and do not go on to develop problems.
- However, young people who use substances – particularly at a young age and frequently – are at higher risk of both physical harm (e.g. damage to brain development and liver function and are at greater risk of school exclusion for offending behaviour, and mental ill health.
- Parents have a key influence over their children's use of substances – positively and negatively.

- Britton (2007);
- Burkhart et al. (2003);
- Health Advisory Service (2001).

Older people

- Generally drink less and use fewer illicit drugs than younger generations.
- Evidence suggests they drink more often than young people.
- Number of older people who experience alcohol- and drug-related problems is increasing as a consequence of our ageing population and changing patterns of consumption.

- An increasing and significant number of older people are at risk from their alcohol use.
- Physical changes in later life mean alcohol consumption can place older people at greater risk of developing acute physical consequences (e.g. heart-, liver- and intestine-related concerns).
- Mentally, older drinkers have an increased risk of memory loss, dementia, depression and suicide.
- Heavier drinkers may also experience specific degenerative brain disorders, such as alcohol-related dementia, Wernicke's encephalopathy and Korsakoff's amnesic syndrome.

- Robinson and Harris (2011);
- Wadd et al. (2011).

BOX 10.1 CONTINUED

Service User and Carer Group	Prevalence	Consequences	Sources
Black and minority ethnic people (BME)	■ BME groups generally have lower rates of substance use when compared with their white counterparts. ■ Individuals from mixed ethnic backgrounds are likely to experience higher than average levels of substance consumption. ■ Substance use varies within BME groups ■ Consumption levels and attitudes towards substances change over time, particularly from one generation to the next. ■ Research tends to over-concentrate on certain ethnic populations; e.g. those of an Indian origin.	■ Cultural or religious prohibition is a protective factor for the use of substances. ■ However, such prohibition can isolate problem users within these communities. ■ Lack of acknowledgement of substance use within some cultures and religious groups makes appropriate service provision a challenge. ■ Families can be left trying to cope, yet ignorant of how to help and to whom to turn.	■ Beddoes et al. (2010b); ■ Hurcombe et al. (2010); ■ UK Drugs Policy Commission (2010).
Physical disabilities	■ Small amounts of UK data and larger amounts of evidence from the USA suggest substance use, and problems with it, are far higher among people with physical disabilities than those without disabilities.	■ Excessive use can exacerbate physical health problems, although some people may be self-medicating through substance use. ■ Problematic use also adds to the isolation people feel through their disability and exacerbate any mental distress, too.	■ Beddoes et al. (2010a); ■ Hoare and Moon (2010); ■ Turner et al. (2006).

161

| Learning disabilities | ■ Very limited data on people with learning disabilities but, generally, levels of substance use are considered to be very low. | ■ Substance use can exacerbate cognitive impairment and other physical and mental health issues.
■ People can be excluded from their existing support services due to intoxicated behaviour and/or face difficulties accessing new services
People with learning disabilities can face increased vulnerability to exploitation when they are using substances and socialising with others who do. | ■ Huxley et al. (2005) |

> ## PRACTICE REFLECTION 10.1
> **Substance use**
> How often do you encounter people who use alcohol and other drugs in your practice? What assumption might this lead you to make about the wider prevalence of substance use among your service user group? To what extent does your experience tally with the evidence base?

Effective interventions for use within social work practice

There is strong evidence in the substance use field for the efficacy of interventions with people with alcohol and other drug problems (Gossop, 2006; Raistrick *et al.*, 2006). The following section outlines five evidence-based interventions which have characteristics that are well-suited to social work practice with individuals, groups and/or families.

Brief interventions: Brief interventions refer to short interventions focused on substance use but that take place within a wider health or social care intervention. They are sometimes referred to as 'identification and brief advice' (IBA) or 'extended brief interventions' (AERC Alcohol Academy, 2010; Lavoie, 2010). Brief interventions are typically 5–10 minutes of discussion and advice, whereas extended brief interventions may last longer – typically 20–30 minutes – and involve the use of motivational interviewing techniques and skills. At their core are good communication skills that advise and/or encourage people to consider reasons to change their substance using behaviour. They offer information about further interventions and services that can support any decisions the person makes about changing their substance use. The existing evidence base for the effectiveness of brief interventions is predominantly for general practitioner, health and criminal justice settings (Moyer *et al.*, 2002; Raistrick *et al.*, 2006). However, social work has been identified as a profession suited to delivering brief interventions and in need of a controlled evaluation of its effectiveness (Raistrick *et al.*, 2006).

Common to brief interventions is the use of a standardised screening tool or instrument to measure the extent of any alcohol and drug use, and its possible consequences. Among tools for alcohol screening, the Alcohol Use Disorders Identification Test (AUDIT) 10-item questionnaire (Babor *et al.*, 2001) is often regarded as the gold standard, but there is also plenty of evidence for the use of shorter versions of this and other tools, including single-item questions (Alcohol Learning Centre, 2012).

Motivational interviewing (MI): MI has an extremely strong evidence base, albeit outside the social work environment in the UK. At the time of writing, social work trials are under way, led by Donald Forrester at the University of Bedfordshire, to determine the effectiveness of MI in a children and families social work practice environment. To date, hundreds of research studies evaluating its effectiveness in a range of settings and with a range of service users have demonstrated that it works at least as well as other treatments, if not better, including studies with non-substance specialist frontline health care practitioners (Lundahl *et al.*, 2010). MI is often used with people who are in the stages of contemplating, or beginning to think about, change – but enhancing motivation to change, or to maintain changes, is essential throughout the process.

MI is not just about interviewing. It is an effective approach to communication that supports people to change behaviours, including alcohol and other drug use (Miller and Rollnick, 2002). It assumes that people will be ambivalent about change, as any significant change in people's lives can have positive and negative effects. Social work is increasingly drawing on the evidence base for the effectiveness of MI as a means to improve social work interventions and encourage service users to engage in behavioural change and substance treatment services (Forrester *et al.*, 2012). In addition to its use in individual client work, the principles of MI have been incorporated into a number of specific family-based interventions. Most notable among these is intensive family support service 'Option 2' in Wales and similar services based on the Option 2 model throughout the UK. It also underpins the Integrated Family Support Services programme being rolled out in Wales (Forrester *et al.*, 2008; Welsh Assembly Government, 2008). These interventions seek to work in partnership with families, using the critical moment of their children's referral to social care as an opportunity to support parents in accentuating the positive reasons for changing their substance use and, at the same time, highlighting the existing strengths they have.

Cognitive behavioural therapy (CBT): Along with the motivational approaches, social work methods have drawn heavily on the evidence base that supports the effectiveness of CBT-based interventions in alcohol and drug work (Forrester *et al.*, 2012). CBT works with how people think and how this impacts on their behaviour. The approach works to support people to change their thought processes and, as a result, change their behaviour. It also helps them to learn new coping responses, rather than relying on a substance as a response or coping mechanism. CBT can comprise individual and group sessions depending on the length of programme and the goal of the intervention, but these can include relapse prevention groups, cognitive skills training, behavioural skills training, abstinence skills training and therapy groups.

Families and networks: A number of approaches for working with families of substance users have been found to be effective in not only helping those using substances to address their use, but also improving the health and well-being of the family members in their own right (Copello *et al.*, 2000a; Orford *et al.*, 2007). These approaches are likely to be particularly effective for social work practice with groups or family members affected by someone else's substance use. Two approaches in particular have been developed in the UK and have been evaluated with non-substance specialist professionals in health care settings: Social Behaviour and Network Therapy (SBNT) (Copello *et al.*, 2002; Copello *et al.*, 2006) and the five-step model (Copello *et al.*, 2000a; Copello *et al.*, 2000b).

SBNT starts with the individual substance user and works with them to build a supportive network of people who would be prepared to help the person address their substance use, both by attending the agency-based intervention and through their actions at home. The network may be one or more family members but also includes friends or others, such as a key worker, who are prepared to take part and offer positive support. The eight sessions that comprise the structure of the SBNT sessions address particular issues (e.g. communication skills), but they also address coping mechanisms and the need for support for both the individual and the network. It has been evaluated both quantitatively and qualitatively, and has been found to be as effective as other methods in reducing substance use, as well as supporting the network members (Copello *et al.*, 2006).

The five-step model recognises that family members of people with substance problems often need support in their own right. It is designed to educate and support family members about substance use and also the options open to them for responding to/living with their substance using relative. The five steps are:

- listen, reassure, explore concerns;
- provide relevant information;
- counsel about ways of coping;
- counsel about social support;
- direct family member to other sources of specialist help.

Two versions of the model are currently available, one session with a professional plus a self-help manual, or the use of the manual across five sessions with a professional. Evaluations have shown the model to have been effective in terms of reducing both the physical and psychological symptoms family members suffer, as well as helping them to cope with their relative's substance use (Orford *et al.*, 2007). In some cases, the approach has also led to a change in the alcohol or drug use by the relative with the problem, as well as improving family relationships.

Peer support: The history of, and evidence for, the effectiveness of peer support and self-help in supporting individuals to make changes to their alcohol and drug using lifestyle is well-documented (Humphreys, 2004; Humphreys and Moos, 2007; Kurtz, 1991). More recently, the discourse about peer support has been assimilated into wider policy discussions about the role of recovery, not only within recovery-oriented systems of care, but also with regard to independent peer-led recovery communities (Wardle, 2009; White, 2009).

Peer support can reflect a range of activities. At one level, this might be support by others who have experienced similar experiences provided within the context of existing service provision, often referred to as 'mentoring'. However, it can also refer to the provision of distinct interventions by service users and carers to their peers. This can be either intervention associated with supporting substance use change, like Alcoholics Anonymous or SMART recovery groups, or those groups associated with helping to maintain much wider lifestyle changes (Livingston *et al.*, 2011). Such groups provide vital support for people away from the formal structures of professional help.

PRACTICE REFLECTION 10.2

Substance use support

How do you currently respond to service users in need of support for their alcohol and/or other drug use? Which of these interventions could you use in your work with service users?

Implications for social work practice

Social workers have the skills to work well with substance problems in a range of practice contexts and a duty to do so. At the core of the evidence-based interventions discussed above are a number of skills and characteristics that are fundamental to good social work practice. While new methods need some training and practice, these interventions use key skills that are used every day by social workers. Indeed, in the case of family-based interventions social workers are more familiar with the skills required for group and family work than most substance specialists.

What the evidence shows is that these successful interventions contain the following skills and characteristics:

- an emphasis on relationship building;
- empathy;
- excellent communication skills, including active listening and reflection;
- an empowering attitude and approach;
- non-judgemental attitudes.

We are not proposing that all social workers need to become substance specialists but we are highlighting that the move towards positive engagement with substance use, by all social work professionals, is not a huge one given the evidence base. Furthermore, social workers already hold the skills to assess people's needs sensitively, ask questions about personal matters and convey information that can sometimes be difficult for people to hear. Working with substance use is no different, yet evidence shows that social workers are ambivalent about engaging with substance use issues among their service users (Hutchinson *et al.*, 2013). The reasons for this are unknown (see Galvani, 2007, for a review) but, as our awareness of the social harms that result from problematic substance use increases, it is clear that we have a duty to engage with it. Working with substance use is a frontline social work issue and requires more than an onward referral to specialist services. Using Case scenario 10.1, we highlight how the evidence base can support social workers to work with substance use.

As in the family in Case scenario 10.1, research evidence indicates that social workers are regularly, if not daily, in contact with people experiencing alcohol and drug issues (Galvani and Forrester, 2011). It further shows that social workers are attempting to ask about substance use, often with very little guidance or professional education on how to do so (Galvani *et al.*, 2013). The roles social workers will adopt in relation to working with substance use will

---

CASE SCENARIO 10.1

Jackie, John and Bob

Jackie and John have two children, both with learning disabilities. Following unsuccessful attempts to meet with them, the children's school recently made a referral to social services as it was concerned about the children's attendance and behaviour.

On working with the family, you establish that both Jackie and John are finding coping with the pressures and demands of parenting difficult and are drinking to cope. John has previously experienced a period of compulsory mental health detention. The psychiatric staff believed his amphetamine use at the time contributed heavily to his poor mental health and expressed concern about future risk of relapse. He continues to receive some support around his mental health. Family members are trying to be supportive but are frequently frustrated by John's return to amphetamine use.

Jackie's parents live nearby and are willing to help but they have some medical issues and feel that, at their ages, they cannot take on much more responsibility for the grandchildren. John's father, Bob, also lives locally and is willing to take on some child care. Bob has finally achieved a sustained two-year abstinence from drinking, which he states was in response to his life in the armed forces and the recent death of his wife. He has some concerns about his own physical disabilities and mental health and is seeking support to address the physical pain and the loneliness he feels.

---

vary widely according to the specialist area of practice and the varying approaches to assessment and intervention. But whatever the role and whatever the approach, it is clear that social workers have to be willing and able to ask about substance use and be able to respond empathically and supportively to keep people engaged with services.

In Case scenario 10.1, it is clear that any social worker working with these family members will have to be aware of, assess for, and work with substance use issues. This may be a children and families social worker responding to concerns about the children, an adult mental health social worker supporting John, or an adults' worker supporting Bob's needs. The research and interventions outlined can support social workers to understand this complex, but not atypical, scenario and how they might most effectively intervene.

Importantly, such evidence shows that substance use is often just one part of a complex mix of social and health problems people face including domestic abuse and mental distress. Add to this poverty, loss or poor physical health and it is easy to see how service users can struggle to identify and address just one of their multiple problems without the positive support and intervention from social and health care professionals. Thus, we can see that John's substance use is entwined in issues of mental health, and both Jackie and John's use is in the context of pressures to parent two children with disabilities. Similarly, Bob's prior use is in the context of his mental and physical distress, and care would need to be taken to ensure Bob avoided relapse by helping him to access appropriate support. Social workers engaged with such a family as this will need to consider these complexities of substance use as both a coping response to situations, as well as possible causes of problems.

Brief interventions are used with people whose use of substances is at the lower levels of risk of harm and not people whose use may be considered substance dependent and high-risk; as such, they have a role in any work with Jackie. If Jackie is not yet drinking at high-risk levels, brief interventions that provide factual information about risk and harm to her and others may be enough for her to change her drinking behaviour, or may lead to discussions about seeking further support. She may benefit from extended brief interventions after which it may be easier to determine her readiness to change and what additional support she needs. John may also benefit from extended brief interventions, but these will need to take account of his potential use of multiple substances.

Motivational interviewing (MI) would be an appropriate approach to use with John to help him reflect on his ambivalence about changing his amphetamine use. It would enable him to be open about the positives of his use, and also the negative impact it has on his mental and physical health and on family relationships. Importantly, MI focuses on reflection and listening and is not advice-giving in the same way as brief interventions. Part of what is motivational about MI is enabling service users to hear themselves identifying the negatives of continued use and the advantages of change. This is done by the social worker enhancing John's motivation to change by reflective listening and skilled questioning, underpinned by a genuine, empathic approach. Through skilled questioning, the worker can highlight the positives of change and influence John's decisional balance and commitment to change. MI techniques are often incorporated into extended brief interventions.

Bob is finding it hard to cope with the loneliness following his wife's death, as well as the physical pain of his disabilities. He has been abstinent from alcohol for two years but the loss of his wife and the physical, emotional and mental distress he is feeling places him at risk of relapse, which would be a return to problematic levels of alcohol use. Cognitive behavioural interventions can be used to help Bob to think through what his triggers might be for drinking and to discuss alternative ways of thinking and behaving in relation to each one. Helping Bob to talk about his fears and concerns is a key element of relapse prevention, as is working with him to have a relapse plan in place.

SBNT would be an ideal intervention for John and the family, given their level of frustration in trying to help him and not knowing what to do next. Helping John and his family to establish more positive family relationships will benefit everyone in the family. Similarly, Jackie and John's parents, who are supportive but concerned about taking on too much, may benefit from SBNT and some supportive and open discussions with them about their role and how to make best use of the support they can give. It would work equally well with Bob, in the context of his apparent need for help in building a social support network to overcome his loneliness and to prevent relapse, possibly by helping him engage with family and friends. The five-step approach may be appropriate for use with Jackie and John's family members, particularly their parents, who are struggling to cope with their behaviour and appear to want to give their children and grandchildren positive support.

Given his loneliness, Bob may well benefit from peer support groups. A social worker could support him to engage in a peer group, if they were aware of the range of local peer and recovery groups. Where no group exists, and in other social work contexts such as residential work, a social worker might help Bob and other similar clients to begin to support themselves. There are also peer support groups available that focus on specific groups of people – for example, women only, young people, and family members – thus Jackie might also find a peer group for support rather than relying on her family for this. For social workers, such peer support can be an important resource for their service users and can offer important 'out of hours' support and motivation in times of need. However, an awareness of the advantages and disadvantages of peer support groups is important, as is briefing service users on what to expect from a peer support group. Thus, preparing Bob or Jackie to attend a support group is an important part of any referral and ongoing support process.

While history has not given social workers clear roles and functions in relation to their practice with substance use, it has long been proposing a range of roles, tasks and functions. As outlined, these include an educator, broker, advocate, case manager (Goldmeier, 1994; O'Hare, 2003) and a self-help group facilitator (Toseland and Hacker, 1982). Others have commented on the ideal position of social workers to engage, assess and support people with substance problems.

PRACTICE REFLECTION 10.3

Interventions

What skills and knowledge do you already have that would enable you to intervene, support and provide services to Jackie and John's family? What additional support would you need to undertake the social worker role outlined above? Do you know if your agency or others provide the interventions outlined above?

Conclusion

In social work, the evidence to support greater engagement with substance use issues is growing. As a profession, we must listen to messages about 'what works' from our specialist substance use colleagues and adapt these approaches to suit our varied work contexts and priorities. Social workers have an important role to play in work with alcohol and drug issues, whether or not this is in partnership with specialist substance use colleagues. The body of evidence to support our interventions is an expanding one.

There remain areas of social work practice that the evidence does not yet fully address. There is a need for more research focusing on ways to support social workers to become more informed and confident about their roles with substance use. There is a demand for more evidence about the impact of alcohol and drug use on specific social work client groups and the most effective responses to these presenting concerns. Finally, there are increasing calls for research to move beyond the standardised approach and limitations of using randomised control trials and other experimental designs to illustrate relative effectiveness of treatment interventions. For example, there is some evidence to suggest that CBT, despite its popularity with policy-makers and commissioners, is no more significantly effective than other interventions, including those outlined in this chapter (Magill and Ray, 2009). There are increasing calls for research to adopt a broader range of methodological approaches that also explores some of the complexities of how individuals influence and form effective working relationships (Orford, 2008).

Thus, as social work research continues to embrace a greater diversity of research designs and approaches (McLaughlin, 2007; Philips and Shaw, 2011), including more qualitative and service user led approaches, it will begin to develop a greater understanding of its role and effectiveness in working with alcohol and drugs in a myriad of practice contexts. For social work to respond effectively to the volume of alcohol and drug concerns it encounters, it needs to remain evidence-based, utilising the evidence which already exists and continuing to develop more of its own practice-based research knowledge.

FURTHER READING

Galvani, S. (2012) *Supporting People with Alcohol and Drug Problems. Making a Difference* (Bristol: Policy Press); Paylor, I., Measham, F. and Asher, H. (2012) *Social Work and Drug Use* (Maidenhead: Open University Press). Both these books provide useful summaries of research evidence.

Gossop, M. (2006) *Treating Drug Misuse Problems: Evidence of Effectiveness* (London: National Treatment Agency for Substance Misuse); Raistrick, D., Heather, N. and Godfrey, C. (2006) *Review of the Effectiveness of Treatment for Alcohol Problems* (London: National Treatment Agency for Substance Misuse). Both these reports provide useful summaries of evidence for the effectiveness of treatment interventions.

CHAPTER 11

Working with People with Mental Health Problems

Nick Gould and Tom Lochhead

Introduction

It is a sad reality that mental ill-health is a pervasive aspect of our lives. Amongst people under 65 years old, nearly half of all illness is mental illness; and it is calculated in a recent report that a common disorder such as depression tends, on average, to be more debilitating than chronic physical illnesses such as angina, arthritis, asthma or diabetes (Centre for Economic Performance's Mental Health Policy Group, 2012). In England, a country with 21 million dwellings, the number of people with a mental illness is estimated in the same report to be around 7 million, from which a not unreasonable extrapolation is that one in three households in England is affected by mental illness. It is also estimated that, in England, 700,000 children have behavioural problems, depression or anxiety, of whom only one quarter have access to treatment (Green *et al.*, 2005) and 700,000 people in the United Kingdom are living with dementia, most of them older people (Knapp and Prince, 2007).

From these illustrative statistics, it can be inferred that mental ill-health is a pervasive issue that will come to the attention of social workers whatever their area of specialism. It is not confined to those who work in designated mental health services. Up-to-date research into the prevalence of mental illness amongst the users of social care services is overdue, but it seems a reasonable expectation that Huxley *et al.*'s estimates still hold true that, amongst all client groups, around two thirds are experiencing some common form of mental disorder concurrent with being helped (Evans and Huxley, 2012; Huxley *et al.*, 1989a; Huxley *et al.*, 1989b). From all of this, it would seem imperative that all social workers have some understanding of key aspects of the evidence base relating to mental health. However, this is a huge challenge, given that the domains of evidence which could be relevant to social work practitioners straddle several substantial fields, such as the epidemiology of mental illness (including social causation), the effectiveness of psychosocial interventions, social implications of biomedical treatments, and the relative merits of alternative modes of service organisation and delivery.

An attempt has been made elsewhere by one of the authors of this chapter to delineate an approach to mapping knowledge for mental health social work, not least to avoid the rigidities of evidence-based medicine's hierarchical ordering of knowledge, privileging the gold standard of the randomised controlled trial which has proven less helpful to social care (Gould, 2006; 2008). A full exposition of this approach is not feasible here but it can be summarised thus:

- What is known about the risk factors for patterns of occurrence of mental disorder, and the social impacts of having a mental illness? Large-scale surveys such as the Office for National Statistics censuses of mental disorder (e.g. Meltzer *et al.*, 2002) can be an important resource.
- What are the experiences of service users and carers of their mental health problems and interventions that have been made to help them? Surveys are again important forms of evidence, but so are in-depth qualitative studies of service user experience.
- Which interventions are effective in helping service users with mental health problems and their carers? Findings from experimental studies, particularly randomised controlled trials are less prevalent in social work, but provide strong evidence about effectiveness, if well-designed and carefully interpreted.
- How can we best deliver effective services to help service users achieve recovery? Organisational research can take many forms, including randomised controlled trials. Also, mixed-methods case studies can be informative because the richness of qualitative data informs and extends analyses based on quantitative evidence.

This chapter will give brief examples of how these types of research have been developed in relation to mental health problems and then a case scenario will be provided through which consideration will be given to the use of research to inform practice. More detail as to the epistemological and methodological aspects of these types of research can be found in Part 1 of this volume, particularly Chapter 1.

Epidemiological studies

Studies in the West find an enduring relationship between rates of mental illness and indicators of social disadvantage including low income, lower educational attainment, unemployment and low social status (Fryers *et al.*, 2003), all leading to trajectories of social exclusion. In England, only 24 per cent of people with long-term mental health conditions are in employment, a smaller percentage than any other main category of people with disabilities (Office of the Deputy Prime Minister, 2004). Financial difficulties accrue with insecure employment and inadequate benefits leading to higher than average levels of debt (Meltzer *et al.*, 2002). Unemployment and financial hardship correlates with deteriorating mental health and suicide, while employment contributes to symptom reduction, fewer hospital admissions and lower levels of service take-up (Drake *et al.*, 1999). Physical health is also impacted by mental distress; a review of research found amongst people with a history of psychosis two to four times the normal rate of cardiovascular disease, respiratory disease, five times the rate of diabetes, eight times the rate of hepatitis C and 15 times the rate of HIV (Rethink, 2008). Higher rates of mortality for people with a mental disorder are partially attributable to suicide and high risk behaviour, but also reflect iatrogenic effects of treatments such as higher levels of diabetes induced by medication and failures of routine health care (Allebeck, 1989; Department of Health, 2004; Rethink, 2008). People with mental health problems are also over-represented in the numbers of people who are homeless (Redmond, 2005).

Qualitative studies

Qualitative evidence about the experience of being a user of mental health services has traditionally been relegated by orthodox evidence-based medicine to a low status. The exception within sociology has been the social constructionist perspectives, such as labelling theory, which tended to treat mental disorder as 'exotic' and deviant. One advance has been an authoritative systematic review and practice guideline published by England's National Institute for Health and Care Excellence, *Service User Experience in Adult Mental Health* (National Collaborating Centre for Mental Health, 2012), based primarily on meta-synthesis of high-quality qualitative evidence collected for existing guidelines. Some of the key messages from the studies synthesised address feelings of stigmatisation and disempowerment by services, problems across the care pathway in relation to assessment, community care, hospitalisation and discharge and, not least, experiences of detention and compulsory treatment. Barriers to accessing services include lack of respect from professionals for the service user's preferences, an absence of information about alternatives, and non-inclusion in significant decisions. Not surprisingly, compulsion under the Mental Health Act is a prevalent theme as it is a unique experience in the health and social care field (with the possible exception of looked-after children) to be subject to curtailment of liberty and treatment against the individual's will (even in situations where the service user may have capacity).

The shadow of the Act falls also on those not compulsorily detained as the implied sanction of compulsion may influence decisions about compliance with treatment in the community, and the regime of in-patient facilities is often dictated by the necessities of a patient population that includes detained individuals (locked doors and windows, and exposure to witnessing treatment administered accompanied by restraint or coercion).

Intervention studies

Although most service users' treatment, for the minority who receive any, will be pharmacological, there has been a significant advance in recent years of evidence for the effectiveness of psychological interventions, in particular cognitive behavioural therapies (CBTs).

Case scenario 11.1 takes as an exemplar an individual living with schizophrenia. In the UK, diagnosis of schizophrenia is usually made according to

Schneider's first rank symptoms, where underlying physical illness has been excluded and the person reports any one of a number of abnormal experiences, including auditory hallucinations, delusions of thought control, other delusions of somatic or psychological control, or delusional perceptions such as interpretations of everyday events having special significance (Gould, 2010).

In recent years, research has shown that some of these diagnostic criteria – for example, 'hearing voices' – are less than clear-cut. Kelleher *et al.*'s research (2012) found that 21 per cent of younger adolescents report hearing voices, and it is hypothesised by Murray and Jones (2012) that, for many people, this phenomenon is more frequently associated with common mental disorders, particularly depression, than the emergence of frank psychosis. Epidemiological evidence shows that even if there is a genetic predisposition associated with schizophrenia, environmental factors also play a significant role in causation, course and outcome. The lifetime risk of developing schizophrenia is about 1 per cent, the risks are higher if a close relative has the illness but, even in identical monozygotic twins, the risk is 50 per cent, showing there are significant factors outside genetic determinants (Warner, 2010). Medication is usually the first line of treatment, but recovery rates have not altered since the introduction of antipsychotic medication (Warner, 2010), and most evidence-based guidelines advocate a combination of medication and psychosocial treatment (e.g. National Collaborating Centre for Mental Health, 2010).

Schizophrenia typically manifests in early adulthood, and evidence suggests the longer an individual remains untreated the poorer the prognosis (e.g. McGorry *et al.*, 1996), though proof that early intervention strategies improve recovery remains somewhat uncertain (National Collaborating Centre for Mental Health, 2010). CBTs seem to help people cope better with managing their symptoms of schizophrenia and increases motivation to remain engaged with treatment (Pilling *et al.*, 2002). Relapses and hospital re-admissions for people living with schizophrenia are also shown to be reduced by interventions with families which enable them to become more understanding of the nature of schizophrenia and the stresses that can be induced by over-critical and intrusive attitudes to the service user (Mari and Streiner, 1999). However, a more recent study found that CBT and family intervention had no impact on relapse and readmission rates (Garety *et al.*, 2008).

Mental health social work research

Research also tells us something about the place of social work in mental health services, and the delivery of services that help recovery. Huxley *et al.*'s (2012) study of mental health teams in England and Wales encouragingly found that inclusion of social workers in teams was associated with greater effectiveness. Community Mental Health Teams (CMHTs) seem to be more effective than other teams in keeping people out of hospital, but other expected benefits have not been found, e.g. higher user or carer satisfaction. Research into assertive outreach teams in the UK have been disappointing with outcomes no better than CMHTs (Burns *et al.*, 2001). However, early inter-vention teams do have better outcomes on a number of measures of social adjustment, though psychotic symptoms were not improved (Garety *et al.*, 2006). These studies highlight the ongoing debate about which indicators of recovery are most relevant for use in research, policy and practice. Tew *et al.* (2012) argue that social workers (and researchers) need to maintain a focus on factors such as empowerment, relationships and social inclusion as well as the more-often measured outcomes such as readmission to hospital.

The design and implementation of services is often, as Huxley *et al.* (2012) found, not based on empirically-deduced principles but on ideologically-based policy. For example, personalisation has become an over-arching policy theme for adult social care, though this is an imprecisely defined term, which has encompassed a number of initiatives including direct payments, self-directed support, and individual budgets. Normative views of personalisation charac-terise this as the promotion of individually tailored services to meet self-assessed need (see Duffy, 2010) while its critics see it as an ideological disguise for cost-cutting and service fragmentation (Ferguson, 2007). An evaluation of individual budget schemes found that people with mental health problems were the smallest user group of this form of provision; most people continued to purchase traditional services (Glendinning *et al.*, 2008). However, central government policy continues to require the widespread, if not universal, adop-tion of personalisation as the norm for funded services in mental health.

Using research to inform practice

If we were to put ourselves in the shoes of Helen (Case Scenario 11.1), how would we go about practising in a way that can be characterised as evidence-based? This takes us to the heart of some of the most fundamental debates that have characterised academic social work (if not frontline practice) during the last twenty-five years.

Social work took a 'reflective turn' with the discovery of the writings of Schon and others on epistemological approaches to practice that rejected the crude deductive models which suggested that theory could deductively be applied to practice in a linear, technical rational way (Gould, 1989; Gould and Taylor, 1996). Instead, Schon argued that practitioners iterated their own theories inductively through engagement with the problems they encountered in practice; their reflections on practice and their attempts to solve problems generated theories of practice that were continuously refined as they succeeded or failed in solving the problems they encountered in their practice. Thus, as an experienced social worker, Helen may have worked with a number of young men who had similar experiences of psychosis and had been detained under the Mental Health Act, from which experiences she had developed a repertoire of approaches that she might find helpful, but reflecting continu-ously on how they might need to be modified as circumstances unfolded.

This is a radically different conceptualisation of practice from the model of practice embedded in evidence-based medicine which implies that there are intervention strategies whose efficacy has been proven through randomised

Paul

We break into Paul's story at a significant point in his history. He is currently an inpatient in an acute psychiatric unit in his home area, having been detained at Heathrow Airport under Section 3 of the Mental Health Act (1983).

Three months prior to this admission, Paul had gone alone to Spain for a two-week holiday, his first proper holiday in the ten years since his first 'breakdown' at age 19. By his late teens, Paul had thought he had achieved well in his life. His mother, a black African immigrant, had raised Paul on her own and Paul had worked hard, with her help, to achieve university entrance, which he viewed as a way out of the limited life he saw in his mother's situation. In his first year at university, Paul had found that cannabis made him feel less stressed and more sociable. He did well in his first year exams but became withdrawn on his return home. He became paranoid, believing others, including his mother, were plotting against him. In response to distressing 'voices', Paul jumped into a canal. This led to his first detention under the Mental Health Act.

On admission, Paul was immediately treated with anti-psychotic medication. Paul felt that the hospital professionals did not really listen to him and only seemed to be interested in reducing the symptoms of his mental illness, which they told him was schizophrenia. Paul hated this diagnosis. He also hated the side-effects of the anti-psychotic medication that he was to be prescribed, in various forms, over the next ten years. He particularly hated the weight-gain and reduced motivation they seemed to cause. But, each time Paul stopped taking this medication, he had ended up in hospital. Paul never returned to university. His mother found she could not cope with both working and caring for Paul, and he moved into supported accommodation.

Paul had been relatively 'stable' for several months when he arranged the holiday in Spain and Helen, his care coordinator and an experienced social worker, had supported Paul's plan to go on holiday whilst urging him to ensure he took regular medication. However, Paul stopped taking medication as soon as he arrived in Spain. He felt alert and excited. By the end of the planned two-week holiday, Paul had a girlfriend for the first time in ten years and felt 'alive'. He decided to stay in Spain, sleeping on the beach and living on his benefits. His girlfriend returned to Germany and Paul's 'voices' and paranoia returned. He was detained to a psychiatric hospital in Spain and given large doses of anti-psychotic medication before being repatriated to England.

Helen had met Paul at Heathrow and accompanied him back to hospital. Paul had been unusually talkative, describing his despair at the thought of his future and guilt at having 'let his mother down', yet wanting to return to live with her. Helen's CMHT had discussed Paul's case at their last team meeting. His psychiatrist had proposed that they should consider putting Paul on a Community Treatment Order as the only way to keep him safe in the future. Helen had been asked to prepare a summary of Paul's case for presentation at his next inpatient review meeting.

Helen felt uneasy about several aspects of Paul's situation and was reflecting on how she could use an evidence-based approach in her presentation of Paul's case and the ensuing discussion with other professionals and Paul himself.

trials, and which can systematically be applied to Paul's situation once a definitive diagnosis of his problem has been agreed. However, these are caricatured representations of reflective practice and evidence-based practice respectively. Reflective practice, in its more nuanced versions, recognises that the practitioner's interventions, while shaped by the particularities of the given 'case', are also informed by the formal research-based knowledge, so-called propositional knowledge, to which he or she has been exposed (Evans and Hardy, 2010). Likewise, revisionist approaches to evidence-based practice have recognised the contributions of qualitative evidence, and that practitioners need to use judgement in determining what evidence is relevant and applicable in a given situation. Taking an anthropological stance in relation to problematising evidence-based medicine, Lambert (2006) has argued that in contrast to positivistic depictions of it as a neutral and fixed set of methodological techniques, it is actually a changing and malleable set of procedures which has been adapted over time in response to internal and external challenges to its authority.

In social work, and its wider constituency of social care, this revisionist approach to evidence-based practice has led to attempts to create alternative taxonomies that substitute terms such as 'knowledge' for the more positivist connotations of 'evidence', and for heuristic categorisations of knowledge that are non-hierarchical (Gould, 2006).

As a social worker, Helen would probably seek to locate Paul's situation in a framework that avoided so-called 'deficit models' that only located understandings of his situation which emphasised pathology and pessimistic prognoses. The 'recovery model' is such a framework – a diffuse value-based approach relating to the principles that should underpin work with service users in mental health, which emphasises hope (expectations of a fulfilled life), agency (gaining a sense of control of one's life) and opportunity (gaining social inclusion). The recovery model, while not in itself an evidence-based approach, provides a values orientation towards implementing interventions which are empirically validated, and which goes with the grain of policy emphases on personalisation:

> How each person reaches their personal goals is a matter for them, and in recovery (rather than feeling themselves recovered) each person has an individual approach, which means that recovery lends itself to current ideas about personalization and inclusive practice. (Evans and Huxley, 2012: 147)

Another influential approach which is indigenous to social work as a meta-framework for orienting practice is the strengths perspective (Rapp, 1998; Saleeby, 2005). Here the emphasis for interventions shifts from a focus on problems and needs, towards identifying and working with the aptitudes, abilities and skills that the individual possesses.

First, and with these perspectives kept in mind, how might Helen's practice be informed by her knowledge of risk factors which potentially make Paul susceptible to interventions that could be oppressive? As a young, black male of African descent Paul is at increased risk of statutory detention. There is a significant body of research showing that people from black and minority ethnic groups are over-represented in the detained population, and under-represented amongst those who are able to access supportive services (Bhui *et al.*, 2003; Cope, 1989).

In 2005 the UK Department of Health launched a 5-year programme to address racism in psychiatry which included a series of surveys, *Count Me In*, to audit the number of people detained in psychiatric hospitals and their ethnic identity, with black and minority ethnic patients detained at three times the national average rate (Commission for Healthcare Audit and Inspection, 2007). This research also shows that people from black and minority ethnic groups are less likely to be referred by their general practitioner for a mental health service, and more likely to come to the attention of services at points of crisis through the police and other emergency services. This cycle of avoidance and compulsion was explored in the qualitative study *Breaking the Circles of Fear* (Sainsbury Centre for Mental Health, 2002) which highlighted the need to make services accessible and appropriate for people from diverse back-grounds. Knowledge of these risk factors associated with Paul's identity will make Helen alert to the particular vulnerability he faces in being accelerated through the statutory mental health services, the need to take an anti-racist perspective to her work with him, and the potential value, if Paul is in agree-ment, to putting him in touch with community-based organisations that offer specific support to black users of mental health services.

PRACTICE REFLECTION 11.1

Restriction of an individual's liberty

In responding to Paul's needs, were the 'least restrictive alternatives' always followed, and can decisions about the restriction of an individual's liberty always be evidence-based?

In anticipating Paul's care planning meeting, Helen is likely to consider the evidence-base for interventions that could be helpful to Paul's recovery. There seems to be an association between Paul becoming unwell and discontinuing his prescribed antipsychotic medication. Some social workers feel uneasy about acting as mediators in encouraging service users to accept psychotropic medication, perhaps because they see this as incompatible with a social model of mental health, or they are aware of the various negative side effects of major tranquillising drugs. As Harris (2002) has suggested, the mental health practi-tioner needs to adopt a way of working that places the service user at the centre of the treatment process and to seek to develop a therapeutic relation-ship with the person. In order to play their part in working in multidiscipli-nary contexts such as CMHTs they also need to have knowledge about neuroleptic drugs and knowledge of medication management, including the need to involve the service user effectively in treatment decisions. This last principle would also apply in any discussion about the appropriateness of a Community Treatment Order in Paul's situation, although the first major UK study of supervised treatment in the community shows no reduction in rates of readmission to hospital, compared with leave of absence from hospital as already available under Section 17 of the 1983 Mental Health Act (Burns *et al.*, 2013).

Helen might also raise with Paul and the team the possibility that he could benefit from CBT. CBT is not a 'cure' for schizophrenia but, given that this disorder is associated with unusual experiences that are interpreted as negative, threatening or external, CBT can help individuals to recognise, manage and reduce the occurrence and distress of these experiences or 'worrying beliefs'. The evidence-base suggests that it could reduce Paul's risk of relapse and readmission to hospital (National Collaborating Centre for Mental Health, 2010). The generic characteristics of CBT which can be helpful to the person living with schizophrenia are that they help the person to recognise the 'activating events' that trigger false or worrying but inaccurate beliefs, and the consequences of these beliefs, such as anger or disengagement (Sullivan, 2010). Therapeutic support with identifying the triggers, and modifying the beliefs that they produce, can lead to less distressing and more productive consequences. Helen might already be trained in CBT and offer this intervention herself, or there could be other professionals in the team, such as a nurse or clinical psychologist, who can offer CBT for Paul.

Helen would also consider Paul within the context of his family and other significant relationships. There is a well-established evidence-base relating to the modification of family interactions to reduce rates of relapse in schizophrenia and subsequent hospital readmission (National Collaborating Centre for Mental Health, 2010). Where the family does not understand that schizophrenia can lead to behaviours that are experienced as problematic by the family, such as withdrawal and apathy, then the resulting criticality that families might express ('high expressed emotion') can impede the person's recovery. Programmes that help the family learn about the nature of schizophrenia can lead to reductions in the expression of critical attitudes towards the person with schizophrenia and, consequently, reductions in relapse rates (Leff *et al.*, 1982; Mari and Streiner, 1999). If the situation arises that Paul returns to live with his mother, Helen might consider with them whether participation in such a programme might be helpful.

PRACTICE REFLECTION 11.2

Evidence-based social interventions

Which evidence-based social interventions would seem to be most helpful to Paul's future mental health?

Not least, but often an overlooked factor in mental health social work, the evidence suggests that Paul's mental health could be improved by interventions that help him to become employed. We have already considered some of the data suggesting that people with mental illness are more at risk of being unemployed, with rates amongst people with schizophrenia exceeding 90 per cent

(Warner, 2010). Amongst psychosocial interventions, some of the strongest evidence for effectiveness (and one of the few social interventions where there are several randomised controlled trials) can be found for individual placement and support services (IPS) to help people find and remain in employment. Studies show that employment resulting from IPS leads to service users having improved confidence and well-being and showing less reliance on mental health services (Sainsbury Centre for Mental Health, 2009). There is a trend for IPS services to be embedded in CMHTs and Helen might investigate whether such a service can be accessed by Paul. Alternatively, Paul may be able to use a personal budget to access specific training and/or equipment to improve his employability.

This overview of interventions that might help Paul's recovery cannot be exhaustive, given the constraints of a chapter of a book, but are indicative of some of the options that could be explored with him.

PRACTICE REFLECTION 11.3

Mental health and compliance with medication: the implications
What are the implications for the social work role in situations where an evidence-based approach indicates that compliance with medication is the most relevant intervention for maintaining an individual's mental health?

Discussion

A concurrent (though not necessarily related) trend alongside the emergence of evidence-based practice has been the integration of mental health services, often involving the integration of health professionals and social workers in mental health teams. This has brought into sharp focus questions about the role and distinctiveness of social work. For social workers, there is insecurity about whether they can make a contribution that is not already provided by others such as community psychiatric nurses, psychologists or occupational therapists. In the UK, this has been compounded by the ad hoc development of integrated teams where there is often no explicit rationale about the professional composition of teams and its relation to service user outcomes (Evans and Huxley, 2012). Yet, a review of evidence about community teams in mental health identified integration of health and social care as a feature of team effectiveness in reducing hospitalisation, despite the development of teams being pragmatic, atheoretical and unresearched (Byrne and Onyett, 2010). A synthesis of reviews reported that multidisciplinary teams and integrated care impact positively on symptom severity, functioning, employment, and housing of people with severe mental illness, compared with conventional services (Huxley and Thornicroft, 2003).

In a climate of economic austerity where mental health services are under threat and there is more pressure than ever for professionals to justify their presence within integrated services, mental health social workers need to be able to identify the distinctiveness of their contribution, and articulate the evidence-base for the effectiveness of that contribution (Webber, 2012). Part of the distinctiveness of social work, if not its main element, is that it brings an eclectic mix of knowledge of welfare law, psychosocial interventions and (though less prominent in recent years in the social work curriculum) foundational knowledge from social sciences, particularly sociology and social policy. Last, but not least, although all professions include, by definition, ethical codes of practice, social work is still distinct amongst mental health professions in requiring student and qualified practitioners to demonstrate an understanding of a value-base that strongly asserts principles of anti-discrimination and anti-oppression. It follows from this that (mental health) social work should assert its evidence-based credentials, not against the conventional standards of evidence-based medicine but, rather, against an indigenous social work model of evidence-based practice. In the United States, this is emerging as 'Multidimensional Evidence-Based Practice' (Petr, 2009) and is a model that incorporates views of service users and professionals, values and qualitative evidence, alongside usual evidence from experimental research in determining what is best practice.

Mental health services seem to be a particularly appropriate context within which to demonstrate the value of multi-dimensional evidence-based practice. As we have seen in earlier sections of this chapter, users of mental health services have demonstrably high risks of social exclusion, and their problems invariably straddle medical and social domains. Social workers, particularly when they adopt systemic perspectives in their practice, bring to the table an emancipatory values perspective, a casework tradition of starting 'from where the client is', as well as their professional knowledge of psychosocial interventions. But, above all, it is important for mental health social work to maintain its criticality towards what constitutes evidence, and to understand that evidence-based practice is an ideological as well as a scientific project. This means continuing to hold on to a pluralistic conception of 'evidence' and one which includes, and possibly privileges, research and other forms of knowledge that capture and communicate the voices of those who experience mental distress and use mental health services:

> Any situation in which some individuals prevent others from engaging in the process of inquiry is one of violence. ... To alienate people from their own decision making is to change them into objects. (Freire, 1972: 66)

░░░ FURTHER READING ░░░

Evans, S. and Huxley, P. (2012) 'What Does Research Tell us About Social Work in Mental Health?', in Davies, M. (ed.), *Social Work With Adults* (Basingstoke: Palgrave Macmillan). A concise overview of the current state of research knowledge in relation to mental health social work with adults by two of the UK's leading social work researchers.

Gould, N. (2010) *Mental Health Social Work in Context* (Abingdon: Routledge). Written for students and practitioners, this book takes an evidence-based approach to social, clinical and organisational dimensions of mental health social work. There are chapters addressing each stage of the life-cycle as well as forensic perspectives.

National Collaborating Centre for Mental Health (2012) *Service User Experience in Adult Mental Health: NICE Guidance on Improving the Experience of Care for People Using Adult NHS Mental Health Services*. (Leicester and London: British Psychological Society and Royal College of Psychiatry). A corrective to a researcher-led perspective on evidence for practice, a systematic review of service users' views on the care they receive, and guidance for improving their experience of care.

Social Care Institute for Excellence (2008) *Research Briefing 26: Mental Health and Social Work* (London: Social Care Institute for Excellence). Research Briefing 26 provides a useful overview of 'mental health and social work' research. More recent SCIE publications address the evidence base in relation to more specific relevant mental health issues.

Webber, M. (2011) *Evidence-Based Policy and Practice in Mental Health Social Work*, 2nd edn (Exeter: Learning Matters). Though written as part of a series of series of books for practitioners on post-qualifying programmes, this book is valuable for students and practitioners at all levels, providing a review of research relating to law, policy and practice together with detailed guidance on the critical appraisal of research studies.

CHAPTER 12

Working with Disabled People

Hannah Morgan

Introduction

This chapter considers the place and purpose of research evidence when work-ing with disabled people. A central concern of the disabled people's movement and of its academic partner disability studies has been to highlight the way in which disabled people have been excluded from the production of research and other forms of evidence, except as passive subjects of research, or as recip-ients of policy and practice based on that exclusionary research. This means that any discussion of evidence to inform practice with disabled people must start with fundamental questions about how disability is understood, how this informs the production of research and, therefore, what the purpose of social work practice with disabled people is (Morgan and Roulstone, 2012; Oliver, 1983; Sapey, 2004).

Disability, disabled people and research

The research used to inform policy and practice with disabled people has been subject to a sustained critique by disabled people and by academics working in disability studies since disabled activist Paul Hunt (1981) labelled researchers Eric Miller and Geraldine Gwynne 'parasite people'. Hunt's paper 'Settling Accounts with the Parasite People' was a response to a research study on residential care for disabled people undertaken by Miller and Gwynne in the late 1960s. Residents of the Le Court Cheshire Home had invited Miller and Gwynne to research their experiences as part of a campaign for greater resident participation in the management of the home. There was sense of 'horror' and a feeling they had been 'badly let down by social science research' (Finkelstein, 2001: 6) when, in their book *A Life Apart: A Pilot Study of Residential Institutions for the Physically Handicapped and Young Chronically Sick*, Miller and Gwynne argued that:

> by the very fact of committing people to institutions of this type, society is defining them as, in effect, socially dead, then the essential task to be carried out is to help the inmates make their transition from social death to physical death. (Miller and Gwynne, 1972: 89)

While the residents and other disability activists agreed that the outcome of residential care was 'social death' for residents, as Vic Finkelstein (2001) put it, 'The issue seemed not so much whether we are or are not "socially dead", but what we can do about it?' (p. 7). According to Hunt, the problem with this type of evidence was that the researchers were:

> profoundly biased and committed against the residents interests from the start ... [this was] evident in their whole conception of the issues, and therefore in their chosen research methods, and in all their analyses, conclusions and recommendations. (Hunt, 1981: 45)

The research was based on disablist assumptions about what it meant to be disabled, and on what appropriate responses were to the predicament of many disabled people.

This critique emerged while the UK disabled people's movement was starting radically to rethink the way in which disability is understood. The Union of the Physically Impaired Against Segregation (UPIAS, 1976) argued that, rather than disability being inevitably created by impairment, instead, disablement was a form of social oppression imposed on top of impairments. This approach was developed by Mike Oliver (1983) as the 'social model of disability', which made a clear distinction between a person's condition or impairment (such as spinal cord injury or learning difficulties) and the socially imposed restrictions and disadvantage they experienced (e.g. inaccessible buildings or presumptions about capacity).

A central element in the development of *disability studies* as an inter-disciplinary area of academic study and research was disenchantment with traditional forms of disability research such as that conducted by Miller and Gwynne. Barton summarised the criticisms that were made which included:

> their misunderstanding of the nature of disability, their distortion of the experience of disability, their failure to involve disabled people and the lack of any real improvements in the quality of life of disabled people that they have produced. (Barton, 1992: 99)

An often cited example of this type of research was the surveys conducted in the 1980s by the Office of Population, Census and Survey (OPCS). Oliver (1990) highlighted the assumptions that underpinned the surveys by contrasting questions used by the OPCS with alternatives that are based on a social model understanding of disability (Box 12.1).

The insight provided by a social model understanding of disability enabled disability studies writers to question the apparently 'commonsense' nature of the questions in the OPCS surveys. Oliver's alternative formulation of the questions demonstrates how a different understanding of what creates disability changes how the problem is constructed or framed. The significance here is the impact that such research had on public policy responses to disabled people because as Harlan Hahn (1985) concluded, 'fundamentally disability is defined by public policy. In other words, disability is whatever policy says it is' (p. 94). Thus, if the research underpinning policy development and practice

BOX 12.1 QUESTIONS BASED ON SOCIAL MODEL OF DISABILITY

OPCS 1986 survey questions	Alternative questions
Can you tell me what is wrong with you?	Can you tell me what is wrong with society?
What complaint causes your difficulty in holding, gripping or turning things?	What defects in the design of everyday equipment such as jars, bottles and tins causes you difficulty in holding, gripping or turning them?
Are your difficulties in understanding people mainly due to a hearing problem?	Are your difficulties in understanding people mainly due to their inabilities to communicate with you?
Have you attended a special school because of a long-term health problem or disability?	Have you attended a special school because of your education authority's policy of sending people with your health problem or disability to such places?
Does your health problem/disability mean that you need to live with relatives or someone else who can help look after you?	Are community services so poor that you need to rely on relatives or someone else to provide you with the right level of personal assistance?
How difficult is it for you to get about your immediate neighbourhood on your own?	What are the environmental constraints that make it difficult for you to get about in your immediate neighbourhood?

Source: Adapted from Oliver (1990), tables 1.1 and 1.2: 7–8.

implementation is based on an individualised personal tragedy understanding of disability that viewed disadvantage as created by impairment (Oliver, 1990), then policy and practice will perpetuate this.

In *Handicapped by Numbers – A Critique of the OPCS Surveys*, Paul Abberley highlighted the significant and frequently negative implications of the ways in which such 'official statistics' were compiled. He noted that:

> It is a political decision, conscious or otherwise, to employ questions of the first type rather than the second. Since state researchers, whatever party is in power, have consistently asked individualising rather than socialising questions on a whole range of subjects it should come as no surprise that they do this on disability, which is as political a subject as any other. (Abberley, 1991: 4)

Thus, as Oliver contends:

> Disability research should not be seen as a set of technical objective procedures carried out by 'experts' but part of the struggle by disabled people to challenge the oppression they currently experience in their lives. (Oliver, 1992: 102)

Disability research should therefore be 'openly partisan and politically committed' (Barnes and Mercer, 1997: 5), with researchers being explicit about 'which side they are on'.

Towards an emancipatory research paradigm

There was considerable discussion within disability studies and the wider disabled people's movement about how this new approach to research should be constructed, with many of the key arguments and proposals brought together in a special issue of the journal *Disability, Handicap and Society* (now *Disability & Society*) in 1992. Here, Oliver (1992) called for a new approach to disability research that he termed 'emancipatory disability research'.

Barnes (2014) summarises the core characteristics of this approach as accountability, the social model of disability, data collection and empowerment. Barnes argues that researchers should develop ongoing relationships with disability organisations so they can 'learn how to put their knowledge and skills at the disposal of disabled people' (p. 39). This requires researchers to work in ways that are accessible and inclusive for disabled people, and that enable a meaningful and honest dialogue about the potential and limitations of research. In particular, Barnes highlights the difficulties raised by the 'market-led environment' in which many researchers work, which can mitigate against small scale user-led research projects that may be viewed as 'political' in nature.

Adopting a social model understanding of disability is frequently viewed as a necessary precursor to emancipatory research. However, there are two key challenges to this. The first advanced by some within disability studies, notably Shakespeare (1996), relates to the first two principles, which for Barnes are inevitably related. Shakespeare makes a persuasive argument that a commitment to a political understanding of disability and accountability to research participants should not automatically translate into formal accountability to disabled people's organisations. He contends disability academics and researchers can produce emancipatory knowledge out with this relationship. However, he makes a distinction between having the intellectual and academic freedom to pursue unpopular or marginalised ideas and presenting such work as 'being neutral or being objective' (Shakespeare, 1996: 117).

A second challenge is the now ubiquitous nature of the social model of disability which has the potential to undermine its effectiveness. It is difficult to find a government department, local authority or disability organisation that does not express a commitment to the social model: as Oliver (2004) put it, 'it is tempting to suggest that we are all social modellists now' (p. 18). However, there is a tendency for organisations and researchers to ape the language of the model without fully adopting its principles (Morgan, 2014; Roulstone and Morgan, 2009). This can make it difficult for user-led organisations and their research allies to compete for research funding with large disability charities and established research institutes who profess a commitment to the social model, but without an accompanying transfer of power to disabled people.

Approaches to data collection methods within an emancipatory paradigm are varied. There has been an assumption that qualitative research is inherently more emancipatory because it allows the voices and narratives of disabled people to be heard; however, Barnes (2014) cautions against such assumptions, reminding us of the potentially damaging nature of 'sentimental biography' that is grounded in individualised accounts of disability. The crucial defining element of emancipatory forms of research lies in a political commitment to challenging oppression, rather than in any particular forms of or approaches to data collection. As Barnes (1996) argues elsewhere, academics and researchers can only be with the oppressors or with the oppressed.

Finally, in response to criticisms that traditional disability research failed to improve the lives of disabled people, Barnes (2014) argues that 'to be truly emancipatory, disability research must be empowering' (p. 42). Research must have – the potential, at least – to generate positive outcomes for disabled people. Barnes and some other disability studies writers contend this is only possible when disabled people's organisations formulate and steer the research agenda, although this remains contested within disability studies. However, these debates should be located within wider discussions about what has been termed 'user-led' research.

User-led disability research

The development of the disabled people's movement took place at the same time, and often in parallel with, the self-organisation of people who use social care and other welfare services, many of whom are disabled. The claim for greater user involvement in and control of research mirrors those made by the disabled people's movement and are summarised by Beresford and Croft (2012: i) as:

- social rather than medicalised individual approaches and understandings;
- the rejection of positivist claims to 'objectivity'; and
- a commitment to personal, social and political change.

As Beresford and Croft acknowledge, there is great diversity and variation in the levels and extent of user participation in research. Initiatives such Involve (http://www.invo.org.uk/), which was established in 1996 to promote public (user involvement in its widest conception) involvement in medical, health and social care research, have had a significant impact on mainstream research activities which much more routinely involve service users. Alongside this, a small but influential body of user-led research has developed. Notable examples include large national projects such as that undertaken on behalf of BCODP (then, the British Council of Disabled People) *Independent Futures: Creating User Led Services in a Disabling Society* (Barnes and Mercer, 2006) and *Supporting People: Towards a Person-Centred Approach*, which was funded by the Joseph Rowntree Foundation (Beresford *et al.*, 2011). There are also numerous small-scale local projects undertaken by disability and other user-led organisations, an example of which is presented later in this chapter (pp. 192–3).

As the majority of user-led research has sought to embody the emancipatory principles outlined, it has been subject to a counter-critique from some quarters. The overtly political nature of this work and its rejection of objectivity and neutrality has resulted in 'problems of credibility and discrimination' (Beresford and Croft, 2012: iii). There remains a suspicion that research commissioned or undertaken by user-led organisations will be partisan and lack the necessary rigour of more 'objective' research. This response fails to acknowledge the strong commitment to transparency demonstrated by user-led research. Such research 'wears its heart on its sleeve' in terms of political commitment and projects such as *Independent Futures* and *Supporting People* provide great detail about their methods of involvement and decisions about research strategy and design. It is also important to bear in mind the relative infancy of such research. As Roulstone notes, social work education and practice is still dominated by research:

> produced for non-disabled professionals by non-disabled researchers each benefiting from the study of 'disabled others'. This picture of a world of 'solutions' created for disabled people by predominantly non-disabled people is noteworthy in the early twenty-first century. (Roulstone, 2012: 146)

The request from disabled people's organisations is not that they should control all research but, rather, that research produced by user-led organisations is accepted on equal terms and valued for the particular contribution it can make to the value base for practice. The development of tools such as the TAPUPAS framework for assessing the quality of knowledge for practice by Pawson *et al.* (2003) for the Social Care Institute for Excellence (SCIE) provides the opportunity to assess different types of knowledge and research within a privileging of particular standpoints or approaches.

PRACTICE REFLECTION 12.1

Is it TAPUPAS?

As discussed elsewhere in this book, Pawson *et al.* (2003) suggest knowledge can be assessed using the following framework:

Transparency: Are the reasons for it clear?
Accuracy: Is it honestly based on relevant evidence?
Purposivity: Is the method used suitable for the aims of the work?
Utility: Does it provide answers to the questions it set?
Propriety: Is it legal and ethical?
Accessibility: Can you understand it?
Specificity: Does it meet the quality standards already used for this type of knowledge?

Revisit some of the research you have considered and ask 'Is it TAPUPAS'? How easy is it to answer these questions based on the format or presentation of the research you are reading?

Research to inform work with disabled people

One of the greatest successes of the disabled people's movement has been to translate its 'big idea' (Hasler, 1993) – the social model of disability – into a rallying cry for change and into innovative mechanisms and practices to support independent living. This included the establishment of user-led disability organisations that provided a focus for campaigning and a location for developing radical new forms of support (Barnes and Mercer, 2006). Many of these initiatives have subsequently been translated into mainstream social care practice under the banner of personalisation.

The impact of the social model of disability has been discussed in some detail already and in key texts such as *Disabling Barriers – Enabling Environments* (Swain *et al.*, 2014) and *Disability Policy and Practice: Applying the Social Model* (Barnes and Mercer, 2004). A significant challenge for policy-makers and practitioners is how to translate the principles of the model into practice. There is no single blueprint or handbook for social model services or practice. Instead, there needs to be ongoing evaluation of the extent to which these principles have been embedded. As this chapter will go on to consider, there is a considerable body of research that emerged to evaluate the effectiveness and efficiency of many of the initiatives associated with the social model of disability. However, there remains less research conducted to assess the extent to which statutory agencies and other service providers have embedded their formal commitment to the social model.

Oliver and Bailey were commissioned by Birmingham City Council to evaluate the impact of its formal adoption of the social model in its services for disabled people (Oliver, 2004). The research sought to evaluate the extent to which this commitment had become embedded in the authority's policies, process and professional practice. They noted that the implementation of the model was varied within the local authority and identified three broad approaches to service provision – humanitarian, compliance and citizenship (Box 12.2). These are not mutually exclusive; different elements of the same organisation or service may embody all or none of the approaches.

PRACTICE REFLECTION 12.2

Typology of welfare

The typology of welfare provision produced by Oliver (2004) provides a framework for evaluating the extent to which organisations are operating in accordance with their commitment to a social model of disability.

Consider a welfare organisation you are familiar with, whether as a user of that service, as a student on placement, or as a practitioner. To what extent do the organisation and the services it provides embody the different elements of Oliver's typology of welfare provision? How might it change to adopt a citizenship approach?

The typology can also be used as a template for the critical appraisal of studies that are researching services and other forms of support that claim to adhere to social model principles.

BOX 12.2 APPROACHES TO WELFARE

Humanitarian	Compliance	Citizenship
Providers	Providers	■ This approach requires older/disabled people to be seen as full citizens with all the rights and responsibilities that are implied
■ We know best	■ Meet laws, rules and regulations	■ Older/disabled people are seen as contributing members of society, both as workers and valued customers (users)
■ Individual/medical model – whereby the older/disabled person is the problem	■ Checklist approach	■ Older/disabled people are recognised as empowered individuals (voters)
■ Doing clients a favour	■ Minimum standards	■ Older/disabled people are seen as active citizens with all that implies in terms of rights and responsibilities
■ Clients should be grateful	■ Lack of commitment or partnership	■ Only when all three dimensions are met will the relationship between providers and users of services be a truly harmonious one.
Older/disabled people	Older/disabled people	
■ Do not like being patronised	■ Rights not fully met	
■ Reject individual/medical model	■ Going through the motions	
■ Not valued as people	■ Still service-led rather than needs-led	
■ Services not reliable	■ Staff tend to own the task not the aim of the service	
Result	Result	
■ Conflict	■ Conflict	
■ Lack of trust	■ Denial of entitlements and expectations	
■ Inadequate services	■ Inadequate services	
■ Poor levels of satisfaction	■ Poor levels of satisfaction	

Source: Adapted from Oliver (2004).

One of the most influential pieces of disability research undertaken was Colin Barnes' (1991) *Disabled People in Britain and Discrimination: A Case for Anti-Discrimination Legislation*. The study was devised by the BCODP and sought to collate existing evidence about the nature and extent of discrimination experienced by disabled people. There was considerable anecdotal evidence about this discrimination but, until that point, it had not been brought together; neither had it been analysed using a social model understanding of disability. The importance of this research was that it provided an empirical basis for the analysis provided by social model writers. As Barnes notes in his foreword to the second impression of the book:

> although today there is no dispute about the extent of discrimination against disabled people, this was not the case two and half years ago. At the start of 1992 the British Government still denied that discrimination against disabled people was a major problem ... [after the book's launch at the House of Commons] the Minister for Disabled People ... admitted for the first time: 'Discrimination against disabled people is widespread'. (Barnes, 1994)

The chapter on 'Health and Social Support Services' summarised the ways in which social care services were structured around traditional understandings of disability that assumed 'disabled people are unable to take charge of their own lives' (Barnes, 1991: 147), that provision was focused on segregated residential settings and that assessment was a professional activity to be undertaken on, rather than in partnership with, disabled people. Barnes concluded that, without significant reform, social care services would remain a barrier to independent living in the community and to disabled people exerting control over their lives. This research provided undisputed evidence that services for disabled people – social care amongst them – was failing to meet the needs of disabled people and that practice would need to look the emerging body of research that was capturing the evolution of new forms of support.

The most influential innovation that emerged from disabled people's organisations is direct payments. Direct payments – in essence, a cash payment in lieu of services – were promoted by disabled people's organisations as a way of transferring power to individual disabled people and enabling them to purchase more personalised and responsive forms of support than the rigid and inflexible services provided by local authorities. *Cashing In On Independence* (Zarb and Nadash, 1994) was commissioned by BCODP to demonstrate the cost-effectiveness of direct payments schemes as part of a campaign for legislation to enable local authorities to make cash payments to service users. The study demonstrated that the use of direct payments enabled greater choice and control and, therefore, resulted in higher levels of service user satisfaction. The study also showed that a perceived disadvantage of the schemes was the time taken to administer them and the additional responsibility taken on by the service user, particularly in relation to becoming an employer. What is significant about these findings is that they have been reiterated by all the major studies of direct payments and more recent iterations of personalised forms of support such as personal budgets.

Personalisation has subsequently become the dominant idea in social care.

It draws on elements of the ideas and approaches developed by disabled people and other service user groups – particularly the emphasis on independent living, and a commitment to greater choice and control for those who use services. These appear uncontentious aims for intervention. However, there is a growing critique emerging from disability studies (Roulstone and Morgan, 2009) and radical social work (Ferguson and Lavalette, 2014; Glasby, 2014) that there are considerable differences and variations in the ways in which these concepts are being utilised and applied. It is also important that a clear distinction is drawn between the principles that underpin the personalisation agenda and the mechanisms that have been deployed to implement them (Gardner, 2012). There has been a tendency in policy and practice contexts to view them as synonymous – that delivery mechanisms such as direct payments or personal budgets are forms of personalisation or independent living, rather than as means to these ends (Beresford, 2014).

There have been two large-scale evaluations of the implementation of personal budgets – the primary delivery mechanism for delivering personalised forms of support (details about direct payments, personal budgets and other delivery mechanisms can be found in Carr, 2012). The IBSEN project (Glendinning *et al.*, 2008) was a national evaluation of the Individual Budgets Pilot Programme (2006–08). The project was unusual in using a randomised controlled trial to consider the costs, outcomes and cost-effectiveness of individual budgets in the 13 pilot local authorities. A key finding of the evaluation was the differentiated outcomes for various service user groups, with people with physical impairments recording the highest levels of satisfaction, and that there are significant 'practical, organisational and cultural challenges' for local authority staff.

The Personal Outcomes Evaluation Tool (POET) was devised by the social enterprise In Control and the Centre for Disability Research at Lancaster University. It seeks to provide a national benchmark on the impact of personal budgets. To date, two surveys have been undertaken using the tool in 2011 and 2013 (Hatton and Waters, 2011; 2013). The surveys reiterated the high levels of satisfaction and positive outcomes for disabled people identified by IBSEN. Similarly, it highlighted the implementation difficulties experienced by local authorities.

While it is clear both these projects have had considerable impact on government policy, there has been concern about the extent to which less positive findings have been addressed. While there was a strong evidence base to support the closure or 'modernisation' of traditional forms of social care provision, particularly segregated institutions such as long-stay hospitals or day centres (Roulstone and Morgan, 2009), research that evaluates new forms of provision has not kept pace with the scale of change. As Beresford asserts, 'the government made the policy move and large-scale associated investment before it had the results of its own research, such as the IBSEN study' (Beresford, 2014: 8). Similarly, Glasby acknowledges that in 'a rapidly evolving policy context, the issues involved are always likely to be far in advance of the evidence base, which has inevitably had to struggle to keep up with such a rapid pace of change' (Glasby, 2014: 4).

There are two important messages to take from this. First, we should question the primacy afforded to 'what works' or evidence-based practice by government when, where it is politically expedient, policy is implemented without this supporting evidence, or in the face of conflicting or disputed evidence. Second, and most importantly in a context of work with disabled people, our starting point should be on embedding values, rather than mechanisms. There is significant evidence that what matters to those who use services and what ensures effective practice is 'a value-based approach to practice and support' (Beresford *et al.*, 2011: 48). There is a very real danger that language of these values – adopting a social model of disability, framing services as independent living – has become ritualised, rather than real (Morgan, 2012). Adopting Oliver's citizenship approach to welfare provision requires practitioners to adopt a critical perspective on their practice and on the research and other evidence that underpins it.

In spite of this, there is a growing recognition that when policy-makers, practitioners and disabled people talk about the social model, about independent

---

CASE SCENARIO 12.1

Mary and Jane

Mary and Jane are both from a large town in the north of England. They both lived in a segregated hospital for people with the label of learning difficulty for over 20 years. The hospital was in a rural area and, at least three times a year, Mary managed to reach a local shop or pub, trying to escape back to the town she was from. Each time, she was returned to the hospital.

The hospital was eventually assessed for closure, after unacceptable restraint practices, sexual assault and lack of privacy were cited in an Inspector's Report. Risk assessments showed some residents to be at worst risk of death, and others at risk of severe distress and mental health service need, given their levels of institutionalisation and the speed of the move that was necessary.

A user-led organisation of disabled people was contracted by the Adult Social Care department to assist with the social well-being of residents, before, during and after the move. Over the next eight months, it put in place support plans with each of the residents for the gradual improvement of options available to the residents.

Members of local self-advocacy groups visited the hospital; residents of the hospital had personal assistants with them and transport to visit the group members in the community centre. The residents began to take an interest in what they would want in the places they might live. Mary asked for her bedside cabinet from the ward where she had stayed to go with her and asked to share a room with her friend in their new supported accommodation. They asked for their curtains in their new room to be made out of the material from the bay curtains in the ward where they had lived. They also took a tea pot and biscuit tray from the hospital. They began to stay in their new homes for short (gradually increasing) periods of time and, eventually, overnight and at weekends. Some of their favourite staff from the hospital transitioned with them to the new accommodation and they helped to recruit their own new support workers. →

living and about personalisation they are not always talking about the same thing (Roulstone and Morgan, 2009). The apparent ubiquity of the social model discussed earlier masks that its impact on social work education and practice is still limited (Beresford and Boxall, 2012; Morgan, 2012; Sapey and Pearson, 2004). Therefore, a key task for any practitioner is to establish what these concepts mean and to understand the implications of the different methods and mechanisms that have been devised to implement them in practice.

Applying research in social work practice

Case scenario 12.1 provides an opportunity to reflect on the preceding discussion about the nature of evidence about disabled people and the policies and practices that seek to support them. Sapey (2004), in his discussion of the place of evidence-based social work practice, reminds us that the use of evidence should be prefaced by a questioning of the nature of the understanding of disability that underpins that evidence, and of the aims of the intervention

→ The advocate who helped facilitate their support plans realised that the choices of food, clothing, activities and relationships generated by self-advocates and the residents represented many indicators of what was good, not so good and poor in housing and community services. These plans were made into checklists, and the residents and self-advocates used them to assess the places they wanted to live. The team leader in the social work department took the checklists and added some more questions, so that she could ask residents to use them as part of her inspections of supported accommodation.

Four years pass.

Mary is engaged to her partner, who lives in another supported home and they will be married next year. She is part of a Reality Checker group, using the checklists that were developed as part of her move to supported living and leisure venues, to assess the suitability and standards of other accommodation for disabled people.

Jane's family were traced through social services and her cousin was delighted to have her join the family for Sunday lunch each week, as long as her personal assistant came to help. Jane formed a bond with her cousin's daughter, and learned to read and write so that she can help her to read, too.

Mary still shields her plate with her hand when she is eating to ensure no-one steals it, a behaviour she learned in the hospital. Mary and Jane still share a house, but have their own rooms in a smaller supported accommodation house.

Mary hopes to get a house with her partner when they marry, but is frustrated when doctors will not give her information about her fiancé when he is in hospital, because they think she will not understand, even though she is listed as his next of kin. Jane has completed a Level 1 childcare course (which was made accessible in Easy Words and Pictures), and now works two mornings per week in the local nursery. She makes good use of the local bus and campaigns to stop disablist hate crime.

being evaluated. The particular value of Case scenario 12.1 is that it demonstrates the multi-faceted relationship practice can and should have with research. The work undertaken by a user-led disability organisation was grounded in a social model understanding of disability and in research either generated by disabled people's organisations, or that evaluating their work. Practitioners recognised and acknowledged the value of the knowledge produced by Mary, Jane and their peers and, through their participation in a 'Reality Checking' group, developed tools for practice and evaluation.

The commissioning of a user-led organisation to support Mary, Jane and the other residents acknowledges the value and contribution user-led organisations make to supporting disabled people. The *Creating Independent Futures* project (Barnes and Mercer, 2006) found that user-led services – that is, those devised and delivered by organisations of disabled people – were more accountable to service users. Additionally, a project that mapped the capacity of user-led organisations in England in 2007 highlighted the specific expertise these organisations have, which include *peer support, mentoring* and *empowerment* (Maynard-Campbell *et al.*, 2007).

An evaluation undertaken by the National Centre for Independent Living (NCIL) (2008) for the Department of Health reviewed the existing literature on peer support. The report cites a range of research that highlights the importance of access to peer support as a crucial element in the effective and sustainable uptake of direct payments. This is supported by the detailed findings of the Supporting People project, which emphasises the 'value of learning from other people's successes' (Beresford *et al.*, 2011: 165) and that 'making choices requires self-confidence' (Beresford *et al.*, 2011: 161). An NCIL review concluded that peer support was an:

> essential element in giving people opportunities to control their own lives and, moreover, where such support does not exist this has had a negative impact on the implementation of self-directed support. (National Centre for Independent Living, 2008: 32)

Peer support is particularly significant for those disabled people who have been subject to institutionalisation, whether in large-scale institutions – such as the hospital described in the case study, or by community-based services that have perpetuated the negative elements of institutionalisation outlined by the *Supporting People* project as:

- people's rigid categorisation;
- being segregated;
- being lumped together;
- the provision of merely physical maintenance;
- group living;
- standardised routines. (Beresford *et al.*, 2011: 156)

The outcome of these situations is that disabled people tend to be marginalised from their communities and wider networks of support, which can limit indi-

> **PRACTICE REFLECTION 12.3**
>
> **Institutionalisation**
>
> Despite the emphasis on closing institutions and supporting disabled people to live in their communities, a considerable number of disabled people continue to live in institutional settings where experiences akin to 'social death' persist. Have you worked with people who have experienced long stays in institutions? What were their experiences?
>
> The needs of lesbian, gay, bisexual and transgendered people are sometimes not met in institutional settings. Reflect on how you can use research to inform working with people who live, or have lived, in institutional settings. How can you best ensure that the needs of all disabled people are met and their unique strengths are developed?

viduals' aspirations for the future. Providing support that went beyond simply physically relocating the former hospital residents in the community enabled Jane and Mary to explore other options for their life and to broaden what can, at times, be a limited 'menu of choices' (Hollomotz, 2012) for those with personal budgets from which to choose.

FURTHER READING

Beresford, P. Fleming, J. Glynn, M. Bewley, C., Croft, S., Branfield, F., and Postle, K. (2011) *Supporting People: Towards a Person-Centred Approach* (Bristol: Policy Press). This text provides rich detail about what matters to people who use adult social care services and how this can effectively be translated into practice.

Carr. S. (2012) *Personalisation: A Rough Guide. SCIE Guide 47* (London: SCIE). This regularly updated report provides an introduction to personalisation and a summary of much of the research that has been undertaken.

Harris, J and Roulstone, A. (2011) *Disability, Policy and Professional Practice* (London: Sage); Roulstone, A. and Prideaux, S. (2012) *Understanding Disability Policy* (Bristol: Policy Press). Both these books are core to understanding more about working with disabled people.

The Disability Archive UK is an on-line collection of material produced by disabled people and disability studies writers: http://disability-studies.leeds.ac.uk/library/

The Social Care Institute for Excellence (SCIE) website has a wide range of resources to support research informed practice: http://www.scie.org.uk/

Blogs provide immediate, powerful and often intimate access to the lived experience of disabled people using adult social care services.

My Daft Life. This blog is written by disability studies researcher Sara Ryan, whose son 'LB' died while in an assessment and treatment unit for young people with learning difficulties. http://mydaftlife.wordpress.com/

Mark Neary's blog provides anecdotes and often fiercely critical analysis of his and his son Steven's experiences of personalisation: http://markneary1dotcom1.wordpress.com/

Kaliya Franklin (http://benefitscroungingscum.blogspot.co.uk/) and Sue Marsh's (http://diaryofabenefitscrounger.blogspot.co.uk/) blogs detail their personal and political disability activism.

You can access the Reach Standards for Supported Accommodation here: http://www.paradigmuk.org/articles/SALE__Reach__Standards_in_Supported_Living_/2946/42.aspx

You can access a training pack to stop disablist hate crime here, which includes the DVD for Holocaust Memorial Day that the group made about the value of disabled people's lives: http://arcuk.org.uk/safetynet/files/2012/08/Hate-Crime-Learning-Together-Training-Pack.pdf

(Case scenario 12.1 was produced by Susie Balderston of VisionSense (a user-led organisation in the North East of England) with the help of Chris Anderson, Brian Baston, George Aitkin, Margaret Cowle, Margaret Purvis, Kay Warren, Graham Newton, Keith Turnbull, Kerry Docherty, Brian West, Linda Richards, John Harbottle, Stephen Watson, Dawn Flockton, Billy Richardson, Anne Tulip, Kevin Stephenson and Stuart Hall at Better Days. We would like to thank Lesley Mountain for supporting the group and wish her a happy retirement.)

CHAPTER 13

Working with Offenders

David Smith

Introduction

This chapter outlines the development over the past 40 years of ideas on 'what works' with offenders. In the 1970s and early 1980s, the dominant view among researchers – and even practitioners – was that nothing worked, or at least that no one knew enough to be confident about what kinds of approach might work better than others. Towards the end of the 1980s, a much more positive view began to emerge, based on extensive research that suggested that some approaches had a much better chance of being successful than others.

This chapter describes the broad characteristics of interventions associated with success, but also shows how a naively optimistic view of how they could be put into practice led to a reversion to a much more pessimistic stance on the part of government officials in England and Wales: they decided that we still knew very little about what worked, and that our knowledge could only be improved by much more rigorous research, of a kind unlikely to be feasible in practice. Drawing on criminology as well as social work, the chapter argues that this pessimism is unjustified, and that research and scholarship can provide helpful guidance on what is likely to work. The point is illustrated by a case scenario and reflections on the prospects for effective practice in the current policy environment.

Research context

Since around 1990, a great deal has been published on 'what works' with offenders, in the sense of helping to reduce the likelihood that they will continue to offend. This work – reports of research, analysis of research findings, and commentaries on their quality and interpretation – constitutes, as a whole, a welcome replacement of what had been the dominant – though not universal – view in the preceding fifteen or so years. This was that 'nothing worked', and that there was no rational basis for preferring any one kind of intervention over any other – at least, if the aim was to reduce offenders' propensity to offend. This gloomy conclusion was most famously derived from the work of Martinson (1974) in the United States, but was reinforced by the interpretation placed on a number of almost contemporary studies in Britain (Clarke and Cornish, 1975; Folkard *et al.*, 1976; Fowles, 1978). As has often been noted (e.g. Nuttall, 2003), all of these studies allowed for a less negative interpretation, and at least one told a much more optimistic story (Shaw, 1974). However, in the prevailing economic, social and political climate of 'late modernity and as a reaction to the perceived crisis of the welfare state faith in rehabilitation lost its appeal for the official discourse' (Durnescu, 2012: 199).

For a time, it seems only to have been in Canada that anyone managed to retain a more positive view of the feasibility of rehabilitation (e.g. Andrews *et al.*, 1990; Andrews and Kiessling, 1980). Then, in the late 1980s, local studies in England and Wales began to suggest cautiously promising results (Raynor, 1988; Roberts, 1989), and news of the Canadian research began to cross the Atlantic (McIvor, 1990). The new, more positive message (crystallised in the collection by McGuire (1995)) has been summarised in various ways, and now follows as bulleted points under the headings *Organisational principles*; *Principles of risk, need and responsivity*; and *General principles* (adapted from Andrews, 2011: 2–3).

Organisational principles

- Community-based programmes will generally do better than programmes run in residential or custodial settings.
- Programmes should be delivered by staff with good relationship skills and skills in structuring their interaction with offenders: motivational interviewing, for instance, will require both types of skill. (These 'core correctional practices' are discussed in more detail in Case scenario 13.1.)
- Staff should be appropriately trained and supported by management.

Principles of risk, need and responsivity (RNR)

- Punitive approaches are ineffective; some 'human service' is needed for rehabilitation.
- Intensity of service should be proportional to offenders' risk of further offending. Work should focus on medium- to high-risk cases. Excessive intervention with low risk offenders can make things worse.
- The main focus for change should be criminogenic needs – i.e. needs that are associated with offending.
- Generally, social learning and cognitive-behavioural methods should be employed; specifically, methods should be adapted to the needs and characteristics of individuals (e.g. preferred learning style, level of motivation, social capital). A range of techniques should be available to ensure as far as possible that each offender will find the programme relevant to their needs and capacities.

General principles

- Programmes should be based on empirically tested psychological theory – especially general personality and cognitive social learning perspectives that allow for an understanding of criminogenic needs and risks, and the processes of learning and behavioural change.

■ All work should be informed by the ethical principles of care and respect for persons, and a commitment to fairness and equity of treatment.

By the late 1990s, at least among some probation managers and civil servants in England and Wales, the wholesale pessimism of 'nothing works' seemed to have been replaced by an uncritical optimism – that we now really knew what worked, and that it only remained for practitioners to get on with the job. If they worked according to principles such as those sketched in the bullet points above, they could expect an 'effect size' of around 25 per cent – for example, a two-year reconviction rate of 45 per cent against the 60 per cent which would have resulted had the offenders not received the 'treatment' prescribed by the research. Even a smaller effect would still be worthwhile – and the most successful programmes could be expected to do even better (Lipsey *et al.*, 2007). While many commentators were sceptical about whether we could actually be so certain about what to do and how to do it (see, generally, the contributions in Mair (2004)), Home Office officials were confident enough on this score to include cognitive-behavioural programmes for offenders in the range of initiatives that made up the ambitious Crime Reduction Programme (CRP), launched in 1998. As with other aspects of the CRP, the offender programmes were to be independently evaluated, and funding for this was built into the design of the CRP.

According to Andrews (2011: 18) the results of the evaluations were 'very disappointing for many correctional professionals and managers throughout England and Wales'. The disappointment was associated not so much with failure on the part of well-implemented programmes to deliver the hoped-for reduction in offending, as with the fact that many programmes were never implemented as intended. Problems of implementation were not confined to the offender programmes within the CRP but arose, more generally, as a consequence of what with hindsight can be seen as a naïve attempt to 'roll out' on a national scale and within a short time-frame interventions that had looked promising as small-scale demonstration-type projects (Maguire, 2004). For the offender programmes, problems included lack of staff commitment (in part, because practitioners felt that the programmes were being imposed on them without adequate consultation), lack of training and supervision, concurrent though unrelated organisational change (the creation of a National Probation Service), and pressure to get the programmes going without adequate preparation (Goggin and Gendreau, 2006). The last factor contributed to a failure routinely to conduct assessments of risk and need and, hence, to inappropriate selection for programmes; this, in turn, meant that drop-out rates for many programmes were high. In the case of the Basic Skills programme, for example, very few of the targeted offenders even started it (Raynor, 2004). In response to these disappointing results, Home Office researchers concluded that, contrary to what had been believed before the CRP (Goldblatt and Lewis, 1998), we actually knew very little about what worked with offenders (Chitty, 2005) and would only improve our knowledge through much more rigorous methods of research – specifically, large-scale randomised controlled trials of a kind often (and for good reason) regarded as impractical (Smith, 2012).

It looked as if the wheel had turned full circle, and that we were back with 'nothing works' – or, at least, with 'We don't know if anything works, and are not close to finding out'. But this pessimism is no more rationally justified than the uncritical optimism of the late 1990s. It would be ridiculous simply to disregard the accumulated evidence of 30 years of research in Canada (Andrews, 2011; Cullen, 2012) that has consistently shown that programmes run according to the principles listed above (pp. 198–9) are likely to produce better results than other approaches – or, assuming that the risk principle is adhered to, would be than doing nothing. The sensible conclusion from the CRP is that more attention needs to be given to issues of implementation, and that to manage this properly requires time, training, consultation and resources. The lesson should be one of realism and modesty, not despair.

Building on the work of Maruna (2001) on how people manage to desist from offending, Fergus McNeill and others (McNeill, 2006; 2009; McNeill and Weaver, 2010) have begun to develop a 'desistance paradigm' for work with offenders. Some advocates of the RNR approach (or, at least, Andrews, 2011) seem to regard McNeill's proposals as fundamentally antagonistic to RNR. It is true that desistance theorists have criticised some aspects of RNR-based programmes as too negative in orientation; too narrowly focused on offending and criminogenic needs; and too concerned with offenders' deficits, rather than their strengths. But it would be a pity if these differences of emphasis led to angry polemics and an outright rejection by either side of every aspect of the other's position. Most of the criticisms of RNR by desistance theorists are more about the ways in which the RNR model was implemented in Britain than about the substance of the model itself. Andrews (2011: 17–18) accepted that there was no inherent contradiction between Maruna's work and RNR principles, and from the other side of the debate McNeill acknowledges, in an email exchange with Andrews that:

> maybe I haven't been clear enough in terms of separating the theory or model from the way it was implemented ... over here at least ... my take on it is that your work (essentially RNR) got mixed up with public sector reforms in the UK (more specifically England and Wales) which were focused on saving costs and reducing the power of the professions – all part of the managerialisation and mechanisation of human services. The result was that ... assessment and intervention systems ... were superficially based on RNR but ... lacked sensitivity to the complexities of offenders' lives and neglected the need for professional reflexivity and ingenuity in individualising the generalised messages from research (and in applying the tools and programmes sensitively). (McNeill *et al.*, 2010: 7–8; ellipses in original)

McNeill *et al.* (2010: 8) went on the say that desistance approaches were 'just as vulnerable to misappropriation and misuse' and that when presenting these approaches he has to take care to prevent practitioners from taking away the message that they '"just" need to have good relationships with offenders and to offer a bit of practical help'.

It is to be hoped that advocates of RNR will accept this olive branch and that what will emerge is a synthesis of the two positions that will be accessible to and usable by practitioners. The implementation of RNR-based programmes in England and Wales undoubtedly did entail a disregard for the 'how' elements of the 'what works' research – its message that the way in which a programme is delivered matters, perhaps even more than the formal content of the programme. But Andrews and others could, and did very reasonably, respond that this was not their fault, and that they had consistently stressed the importance for success of the 'core correctional practices' summarised above (p. 198).

Case scenario 13.1 is an attempt to show how both 'what' issues (about the content of programmes) and 'how' questions (about the quality of the relationships between helpers and helped) matter for success. It also attempts to show how complex it can be to establish the motivation for an offence and to infer from it what the focus of intervention should be. The offence described seems to have an element of racist motivation, but it should not be assumed from this that it can conveniently be categorised as a 'hate crime'. As with most people convicted of racially aggravated offences, the young man in the case study is not a specialist racist offender (Palmer and Smith, 2010; Ray et al., 2003; Ray et al., 2004); and, again – in line with research findings, and contrary to the 'classic' hate crime in which the victim is a stranger to the offender – he and his victim knew each other, though not well. Again typically, the offence – facilitated by alcohol – arose from a dispute in which racial hostility was not the only motive. Indeed, it is common for people convicted of such offences to deny any racist motivation, even when the evidence suggests otherwise.

As Darren's offender manager, you judge that he has good social capital in the form of stable and supportive relationships that seem more likely to promote law-abiding behaviour than to encourage further offending – for the importance of this, see McNeill (2009) and McNeill and Weaver (2010). He is clearly capable of working regularly and reliably, and of earning a reasonable income. On the other hand, this latest offence has worrying features. It shows that he is capable of seriously aggressive behaviour, and the element of racist hostility is also a concern: if he had been convicted of a racially aggravated offence, he would have been at serious risk of a custodial sentence. Darren denies having any racist views or attitudes, but agrees that he used racist language in the takeaway. If a programme specifically for racially aggravated offenders were available, you would certainly have considered it for Darren but – as in most areas – no such programme exists locally (Iganski et al., 2011).

PRACTICE REFLECTION 13.1

Intervention in attitudes

Darren's latest offence involved the use of racist language, suggesting underlying racist attitudes. Is there a case for a specialist intervention to tackle these attitudes? What might the advantages and risks of such an intervention be?

> ## CASE SCENARIO 13.1
>
> **Darren**
>
> Darren, aged 22, has just been made subject to a 12-month community order, with a supervision requirement and an activity requirement, which in your area normally means that he will be required to undertake a group work programme. He was convicted of an offence of criminal damage. The police flagged the offence as possibly racially motivated but, in the event, Darren was prosecuted and convicted for the standard offence, to which he pleaded guilty. (He said he would have pleaded not guilty if he had been charged with a racially aggravated offence).
>
> Apart from the presence or degree of racial motivation, the facts of the case were not disputed. The offence took place just before midnight at an 'Indian' take-away shop at which Darren was a regular customer. He and a male friend arrived after spending the evening in a pub and tried to place an order, but were told by the manager that he was closing up and could not serve them. Darren argued that since other customers were waiting for their orders he was being treated unfairly in being refused service. He began to behave aggressively, swearing and shouting that he was the victim of discrimination. He did not respond to efforts by his friend and other customers to persuade him to calm down, and the shop manager said that he had 'had enough' and was going to call the police. Darren swore at him and abused him, using obscene and racially-charged language. He then went outside and began kicking the shop window. When it did not break, he crossed the road to a building site and returned with a large stone, which he threw at the window, causing damage later estimated at £300. Darren finally began to walk away, still shouting abuse. The whole incident →

The most suitable activity for Darren therefore seems to be the Thinking Skills Programme (TSP), which should be an appropriate focus for work on Darren's offending. This is what was proposed in the court report, and Darren says that he understands what the programme involves and is prepared to undertake it. He will be able to start in two weeks' time, when one of the three group work modules, each of five sessions, that make up the programme is due to begin. It runs in the evening as well as during the day, so Darren will be able to continue working. You are relieved that he will not have to wait for many weeks before starting the programme; it is helpful that the programme is structured to allow people to join it at the start of a module, rather than only at the start of the programme as a whole (one of the implementation problems that led to the disappointing results of the Crime Reduction Programme (Raynor, 2004)).

Thinking skills

TSP is a nationally accredited programme which was introduced in 2009 and replaced two long-established programmes – Think First and Enhanced Thinking Skills – both in prisons and in the community. The use in prisons of the Enhanced Thinking Skills programme was evaluated with promising results by Sadlier (2010). The new programme covers many of the same

→

lasted about 15 minutes, and the police arrived before Darren had gone far down the road. He and his friend were arrested, but only Darren was charged.

You have seen the report prepared for the magistrates' court at which Darren was sentenced. From this, you learn that he is at medium risk of further offending according to the Offender Group Reconviction Scale (OGRS) (Howard et al., 2009) and that he has been convicted on four previous occasions for offences of criminal damage and assault. Drinking has usually been a factor in these offences, but Darren's use of alcohol is probably not unusual in his peer group. He served a short custodial sentence for assault as a 16-year-old, and since then has received a community order with a community payback requirement (which he completed successfully), and several fines (which he seems to have paid off). His last conviction was almost a year ago.

Darren grew up on a run-down council estate on the outskirts of the large city in which you work. The area has an almost exclusively white population. The report says that Darren's early years were spent in a supportive family in which he was the youngest of three children. His school record was undistinguished but uneventful and, after some experience as a trainee warehouseman, he began working with his brother on building sites when he was 17. He has continued to work mainly in construction and demolition, and can earn what he regards as a reasonable wage when he is in employment, though it is in the nature of the building trade that work is not always available. About one year ago, Darren left his mother's house and went to live with his brother and his family. He says he is reasonably settled and content with this arrangement but would like to get a flat with his girlfriend, who he says is a good influence on him.

themes – problem-solving, goal-setting, emotional self-management, perspective-taking and the development of positive relationships. The programme consists of 19 sessions, each lasting two-and-a-half hours; 15 are group work and 4 are individual sessions, one before the start of the group work, the other three between the group work modules; these are used to assess progress and to reinforce learning and motivation. There is also a requirement to undertake psychometric tests before and after the programme, and to attend a review meeting with the offender manager at the end of the programme.

PRACTICE REFLECTION 13.2
Separation of responsibility
The requirements of Darren's order are fairly typical of current practice in that they include attendance at a group work programme run by staff other than the offender manager who has overall responsibility for the order. The court report has been prepared by another staff member who will not be involved in any aspect of Darren's supervision. What does this separation of responsibility imply for continuity and consistency of approach, and for the possibility that Darren will be able to establish a good relationship with the staff involved?

As with all such programmes, there is the possibility that it may prove too demanding in terms of time and commitment, especially when participants have to attend after work. They are expected not only to turn up, but also to participate actively in the programme activities, undertaking exercises and contributing to discussions. There is some leeway under the 2011 interpretation of national standards (Ministry of Justice, 2011) to allow for participants to catch up if they miss a session (one session per module is allowable). However, the more demanding the requirements of a community order are the greater the likelihood of a breach of these requirements (Mair *et al.*, 2008). The programme staff have the difficult task of ensuring that the prescribed sessions are delivered and the learning associated with them is reinforced, while avoiding repetitiveness and the risk of boredom and disenchantment.

This means that the staff who are delivering the programme need to be capable of doing so in a lively, open, active and enthusiastic style – in the jargon, they are aware of the importance of the 'core correctional practices' described by, among others, Dowden and Andrews (2004) and summarised above. This is because the way in which a programme is delivered is as important for success as its adherence to the principles of risk, need and responsivity (and, according to some scholars (Marshall and Marshall, 2012), it may actually be more important). Therefore, what Dowden and Andrews (2004) call the principles of *relationship* and *structuring* are central to success. The relationship principle refers to the workers' capacity to show warmth, interest, enthusiasm and respect, and to communicate in ways that do not come across as blaming and condemning the offenders with whom they are working. The structuring principle involves consistent reinforcement of pro-social attitudes and behaviour, effective modelling of these characteristics and the provision of clearly structured opportunities for learning. It may also entail the expression of disapproval and the appropriate use of authority – both much more likely to be accepted and acted on by those on the receiving end, if the relationship is a positive and respectful one (Raynor *et al.*, 2010). These core correctional practices are important not only for the staff running a group work programme, but also for the individual work undertaken by the offender manager (see McNeill *et al.*, 2010, especially the chapters on compliance in pt IV).

The programme staff will have much more frequent and intense contact with people on community supervision than the offender manager, so it is important that they communicate regularly about offenders' attendance, participation and attitude. There should be a formal report at the end of the programme, including re-run psychometric tests that allow for an assessment of change in attitudes (with luck, in a pro-social direction), receptiveness to ideas on changes in behaviour and emotional control, and the development of victim empathy (in Darren's case, for example, how far he accepts that his behaviour caused distress to the manager of the takeaway and to the other customers).

What should the offender manager expect of someone like Darren? It is normal for people made subject to a community order with a programme requirement to start off feeling somewhat sceptical about it, and to say that they are only attending the programme because they have to. As time goes on, however, if the programme is delivered according to the core principles, they are likely to acknowledge that they have learned something useful from it (e.g. Palmer and Smith, 2010). On the whole, people on community orders tend not to see themselves as, in some sense, essentially offenders: they dislike the part of themselves that leads to offending, and would rather see themselves as basically good and likeable people than as frightening and aggressive ones (Maruna, 2001). If, as is plausible in Darren's case, they believed that they were at real risk of a custodial sentence, they are likely to start the order feeling relieved that this did not materialise and grateful – as in this case – that the court report proposed a community order, allowing them to keep a job and maintain valued relationships, which may well be supportive in encouraging a commitment to successful completion of the order and, in the longer term, to a stronger commitment to pro-social values and behaviour.

In the terms used by writers on desistance, which are not very different from those long-used in social work (Porporino, 2010), one can think (hopefully) of someone in Darren's position as having a motive to stop offending (his desire to see himself as a good person); some means of achieving this aim (the enhanced skills and changed attitudes derived from his participation in the Thinking Skills Programme); relevant experience of himself as someone behaving in pro-social ways (success in keeping a job); and acceptance by valued others (his girlfriend, members of his family, and friends who would rather not have the responsibility of controlling him when he becomes aggressive). Given all this, there should be a good chance of avoiding a long-term criminal career (Barry, 2010).

> ## PRACTICE REFLECTION 13.3
> **Responses to non-compliance**
> Darren complied reasonably well with the requirements of his order. What would have been the most constructive response of the offender manager if he had not done so – for example, if Darren had missed more than one session without a good reason, or refused to participate in group work tasks?

Reflections

The reader may be thinking that this is a rather bland and comforting conclusion, and of course it is true that, for example, the Thinking Skills programme will not always be delivered as well as it should be; and even apparently well-motivated people, with positive social and personal capital, do not always manage to desist from offending. But, given the availability of resources of the kind that evidence suggests are most likely to be helpful, community supervision can succeed, and it is important to remember this at a time when probation is the subject of much political and media criticism – as indeed it has been since at least the early 1990s.

Government rhetoric in Britain – less so in Scotland than south of the border, but the same tendency is present – has from the early 1990s emphasised the need for supervision in the community to keep 'offenders' under surveillance and ensure that they are suitably punished, but this does not mean that committed, forward-looking, optimistic practice has evaporated (for an example, see Palmer and Smith, 2010). The rhetoric may present people who offend as liabilities, rather than potential assets to their communities (Travis and Petersilia, 2001), and as in essential respects quite different from us, the law-abiding, but it is still the case that most people who offend have much more in common with the rest of us than this rhetoric suggests. Garland (1996: 461–2) identified in official discourse a 'criminology of the self' and a 'criminology of the other', and discussed their political implications – respectively, to 'routinise crime, to allay disproportionate fears and to promote preventive action' and 'to demonise the criminal, to excite popular fears, and to promote support for state punishment'. For Garland, what is missing is the 'once-dominant' image of offenders as disadvantaged and deprived people for whom the state has a responsibility to take 'remedial' action in the form of some kind of rehabilitation. Garland suggests that the criminology of the self constructs offenders as 'rational consumers', but the idea could be interpreted in other ways: we are not only rational consumers (and neither is Darren). Rather, as Christie (1997: 14–15) reminded us, much of the subject matter of criminology is ourselves: 'There is so little in the field of criminology that we have not yet experienced. The problem is access to ourselves. Access, and respect for what we find'. Respect for what we find in ourselves may well be necessary for a respectful attitude to 'offenders' such as Darren – and such an attitude is likely to be a prerequisite for successful intervention (Dowden and Andrews, 2004).

FURTHER READING

Brayford, J., Cowe, F. and Deering, J. (eds) (2010) *What Else Works? Creative Work with Offenders* (Cullompton: Willan). This has chapters on aspects of effective practice not included in the standard 'what works' agenda, and a chapter by Frank Porporino, one of the pioneering Canadian researchers who developed the RNR model, which argues for a broadening of the research agenda.

Cullen, F.T. (2012) 'Taking Rehabilitation Seriously: Creativity, Science and the Challenge of Offender Change', *Punishment and Society* 14(1): 94–114. A review article that mounts a strong defence of 'the Canadians' and the RNR model.

McNeill, F., Raynor, P. and Trotter, C. (eds) (2010) *Offender Supervision: New Directions in Theory, Research and Practice* (Abingdon and New York: Willan). Very comprehensive in terms of topics covered and approaches represented. The introduction includes an interesting dialogue among members of the Collaboration of Researchers on the Effective Development of Supervision (CREDOS), out of whose work the book was developed.

McNeill, F. and Weaver, B. (2010) *Changing Lives? Desistance Research and Offender Management*, Glasgow, Scottish Centre for Crime & Justice Research and Glasgow School of Social Work. A useful review of the literature on desistance and offender management.

CHAPTER 14

Working with Older People

Jill Manthorpe

Introduction

Social work practice with older people is an emerging area of specialism, not least because the world's population is ageing. However, there has not been a strong interest in gerontological social work in the UK, although some social work educators have argued recently that social work with older people is on the verge of a new frontier (Richards *et al.*, 2013). Nonetheless, the same educators admit that evidence from current UK social work post-graduate training programmes suggests that there is overall neglect of ageing in teaching content and practice learning.

Policy-makers, the media and most people are well aware of the ageing population and, in particular, the increased incidence, prevalence and recognition of dementia, which is a disabling and life-limiting condition (for general demographic information, see Alzheimer's Society, 2012; Alzheimer Disease International, 2012). This means that this area of social work practice among older people will continue to expand – old age itself does not require social work support or advice.

In this chapter, the impact of personalisation will be the central theme, as social work is renegotiating its role and function in this context. Because there are many possible groups of older people to consider in this context, the chapter further employs the lens of personalisation to focus on practice and research with older people with dementia.

Naturally, social work with people with dementia overlaps with several other practice areas (Cox, 2007). There is overlap with social workers' roles in assessing and arranging support for older people and supporting family carers of any age. The international definition of social work states that:

> It is driven by the need to challenge and change those structural conditions that contribute to marginalization, social exclusion and oppression [and] a major focus of social work is to advocate for the rights of people at all levels. (International Federation of Social Workers, 2013)

Older people, especially those lacking mental capacity or those who are cognitively impaired, have not always been well-served by care and support services, or society generally, so the international definition of social work is helpful in thinking about practice beyond individual casework to wider social movements and values. (It also cautions against a 'rose-tinted spectacles' view of the past; Meacher (1972), for instance, shows a dismal picture of social workers peremptorily taking older people into care homes.) The stigmas of ageing, disability and dementia may be something that social workers can help reduce without giving the sense that their effects are not empathised with, or are under-estimated and misunderstood.

Personal budgets and self-directed support may offer increased opportunities for older people to have greater choice in terms of how they spend their time, or how they are cared for (Netten et al., 2012), although it is as yet unclear whether this leads to a greater sense of independence and control for everyone (Callaghan and Towers, 2013). Briefly summarised, in England a person eligible for publicly funded social care support receives an individual or personal 'budget' which they can spend themselves, or have spent on their behalf. In England, the form most favoured by politicians is where people manage their own budget, through Direct Payments, although many older people will have these managed by the care provider or local authority on their behalf.

Gridley et al. (2012) have pointed to the value of personal budgets in providing continuity of care across social care services and over time for people with complex needs, such as dementia accompanied by other long-term conditions (illness and/or disability related). They found that having a personal budget could mean that a person receives care at home that is timely and even proactive in minimising problems. While people with complex needs may not necessarily find personal budgets are the only way to fund good quality care and support, it seems to be a promising approach.

Gridley et al.'s (2012) literature search found 35 papers that supported the effectiveness of person-centred support. Among these, approaches that promoted the individualising of services – not necessarily personal budgets – were promising. They noted that, while there are no high-quality evaluative studies, people who might best benefit from personalised approaches require significant support when planning, setting up and managing care arrangements, particularly when a person's needs change, or become more complex. Older people with dementia are a good example of this group, since they may have fluctuating health care needs as well as over-stretched or fragile support systems. Managing the impact for social care support of these fluctuations is likely to be a key task for social workers in revising the person's support plan, amending the budget, revising risk assessments and changing care providers. This research evidence could be useful in practice when thinking about the amount of monitoring that should be extended to people with personal budgets themselves or their carers.

The ways in which personal budgets for people with dementia are developing offer a sort of natural experiment in which different approaches are being taken in different contexts. There is no agreed template for social workers to follow and they need to be mindful of the limited evidence on outcomes and the seduction of the rhetoric of personalisation, as well as avoiding general cynicism. In this section, the key evidence on personal budgets is presented and applied to people with dementia (though these do not of course form a homogeneous group).

Clearly, two important matters need to be recalled. First, not all people with dementia are eligible for publicly funded social care and support, and social workers will need to be able to work with people who feel aggrieved that there is no help for them. Second, not all people who might be eligible on the grounds of their needs for care and support are eligible for public funds to meet these needs. Means-testing applies to people with dementia and it will take time for the provisions of the Care Act (2014) to reduce some of the amounts that some people are required to pay for their care. Social workers need to be sufficiently financially and legally 'savvy' to be able to explain the eligibility and funding systems of their localities. This requires knowledge of general principles, local intelligence about good sources of advice and advocacy, and the ability to work with people who are confused and angry about service restrictions and limitations. At a time when the numbers of self-funders (people paying for their own care) are growing, there is much to learn from their experiences and those of their families of managing care.

Personal budgets: the evidence emerges

This section considers the research evidence about personal budgets and their use by people with dementia and by their family carers. There has been less focus on the experiences of people with dementia compared with other client groups, such as people with physical disabilities and learning disabilities, or people with mental health problems more generally. In part, this is because the category 'person with dementia' does not sit comfortably in UK social care services recording systems and so many people with dementia might be classified as older people and not easily distinguished.

Many older people who are eligible for publically funded social care have complex needs (physical disabilities or long-term conditions that are more debilitating than early dementia) and support networks that are at risk of being affected by stress (Jolley, 2005). Their contact with social care services may therefore pre-date a diagnosis of dementia. A further dimension affecting people with dementia is that their abilities to manage decisions associated with personal budgets may be affected by their cognitive impairments, and their own rising apprehension about managing money may mean that they shy away from taking on further financial or practical tasks associated with employment (Alzheimer's Society, 2011). Other debates have arisen from research about how best to safeguard the interests of people with dementia who are possibly more vulnerable than others to undue influence and fraud while not infantilising them (Manthorpe and Samsi, 2013). There are current debates about how to enhance the ability of people with dementia and those in contact with them to be more alert to the risks presented by false 'friends', explorative social contacts, and electronic crimes (e.g. scams) that might be attracted by the opportunities presented by Direct Payments.

For people with dementia who do not have the capacity or ability to consent to the most prominent form of personal budgets, Direct Payments (money paid directly to the individual), local authorities may appoint proxies to access them, if they regard them as 'suitable people'. Regulations have been amended to enable people supporting individuals who cannot consent to Direct Payments to receive them on their behalf (Department of Health, 2009). This builds on the English legal framework for decision-making for adults whose capacity to make decisions is impaired. The Mental Capacity Act 2005 (MCA) confirmed and extended the rights of people to appoint proxy decision-makers and set out the legal principles and authorities underpinning best-interests decision-making (see Code of Practice, Office of the Public Guardian, 2007). If a person has not given Lasting Power of Attorney to anyone (which they can do prior to losing decision-making capacity), the local authority is able to set up proxy arrangements. Recent research has identified that practice varies within and across local authorities, so carers and even practitioners may find this confusing (Mental Health Foundation, 2014). One of the advantages of recent research is that it does not only identify problems but it offers ideas about practice solutions. The Mental Health Foundation research is a good example of this – offering phone apps to give instant guidance to social workers on what needs to be considered – all on the basis of practice experiences.

Whether or not a carer is acting as a proxy, the use of personal budgets to support people with dementia may extend choice and control and, more importantly, may lead to positive outcomes for the person involved. The agreed support plan should cover planned support and arrangements for contingencies and the proxy budget holder takes on the task of realising these ambitions. While some people may spend part or their entire personal budget on paying for a day centre place or an activity beyond the home, for older people the size of the personal budget may be small and this may have to be concentrated on expenditure for care in the home (Netten *et al.*, 2012). This exposes the underlying problem of ageism and the ways in which support for older people has often been lower in amount and quality than for other age groups. Research has generally been better at identifying this problem, rather than offering practice solutions – although the Equalities Act 2010 outlaws overt discrimination (see Moriarty and Manthorpe, 2012) and offers opportunities for legal challenge.

This purchasing process and arranging of long-term care for older people who have often striven hard to be independent may benefit from social work advice, especially in respect of people who have limited social contacts. There is evidence that recruitment of directly employed care and support workers relies heavily on personal contacts or social networks. The Office for Public Management (2007) found that disabled people sometimes knew whom they wanted to employ but that others had to make enquiries among extended social networks, or even further afield by advertising. People with strong support networks and local connections may find this easier than those with weaker networks who may have to rely on 'unproven' personal assistants whom they have not known previously, or who are not known to others close to them, such as recruitment through international websites whose use is growing in this area of employment. This may particularly worry the relatives of people with severe dementia, who fear they are vulnerable in many ways.

It is emerging that carers who manage the personal budget on behalf of a relative and undertake tasks of administration may accept this as their responsibility, but it is work nonetheless (Carers UK, 2008).

More recently, Williams *et al.* (2013) found that whether social workers or voluntary or third-sector advisers were helping with support plans or not, some people need more help initially with this than others. They argued that support for Direct Payments should be flexible, to allow people to move towards independent planning at their own pace. Carer groups and disability/user advisory groups may often be the best source of support and information around such issues, even though a social worker may think that they have provided all the necessary information.

Local authority responsibilities still lie in commissioning and market development. While people with dementia and their carers have considerable purchasing power, in many areas local markets or providers are not yet sufficiently developed to offer personalised, flexible services for people with dementia. The Mental Health Foundation (2011) acknowledged that this is not unique to dementia care but could be seen as a 'chicken and egg' situation: if people with dementia do not access personal budgets, then local providers of care services will likely stick with traditional models of social care services. Practitioners' views about what the local care 'market' cannot meet may be able to influence commissioning strategies and local market developments.

PRACTICE REFLECTION 14.1

Local support for dementia sufferers

When you look at what is available to people with dementia locally, what areas do they tend to cover? Are there any types of activities that are few and far between? If you do not know this yourself, what do your colleagues, friends and voluntary sector or community groups say?

When I asked some friends supporting older parents in this situation, they mentioned receiving help with gardening, finding care workers who would be prepared to go out with their parent to the shops or park, and good-humoured taxi drivers. I was interested to hear of developments in another city where all taxi drivers were being told about dementia and how their customers might have special needs.

In current social work practice, there is less debate about the effectiveness of personal budgets and more about the means of implementation and sustainability as budgets are scrutinised to reduce local authority expenditure. Fundamentals of trusting relationships remain, however, and one important cautionary point of work with people with dementia is that focusing attention on physical care may overlook emotional and other needs. There is growing evidence that some activities are beneficial for people with dementia, if they are implemented properly – such as cognitive stimulation, a brief intervention that can be run by any professional who has undertaken training in these themed activities (Spector *et al.*, 2003) (see http://www.cstdementia.com/ for additional information). Social workers need to consider this type of evidence, as well as evidence about meeting social or personal care needs. Such interventions may be beneficial for carers in helping the person with dementia to communicate and be more alert. The next section of this chapter moves to consider the implementation of research on personal budgets for an older person with dementia in practice.

A case scenario

A case scenario of a person with dementia could cover several years, or very few. One of the key points that is emerging from studies of the progression of dementia is that it is a variable, and often unpredictable, disability. Case scenario 14.1 covers several different points of the dementia trajectory – the period before symptoms give rise to concern, a feeling that something is wrong, going through the process of diagnosis and accommodation to this, the growing disabilities that affect everyday life and decisions that need to be taken, and finally end of life care. And, even after death, the potential for family carers to feel guilty may make bereavement itself more difficult.

Many different types of knowledge – research, theory, emotional, law, policy and procedural – are needed in social work; working with older people and their carers demands these, but extra knowledge is required, too. Here, there is great need to understand the disabilities and long-term conditions

---

CASE SCENARIO 14.1

Mrs Hill: introduction

Mrs Hill used to work in the very office where the Ington adult services office is now located. Not many people saw her, however, since she was one of the silent army of office cleaners who arrive and leave before other people start work. She is now in her late 70s and was widowed 20 years ago. Her husband had a manual job, too, working in the building trade. They bought their council house as soon as they could and he spent much time renovating their home while Mrs Hill cleaned for the council, at other times for older neighbours, and quite often for her adult children and their families. The couple were both cigarette smokers and spent time socialising with neighbours and family in the local pub. This has now become a rather smart gastro pub but it is still open.

Mrs Hill's daughter Janet sees her mum every week and phones her most days. Her other daughter, Gemma, is a nurse in Canada. Janet, who lives on her own, has been noticing that her mother is not looking after her house as well as she used to, the cups are a bit grubby, and her mother does not seem to do any baking any more. Occasionally Janet wonders if the rubbish is getting put out properly and if her mum is having a shower as frequently as she used to do. Janet finds that her mum does not seem able to manage her bills as well as she did and Janet has suggested that they are moved to direct debits.

CASE SCENARIO 14.2

Mrs Hill: assessment

Janet arranges for her mother to see her GP. At this consultation, the GP talks to Mrs Hill and to Janet and arranges for some physical tests to check her general health. When the results of these come back and other possible problems have been effectively ruled out, the GP arranges for Mrs Hill to attend a local memory service (sometimes called a 'memory clinic'). Here, other tests, and possibly a scan, are carried out by nurses and other professionals. While this might take some time, our story unfolds quickly to the time when Mrs Hill is told that she has a likely dementia – of a type for which there is currently no 'anti-dementia' (symptom containing) medication available in the early stages. Follow-up after the diagnosis is promised but Mrs Hill is suffering from a bout of flu and does not attend the post-diagnosis group.

affecting later life so that care and support plans can be tailored to the individual. One of the syndromes where such knowledge is required is dementia and this is the focus of Case scenario 14.1. Many older people, however, do not have dementia on its own; they are very likely to have other impairments, particularly hearing and sight loss, and also mobility problems and pain. In this scenario, the potential for such problems to be overshadowed by dementia is discussed, as the situation where other conditions might mask an emerging cognitive problem, such as dementia.

The research evidence currently suggests that many people manage this period of uncertainty for quite a considerable period (Samsi *et al.*, 2014). Janet might feel that this is part of normal ageing, or that her mother is feeling a bit tired and lonely. She knows that her mum gets seen by the practice nurse and hopes that this means that the nurse would pick up anything that is wrong, or would pass on any changes in Mrs Hill to the general practitioner (GP). For many people this will, indeed, happen.

The role of a social worker at this time is likely to be opportunistic. There is little way that Mrs Hill or Janet will be in contact with one directly. Importantly, any contact that might occur – for example, Janet could seek advice about a fall alarm for her mum – provides the opportunity to listen carefully to Janet's broader concerns and to suggest that she talks to the GP. While this case study is going to suggest that Mrs Hill has a dementia, other things need to be considered – such as depression, or a physical problem. Such is the interest – in policy and professional terms – in dementia or Alzheimer's disease that there is a risk that people might jump to conclusions that this is the problem without proper investigation.

Assessment and communication

We are beginning to know more about the experiences of people with problems, like Mrs Hill, who attend memory clinics or related services, or those of their carers and supporters, like Janet. Information provision and communication by professionals are reportedly variable and not generally evidence-based.

In only a few memory services are there very close links with social workers and wider adult services.

The importance of providing advice and information to individuals before during and after diagnosis was highlighted in England in the National Dementia Strategy (Department of Health, 2009b). Current consensus on best practice around the provision of information to people with dementia, or suspected memory problems, following a diagnosis, recommends that they are offered individually tailored information and support over time and several encounters. But answers to questions such as what information, how much and when to provide it are not clear. Some relatives (who end up as carers) wish to have as much information as possible, but some wish information provision to be staggered, while other studies reveal carer frustration at a lack of information at such an important time. Regarding the nature and type of information desired, carers most commonly want information around disease progression and what to expect, and the availability of therapies and services. However, research exploring what information people with dementia themselves want is very limited (Abley *et al.*, 2013). Social workers may find that by the time the person with dementia and their carer approaches them for social care, the information they received at diagnosis is out-of-date, or that they are distressed by a lack of timely information to the extent that this sours relationships with professionals and services.

But this is to jump ahead, let us presume that the memory service in Ington is well organised. We would be able to conclude, if key information has been

CASE SCENARIO 14.3

Mrs Hill: declining health

Mrs Hill's ability to cope declines rapidly. She becomes increasingly forgetful and unable to manage her own home and personal care; her physical disabilities worsen, too. For a while, Janet takes on various tasks, such as paying bills, cleaning her mother's home, doing the washing, shopping and providing companionship. She keeps quiet about the distress that some of her mother's symptoms are causing her – the shouting, swearing and accusations.

Things reach a crisis point when Mrs Hill falls and breaks her hip. In hospital, a hugely upsetting time for Janet in which her mother seems to get noticeably more frail, discussions about discharge are led initially by the nurse who calls in the hospital social worker as soon as it emerges that Janet is the main carer and is struggling.

It is some time after the diagnosis was initially made that a social worker, Andrew Lodge, encounters Mrs Hill and Janet. Conversation quickly turns to Janet's fears, her distress, her guilt and her relief at telling her story. Mrs Hill is not well and the social worker's assessment of her mental capacity is that this is substantially impaired. The social worker starts the assessment process but tells Janet that this will take a while and that he will give her time to think about matters and to make arrangements. The option of Mrs Hill moving to a care home is also discussed, on a permanent or temporary basis, but Janet feels it is too early for this.

provided and understood, that the worries of Mrs Hill and of Janet have been listened to, and that the care of Mrs Hill is taken up by the GP as part of the health centre's organised response to all its patients with dementia and to all family carers. It is important for social workers to know what 'good' looks like, which includes being aware of the NHS primary care commitments to people with dementia to undertake reviews, to keep a dementia register (of patients), and to refer carers to adult services, if appropriate. Some social workers have well-developed links with primary care colleagues in which communication is a mutual responsibility. Both social work and primary care professionals also need to be well-acquainted with local third-sector or voluntary sector groups, which may vary hugely in what they are able to offer to Mrs Hill and her family. Similarly, social care and primary care commissioners need to become aware of gaps in provision and the effectiveness of commissioned services. Supervision offers one way to communicate this information to managers but so, too, can audits and case reviews be used to make observations on service capacity.

Assessment and support planning

In the UK, three pieces of legislation: the Carers (Recognition and Services) Act 1995; the Carers and Disabled Children Act 2000; and the Carers (Equal Opportunities) Act 2004 provide those defined as providing 'regular and substantial' care with the rights to have their needs assessed and, if eligible, to receive services (or a personal budget) in their own right. The carers' assessment needs to identify, first, what support carers are providing and, second, their feelings about how they are managing their caring role. Essentially, this is Andrew's task and the Care Act (2014) means that more carers will be entitled to such assessments. Regulatory changes (as mentioned earlier) mean that it is possible for Janet to be the 'suitable person' to take on the management of her mother's personal budget, if she would find this helpful in arranging her care and support (see Mental Health Foundation, 2014).

This case scenario illustrates the interconnectedness of the lives of many carers and the person for whom they care (Moriarty, 2012). This means that services ostensibly aimed at an older person, such as home care or day centres, should also be beneficial for carers. Assistive technologies may be particularly valued by carers such as Janet who do not live in the same household as the person for whom they care (such as alarm systems, reminders or memory aides). But, as this scenario suggests, it tends only to be at times of crisis, such as hospital admission and discharge, that carers are asked to make important decisions about the sort of services they want, and they are very often reliant on professionals to explain what help is available to them, its costs and its availability.

Moriarty (2012) notes that although the majority of carers will not experience difficulties with their caring role, a substantial number will. This is usually influenced by the amount of care that they provide and the emotional context in which it is given. Interventions increasingly use a combination of methods and may be based on the use of new technologies combined with some of the most traditional of supports, such as home care and residential

---

CASE SCENARIO 14.4

Mrs Hill: personalising care and support for Mrs Hill

During Mrs Hill's time in hospital, Andrew is able to talk to Janet and they think about what Mrs Hill would need to have in place on her return home and what might be the options for the future. Andrew is familiar with situations where re-ablement or temporary support after a hospital stay is gratefully received but may not be enough in the long term. He works with Janet to think about what Mrs Hill needs and how a support plan could not only meet her needs, but also maintain her quality of life. He talks to Janet about having a regular break, making arrangements for sudden eventualities and recommends she talk to someone at the local Carers' Centre. Together, they agree on a support plan that swings into place when Mrs Hill goes home and this complements the re-ablement service during its four-week involvement.

'Choice' and 'control' were not the words that Janet used in her discussions with Andrew but they were behind many of her concerns. She described her mother's attempts to do housework and how important it was for a care worker to involve her mum in this, even to a minimal degree. She thought that her mum would like to walk to the local pub and could probably manage to have her lunch there one day a week. She wanted a care worker who would be discreet about changing her mother's clothes and making sure they went into the wash.

All this seems to be focusing on the practicalities of care but the underlying discussion with Andrew was one where Janet could voice her fears that only she would be able to care for her mother well and that only she could validate her mother by 'knowing' her and presenting her to the world not just as a person with dementia, but also as a person with a past and a future. Andrew listened, affirmed, reframed Janet's views on occasion, and listened some more. His knowledge of the promising results from Cognitive Stimulation Therapy (CST) research enabled him to suggest that this could help Mrs Hill; he described this approach to Janet and described what was available locally.   →

---

services. For Andrew, the assessment process is the opportunity to find out what Mrs Hill wants (or may have wanted), what Janet wants and the prognosis for Mrs Hill. Andrew uses a strengths- or assets-based perspective to help Janet see both problems and resources, such as her love for her mother and the strength of their relationship.

PRACTICE REFLECTION 14.2

Care Act (2014): the concept of balance

The Care Act (2014) affords more freedom for practitioners to make decisions about support planning that go beyond traditional methods of meeting needs and usual care management tasks. It also requires social workers (and others) to seek to achieve a balance between the individual's well-being and that of any friends/relatives who are involved in caring for the individual. How far do you think Andrew achieved that in this case? Can you foresee any problems associated with moving to this concept of 'balance'?

→   Andrew helped to set up a personal budget for Janet to manage on her mother's behalf to fund a care plan that provides Mrs Hill with care from her neighbour, from Janet and to pay for a good alarm system that can be adapted to changing needs. Andrew monitors this – not simply for accounting reasons, but to ensure that the workload placed on Janet is not becoming too onerous. A CST group is available at a local day centre but there is a long waiting list, so this is not accessed.

Mrs Hill talks to Andrew, too, but communication is getting hard. In his mind, Andrew expects that he will be talking to Janet about a care home for Mrs Hill as another element of choice. He has already talked to her about a form of advanced care plan so that decisions about care at the end of life may be considered when time is not pressured. He has said that this needs to be discussed with Mrs Hill's GP but that he will collect some information for Janet and will go with her to the GP if she would like. If asked to make predictions, reluctantly Andrew says that he expects that if Mrs Hill's support plan begins to fray at the edges then Janet may consider a care home place for her mum. But he would not be too distressed if Mrs Hill died in her sleep one night – he has considerable admiration for how Janet has surrounded her mother with love and support, and thinks this is what both would want.

Personal budgets in this case have been part of a generally successful social care plan. Andrew's social work skills have been used subtly yet constructively and, while matters are generally not perfect in social care, older people such as Mrs Hill may be able remain at home as they wish with the help of carers like Janet to make this possible. Following Mrs Hill's death some months later, Janet is saddened but proud that her mum was where she wanted to be when she died, in her own chair, holding a tea cloth that gave her some comfort with its familiar texture and memory. Andrew attends the funeral – a practice that his manager approves for the team.

Conclusion

Social work with older people may be coming of age and the personalisation of social care is one way in which the voice of older people is better able to influence social care provision and social work support than previously. This may help to reduce ageist practice and resource allocations, as well as acknowledging the great diversity of older people and their carers and the multiple exclusion that some experience. This chapter has focused on evidence about personalisation and on the unfolding example of the case of a person with dementia to illustrate the potential for social work with older people to make a difference. It has pointed to the use of research – illustrating this with examples of cognitive stimulation therapy (CST) and 'proxy' budget holding. The former example is used in order to suggest that social workers should feed their research and experience (in this case, that CST services are insufficient locally) to local funders. The second example, research on proxy budget hold-ing, is an illustration of how quickly research findings can be made available to practitioners – here, through the use of new technology. Social work with older people therefore needs to be research-minded not for abstract reasons, but because it can make a difference to people's lives.

FURTHER READING

Newbronner, L., Chamberlain, R., Bosanquet, K., Bartlett, C., Sass B. and Glendinning, C. (2011) *SCIE Report 40: Keeping Personal Budgets Personal: Learning from the Experiences of Older People, People with Mental Health Problems and their Carers* (London: SCIE). This study reports on users' experiences of personal budgets and offers suggestions for good practice.

Ray, M. and Phillips, J. (2012) *Social Work with Older People* (Basingstoke: Palgrave Macmillan). This policy-informed text book covers theory and practice knowledge relating to older people. It draws on key gerontological theories and evidence.

Sanderson, H. and Lewis, J. (2011) *A Practical Guide to Delivering Personalisation: Person-centered Practice in Health and Social Care* (London: Jessica Kingsley Publishers). This practice guide takes a broad view of personalisation, and covers health and social care-related principles and practice.

Here are some of the key websites and online resources that may help to extend your understanding of the ideas presented in this chapter:

Rethink Mental Illness – Personal Budgets Free Guides: http://www.rethink.org/living-with-mental-illness/personal-budgets

Think Local Act Personal: http://www.thinklocalactpersonal.org.uk/

Self-Directed Support in Scotland: http://www.selfdirectedsupportscotland.org.uk/

Age UK – personal budgets in social care: http://www.ageuk.org.uk/documents/en-gb/information-guides/ageukig26_personal_budgets_inf.pdf?dtrk=true

Personal Health Budgets Evaluation: https://www.phbe.org.uk/

Carers Trust Progression Personalisation: http://www.carers.org/sites/default/files/progressing_personalisation.pdf

CHAPTER 15

Increasing the Synergy between Research and Practice in Social Work

Martin Webber

Introduction

This book has featured contributions from leading experts in social work. We have gathered thoughts from academics, researchers, practitioners and people with experience of using services on the research–practice interface in social work. Some embrace notions of evidence-based practice, while others eschew it. What is of key significance, though, is that they share a desire to see research informing social work practice.

This final chapter reviews some of the key themes, debates and tensions which have been discussed during this book. These are situated within the context of contemporary social policy which simultaneously welcomes and ignores research findings, sometimes at the convenience of policy-makers and sometimes for political purposes. Research on the use of research in practice, and the current state of evidence-based practice in social work, is then reviewed to further understand some of the challenges of applying research evidence in social work practice. Finally, looking to the future, I consider some of the opportunities for practitioners to engage both with, and in, research to help shape the agendas for practice and research in social work.

Evidence-based policy

Social work practice is both constrained and enabled by the policy framework in which it operates. This is evident in the UK at present – and in England, in particular – where, on the one hand, there are moves within UK social policy to constrain social work practice within a bureau-technocratic framework. Bureaucratic measures which focus on procedures, rather than outcomes, have frustrated the professional development of social workers in the UK. For example, the Common Assessment Framework (CAF) was heralded as an evidence-based tool but practitioners in child welfare agencies appear to make strategic and moral decisions about whether to use it (White *et al.*, 2009), partly because of the workload involved, and implementation is varied such that it has been observed that the 'CAF of policy' is quite different from the 'CAF of practice' (Pithouse *et al.*, 2009). The Care Programme Approach (CPA) has similarly impacted on social work in mental health services as it has constrained social work within a bureau-medicalised system which squeezes out psychosocial intervention in favour of risk assessment and management (Nathan and Webber, 2010). The result has been for some local authorities to remove their social workers from integrated mental health services to focus on 'core' social work activities, such as personalisation and safeguarding, and others to review their partnership agreements (McNicoll, 2013).

On the other hand, there have been renewed calls for a focus on advanced reflective practice and relationship-based practice in social work (e.g. Ruch, 2012; Webber and Nathan, 2010). This is echoed in the Munro Report (Munro, 2011) and the work of the Social Work Reform Board (2010), which led to the creation of the College of Social Work to lead the professional development of social work in England, and the posts of two Chief Social Workers (one for social work with adults and one for social work with children) to champion social work at ministerial level within government. Reforms since 2010 have provided social work with the opportunity to shape its own practice and influence its own future, rather than be at the whim of policy-makers. Change may be slow in coming, but the structures are in place to make it happen.

These developments are occurring in the context of waning interest in evidence-based policy-making. Although heralded by the New Labour government in the UK in the late 1990s, evidence-based policy-making has been a concern of governments of different political colours before and since then. New Labour were concerned about 'what worked' across all domains of public policy (Nutley *et al.*, 2000). Their *Modernising Government* (Cabinet Office, 1999) agenda explicitly cited the better use of evidence and research in policy-making. When it came to social work and social care, we were asked to 'learn' from the developments in evidence-based medicine; hence, the development of evidence-based practice as discussed in Chapter 1.

The National Service Framework for Mental Health (Department of Health, 1999) was an example of evidence-based policy-making. An External Reference Group was tasked with searching for the best available evidence according to the hierarchy of evidence discussed in Chapter 1 and mental health policy was constructed on this basis. Systematic reviews of randomised controlled trials, particularly those conducted by the Cochrane Collaboration, were highly influential in shaping mental health services in England and Wales for a decade. New services such as Crisis Resolution and Home Treatment teams, Early Intervention in Psychosis teams and Assertive Outreach Teams owed their genesis to evidence-based policy-making.

Assertive outreach teams, for example, were established because the US model of assertive community treatment (ACT) was found by a Cochrane review to be effective in reducing hospital admissions and time spent in hospital, and increased the engagement with services of people with psychosis in contrast to standard community care (Marshall and Lockwood, 1998). ACT, which originated out of community mental health practice influenced by social work principles of seeing people within their own homes rather than within clinics (Stein and Test, 1980), has not been successfully replicated in the UK. Trials in the UK have not found any evidence that it improves outcomes for people with psychosis in comparison with community mental health teams (CMHTs) (e.g. Burns *et al.*, 1999; Killaspy *et al.*, 2006). This is partly because the comparison groups in these trials received CMHT care, which is substantially better than the control groups in the US ACT trials, whose community care provision was very limited or non-existent. Also, a later systematic review found that trials with less fidelity to the ACT model (where it was not being implemented fully) had poorer outcomes (Burns *et al.*, 2007). The lack of convincing evidence in support of assertive outreach in the UK has led to the conclusion that CMHTs are the most cost-effective and evidence-based provision of community care for people with severe mental health problems (Burns, 2010). This example illustrates that simply basing policy on evidence without a full appreciation of either the context of the original research, or the context in which new interventions are being introduced, has limited positive impact.

An example to the contrary – of policy-making in the absence of evidence – can be found in Community Treatment Orders (CTOs). Compulsory community treatment of people with severe mental health problems was introduced in England and Wales by amendments to the Mental Health Act 1983 in 2007. A feature of mental health law in many jurisdictions throughout the world such as Scotland, Australia, Canada, New Zealand and the US, a systematic review commissioned as part of the review of the Mental Health Act found no evidence that CTOs improve outcomes for people (Churchill, 2007). As discussed in Chapter 11, a recent trial of CTOs in England also found no improved outcomes for people receiving compulsory treatment in the community (Burns *et al.*, 2013). However, in spite of evidence that they are no more effective than placing someone on leave from hospital, CTOs are popular amongst psychiatrists (Coyle *et al.*, 2013) and there appears to be no appetite to revise the Mental Health Act despite randomised controlled trial evidence to the contrary.

These examples illustrate the difficulties in using research to generate policy and how easy it is to ignore when it tells inconvenient truths. To resolve some of the difficulties with complexity, context and the reliability of research use, Pawson (2006) developed a realist approach to evidence-based policy-making. He and his colleagues argued that the process of appraising and applying evidence should acknowledge complexity 'in the task of scouring the evidence base. The success of an intervention theory ... depends on the individuals, interpersonal relationships, institutions and infrastructures through which and in which the intervention is being delivered' (Pawson *et al.*, 2004: iii). So this makes the simple 'what works' appraisal question more complex: 'what counts may be what works; but understanding and identifying what works is not a simple technocratic task, but a tellingly reflexive one' (Wells, 2007: 27). In considering the use of research for public policy and for social work practice, it is important to bear in mind the following contention:

> Rather than seeking generalisable lessons or universal truths [we should recognise] ... the fact that the 'same' intervention never gets implemented identically and never

has the same impact, because of differences in the context, setting, process, stakeholders and outcomes. Instead the aims of a realist [approach] is explanatory – 'what works for whom, in what circumstances, in what respects and how?' (Pawson *et al.*, 2004: v)

A realist approach to policy-making is perhaps most appropriate when applied to local decisions or local policy-making where an appreciation of the context is important. It is less often applied to national policy-making but finds favour amongst practitioners and managers who seek to draw on research findings in their decision-making.

PRACTICE REFLECTION 15.1

Evidence-based policy making

Consider Pawson's realist approach to evidence-based policy-making. What do you think are its benefits? Can you apply it to policy-making within your agency? Do you think it will improve experiences and outcomes for your service users?

Implementation of evidence-based practice in social work

The Social Care Institute for Excellence (SCIE) was set up to inform social care and social work with findings from research. Its equivalent in health, the National Institute for Health and Care Excellence (NICE) (its name was changed in 2013 to reflect a new role providing guidance to social care staff) was set up in 1999 and issues clinical guidance to health service practitioners about which interventions they should be using on the grounds of effectiveness and cost-effectiveness. SCIE and NICE undertake similar roles though their outputs vary, reflecting differences in their respective evidence bases and in the way in which research is applied in health and social care contexts.

As has been discussed throughout this book, discovering 'what works' in social work and social care (if that is, indeed, possible), and then simply exhorting practitioners to implement it, does not work and is not desirable. At the very least, practitioners need to consider the complexity of the circumstances in which evidence is produced, and the situation in which it is appraised and applied. Even then, there is no clear link between the production of evidence, its use in practice, and outcomes appearing or being improved. However, as Victoria Hart argued in Chapter 6, practitioners have been unfairly blamed for the inability of research to translate into improved outcomes for service users. In part, this is because they have been ill-equipped for the role.

Social work education in the UK places much less emphasis on critical interrogation of research than it does on understanding and using theory to inform practice. It arguably does not equip social workers with a robust understanding of research methodology, which is crucial to the successful integration of research into practice (Mullen *et al.*, 2008). As discussed in Chapter 1, proponents of evidence-based practice argue that practitioners require an ability to understand and appraise the quality of research in order to make a judgement about its usefulness for their practice (Gambrill, 1999; Mullen *et al.*, 2008; Sheldon and Chilvers, 2000). However, the social work profession suffers from endemic research illiteracy (Marsh and Fisher, 2005) and social work qualifying programmes are limited in their capacity to develop evidence-based practitioners (Caldwell *et al.*, 2007). But this is not a new problem. It appears that social work students have struggled with learning research methods since they were first introduced into curricula in the US over 25 years ago (Epstein, 1987). A recent audit of research teaching on UK social work qualifying programmes (MacIntyre and Paul, 2012) indicates that students continue to struggle to learn (and lecturers to teach) research methods effectively.

Entrants to social work programmes are more likely to have a background in the humanities, rather than the sciences. This makes them less familiar with empirical research methods at the beginning of their social work training than those entering professional training in clinical psychology or psychiatry, for example. When they are included in social work curricula, empirical research methods are taught alongside other methods, such as participatory research, reflecting the discipline's diverse epistemological paradigms (Shaw *et al.*, 2010b). Therefore, teaching research methodology to social workers frequently takes them beyond their 'comfort zone'. Additionally, the discourse of evidence-based practice has itself deterred social workers from enhancing their understanding of research methods. It is perceived as being associated with medicine and not applicable to social work, although it appears to be equally problematic for some doctors (Straus and McAlister, 2000).

Evidence from international studies suggests that social workers support the idea of using research in their practice but many report barriers to doing so (Booth *et al.*, 2003; Gray *et al.*, 2013a; Gray *et al.*, 2013b; Mullen and Bacon, 2004; Sheldon and Chilvers, 2000; Sheldon and Macdonald, 1999). In general, these studies found that understanding of research terminology was low, practitioners felt that keeping up to date with research was important but there were organisational barriers to this and training courses contained few references to research. Practitioners rarely consulted research when making practice decisions and were unaware of evidence-based practice guidelines. These studies conducted since the late 1990s suggest that there remains a long way to go to 'catch up' with health colleagues (Cooke *et al.*, 2008; McCrae *et al.*, 2005) and that knowledge of evidence-based practice remains variable amongst social workers (Pope *et al.*, 2011).

A recurring theme throughout this book is echoed by Davies and Nutley (2002), who argue that the translation of research into practice requires more than exhorting practitioners to implement practice guidelines based on research findings. Unless the organisational context for practice is changed, it is unlikely that research can be effectively implemented. At present, as discussed, it appears that the organisational culture in which social work is practised is a prominent barrier, as it is not oriented towards embedding research into its practice. Agencies focus more on processes than outcomes; commonly provide insufficient time for practitioners to read research papers; and there is generally not a culture of research implementation within social care agencies, perpetuating a circle of resistance to the development of a social work research culture (Orme and Powell, 2008). For effective implementation, evidence-based practice requires organisational change with leadership from the top and the engagement of staff across the organisation (Plath, 2013), but in the Age of Austerity this is possibly unlikely to be forthcoming unless there are clear cost-benefits of doing so.

This book has taken a positive, proactive stance towards research utilisation in social work and is not going to end on a despondent note. Indeed, there is much to be hopeful about. There are strategies for professional development which we can adopt to facilitate a greater synergy between research and practice in social work. In closing, I shall suggest three, starting with the research training we provide to social workers.

Research training

A case could be made that it is possible to apply research findings in social work practice with little or no understanding of research methodology. If a practitioner were to follow a practice guideline which has been developed from the findings of a robust research project, and implement an intervention with proven evidence of its effectiveness then, arguably, they are embedding research findings in their practice and (hopefully) improving outcomes for service users. They do not necessarily need to know about, or understand, the research on which it was based; they 'just' implement it.

If one were to accept this perspective, however, it fundamentally negates the principles of evidence-based practice or evidence-informed practice. As all the authors have repeatedly argued throughout this book, it is essential to engage critically with research findings in order to appraise their strengths and weaknesses, understand the context in which they were produced and consider their relevance for the particular practice question you seek to answer. Social workers should not be automatons who blindly implement guidelines without critically engaging with the research which underpins them. Their professional training equips them to make complex decisions in the best interests of the individual or family with whom they are working. Evidence-based or evidence-informed practice supports professional decision-making, and to do this without critical engagement is short-sighted and potentially damaging.

As we have discussed, though, social work education does not always equip practitioners with the skills to engage critically with research findings. Some qualifying social work programmes provide good training in critical appraisal skills and research methodology but, because of other curriculum requirements, many programmes struggle to find the space to do more than a quick introduction. Research teaching is frequently focused on supporting students to write their dissertations, rather than on preparing them to interrogate research papers to answer their practice-based questions. There is a greater opportunity on post-qualifying programmes for this but, in my experience, it has been a challenge to convince employers (who typically fund practitioners either through the payment of fees, or by permitting them time to attend university) that it is a valuable aspect of a social worker's professional development. The focus on procedural competence, rather than professional capability, has held back the development of social work research literacy, though I remain optimistic that the advent of the Professional Capabilities Framework (College of Social Work, 2012) for social workers in England may help to change this.

On an advanced level post-qualifying programme I used to lead, we provided critical appraisal training and teaching on research methods. We taught both quantitative and qualitative research methods, though the emphasis was on the former to address a frequent absence of this on qualifying programmes. As our programme was in mental health social work, it equipped practitioners with the ability to read and critically to appraise the research which also underpinned the practice of psychiatrists and psychologists. This training provided practitioners with the confidence to challenge health colleagues about the research evidence they cited in support of their practice. Quite frequently, they were able to ask 'Where is the evidence for that?' and be able to discuss the strengths and limitations of the research methodologies which were used without fear of feeling out of their depth. This enhanced their professional competence and ability to be equal members of multi-disciplinary community mental health teams (which are frequently health-led and dominated) (Webber, 2012).

Our students – all experienced practitioners – conducted an empirical research study as part of the Masters programme. They were supported and supervised to undertake research within their agencies, frequently using techniques akin to clinical data mining (Epstein, 2001; Epstein, 2010), or the collection of original data. Their research projects answered practice-based questions which informed their work and that of their agency. Some were published in international peer-reviewed journals (Bookle and Webber, 2011; Dunn, 2001; Dutt and Webber, 2010; Furminger and Webber, 2009; Kingsford and Webber, 2010; Slack and Webber, 2008), making a modest contribution to the evidence-base for mental health social work practice in the same way as the work conducted by Joubert, Epstein and colleagues has (see special issues of *Social Work in Health Care* (vol. 33, issue 3/4) and the *Journal of Social Work Research and Evaluation* (vol. 6, issue 2)). Practice research both challenges the notion of research expertise as residing with social work academics and creates new forms of practice-knowledge, contributing to removing perceived barriers between research and practice in social work.

University partnerships with employers which help to deliver practice learning on qualifying social work programmes can provide the context for enhanced research-practice partnerships. This could include social work academics delivering research training to practitioners and supervising practice-research projects in return for practitioners providing practice education and contributing skills teaching to social work programmes, for example. As practitioners have limited time to attend university training, it is possible to deliver research methods and critical appraisal training by means of e-learning. Our evaluation of a pilot e-learning course of post-qualifying research methods training found practitioners can learn equally as effectively as a classroom-based cohort (Webber *et al.*, 2009). Similarly, practitioners can learn the skills involved in writing a research protocol online if they are not able to attend classroom based study (Webber and Currin Salter, 2011). The increased involvement of practitioners in research activities could potentially play a role in re-shaping agencies' engagement with research findings.

PRACTICE REFLECTION 15.2

Practice research

Consider the opportunities for you to undertake practice research in order to answer practice questions that arise in your agency. Talk to your supervisor about how your agency could support you with this. Talk to university colleagues to see how they can help to support and supervise practice research projects.

Learning organisations

Newly qualified social workers (NQSWs) and experienced practitioners alike who are enthused about applying research findings in their practice can quickly become frustrated by the agency which employs them if it does not encourage learning from research. As we have discussed, practitioners can only successfully apply research findings in their practice if their agency permits or supports them to do so. Many social work employers do not actively encourage research literacy, considering time spent on reading journal papers as a luxury. Transforming social work agencies into learning organisations (which readily embrace learning and new ways of working) is challenging (Orme and Powell, 2008), but the current economic climate presents a unique opportunity.

Public sector spending cuts mean that there is less money available for social work and social care services. The global recession has ensured this to be the case for many countries, not just the UK. As a result, Directors of Adults or Children's Social Care Services face increasing pressure to deliver or commission better services at a lower cost. They have difficult decisions to make about which services to cut and which to retain. Some are turning to researchers to see whether they can help. They are interested to learn whether there are cost-effective ways of delivering the same services or new services which can be commissioned which produce the same outcomes at a lower cost. This sudden interest in research is unlikely to represent a sea-change in attitudes, or the transformation of local authority social care departments into learning organisations. However, this window of opportunity may permit practitioners who are research-literate to search, appraise and evaluate the research literature to assist decision-making about the future of the services in which they work. There may also be opportunities to undertake practice-research to inform these decisions.

A further opportunity is provided by the social work reforms in England which have introduced continuing professional development (CPD) as a requirement of registration with the Health and Care Professions Council. Reading, appraising and applying research findings is a valid CPD activity and employers should provide practitioners with the time to undertake it. If practitioners share the findings of their reading or practice-research with their colleagues, they can subtly inform policy and practice within the agency at no additional cost. In doing so, they could influence the agency's attitude towards research. Combined with an effective practice–research partnership with a university, there is potential to transform social work agencies into learning organisations from within over a period of time.

PRACTICE REFLECTION 15.3

Influencing decision-making

What are the opportunities for influencing decision-making within your agency? Consider how you can apply some of the learning from this book to decisions about the future services within your agency. Although you may not be in a position to make these decisions, can you undertake a systematic literature review or piece of practice-research as part of your CPD that can inform this decision-making?

Making research relevant

As this book is written for practitioners, rather than researchers, we have not considered in depth the implications of the practice–research interface for social work researchers. It is clear, though, that research cannot have an impact on practice without it being relevant to the concerns and needs of practitioners. Unfortunately, this is not always the case as sometimes social work academics focus more on research of interest to them than addressing practice-based questions. Additionally, our intervention research does not always adequately consider the context from which it was derived, or that to which it is to be applied, making it difficult for practitioners to apply it in their practice. In finishing this book, I provide an example of research I am undertaking which, although far from perfect, attempts to account for the context in which social interventions are applied.

The Connecting People study

Standardised psychosocial interventions are accompanied by a practice manual which guides practitioners how to implement them. Evaluations of interventions consider how faithfully manuals have been implemented in practice. This helps to ensure that the outcomes measured have been produced by the intervention being evaluated and not something else. Quite often though, as has been mentioned throughout this book, it is not possible to implement an intervention according to the manual. Either the context or the service users' problem requires flexibility in the way in which the intervention is applied. A lack of fidelity to the intervention can mean poorer outcomes for the service user, and practitioners are subsequently blamed. But if flexibility and an understanding of different contexts are considered within the intervention itself, it may be possible to develop approaches which can be both rigorously evaluated and readily applied in practice.

The Connecting People Intervention (CPI) articulates the processes involved in supporting people to connect with others (Webber *et al.*, under review). It describes what a worker and the individual with whom they are working should be doing together and, arguably just as importantly, it articulates the features of the context in which this practice is to be supported. The intervention model has the agency at its base (representing the context for the practice) and running up through the middle (supporting the co-production of the worker and the individual). The CPI includes the practice context because it needs to be oriented towards the community of the individual or family with whom the worker is working, and not all social care and social work agencies are set up to do this.

The CPI model was developed out of existing good practice, as captured by qualitative research methods including observations, interviews and focus groups (Webber *et al.*, in press). The findings of the thematic analysis from this qualitative study were modelled by practitioners, service users and the research team during focus groups to describe the processes involved in connecting people. It emerged through this process that the context in which the practice occurred was inseparable from the practice itself. Perhaps as a result of this, the context of the intervention is crucial to it producing favourable outcomes.

The pilot of the CPI found that outcomes are better for service users (adults with a mental health problem or a learning disability) in agencies which more fully embody the practice model (Webber *et al.*, under review). Agencies which are more faithful to the CPI model are more effective at increasing their service users' access to social capital and perceived social inclusion, at lower cost than those with lower fidelity. Whole-team intervention training is provided at the beginning to help practitioners consider their existing practice, and that of their agency as a whole. This initiates conversations in the agency about the changes which need to be made to adjust its way of working to be faithful to the model. Instead of practitioners struggling to fit the intervention into their practice context, the context of their practice is supported to adjust to accommodate the intervention model. This shares the onus of intervention fidelity between practitioners and the agency as a whole, and improves the transferability of the CPI from one practice setting to another.

Concluding thoughts

Research into effective ways of translating research findings into practice is a burgeoning area of enquiry in health disciplines. In contrast, translational research in social work is in its relative infancy. This is partly due to ambivalence about the paradigm of evidence-based practice in social work, but also partly due to a relative dearth of intervention research in social work. Although many social work academics aspire to conduct research of real-world relevance for practitioners and of intrinsic value for its scholarship

(Parker and van Teijlingen, 2012), more is required.

To facilitate the translation of social work research findings into practice, practitioners need to be supported to develop their research literacy. This includes being given the opportunity to interrogate research findings and/or conduct their own research to answer practice-based questions. Social work researchers need to retain their connections with practice and respond to research questions arising from it. Social work academics need to foster the development of practice–research partnerships. And employers need to support the professional development of their social workers and be open to new ways of working as informed by the latest research findings.

There is something for us all to be doing, so let's get on and do it.

FURTHER READING

Epstein, I. (2011) *Practice-Based Research in Social Work: A Guide for Reluctant Researchers* (London: Routledge); Epstein, I. (2010) *Clinical Data-Mining: Integrating Practice and Research* (New York: Oxford University Press). Two excellent introductions to practice-research for practitioners.

Pawson, R. (2006) *Evidence-Based Policy: A Realist Perspective* (London: Sage). Essential reading for anyone interested in exploring how research can be used to inform policy.

Glossary

Bibliographic database Extensive online collections of (typically) peer reviewed journal articles; the best place to search for research evidence.

Boolean operators Small words (AND, OR, NOT) placed in search strings in bibliographic databases to refine searches for research on a particular topic.

Campbell Collaboration Publishers of high-quality systematic reviews of interventions in education, crime and justice, social welfare and international development.

Cochrane Collaboration Publishers of high-quality systematic reviews of interventions for health problems.

Cohort study A longitudinal study that explores cause–effect relationships.

Cost-effectiveness The effectiveness of an intervention or service in relation to how much it costs to be provided.

Critical appraisal The process of assessing the strengths and weaknesses of a research study.

Cross-sectional survey A snapshot of a population or a group at one point in time to measure the prevalence of a particular phenomenon.

Empiricism A theory of knowledge that gives primacy to sensory experience and the role of experiments in deriving our knowledge about the world.

Ethnography A research method that involves a researcher becoming immersed within the social environment they are studying and often includes observations, interviews and focus groups.

Evidence The available facts or information that are provided in support or refutation of an assertion.

Evidence-based practice A systematic process of applying research evidence to practice by developing a practice question; searching for the best available evidence to answer it; appraising relevant studies for quality and usefulness; considering unique needs of the service user and applying the best available evidence to practice decisions; and evaluating the outcome.

Evidence-informed practice This does not privilege particular types of research over others and equally values practice wisdom as a form of knowledge that informs practice.

Experimental study   A study that evaluates the outcomes of an intervention, sometimes involving randomising participants to an intervention or a control group, but not always.

Focus group   An interview involving a group of people; useful for gaining additional insights from the interaction between group members.

Generalisation   The formulation of general concepts, from specific instances, that can be applied to circumstances beyond those in which they originated.

Hierarchy of evidence   A ranked list of types of research methods and forms of evidence from systematic reviews of randomised controlled trials at the top to practitioner's opinions at the bottom.

In-depth interview   A method of capturing a respondent's detailed thoughts on a particular topic.

Intervention   The act of 'doing' practice; what a social worker does in practice with the individuals and families with whom they work.

Manual   A step-by-step guide to implementing an intervention.

Outcome   The specific goal of practice or an intervention; what you want to achieve.

Positivism   The idea that scientific knowledge is built up by the accumulation of facts about the world.

Practice question   A query that arises out of practice shaped into an answerable question.

Pragmatism   The regarding of knowledge as a means of problem-solving so as to achieve specific ends.

Prevalence   A measure of 'how much' a particular phenomenon is present within a particular group or population.

Psychosocial intervention   Something a practitioner does to ameliorate the social environment of an individual to improve their psychological wellbeing.

Qualitative study   A generic term for studies that investigate *why* and *how* questions and typically explore experiences, values, attitudes and processes.

Quantitative study   A generic term for studies that measure phenomena and analyse data with the help of statistics.

Randomised controlled trial   A research method viewed as the most reliable way to test the effectiveness of an intervention whereby participants are randomised to receiving either the new intervention or an existing one.

Reliability   The ability of a measurement tool or an intervention to produce consistent results under similar conditions.

Research evidence   The findings of a research study that can support the development of social work practice.

Risk factor   Typically, this is something that causes problems to occur, but positive risk factors are those that bring about change for the good.

Service user   A term used to referred to the person or people who receive social work services. Although many other terms are preferred or used interchangeably throughout the book – such as 'client', 'consumer', 'patient' or 'survivor', for example – this term is used most frequently.

Systematic review   A transparent and rigorous literature review that finds, evaluates and synthesises the results of research relevant to a particular practice questionnaire.

Tacit knowledge   Acquired through practice experience and seldom written down, this is the 'practice wisdom' that guides much of social work practice.

Validity   The extent to which a concept, measurement or method is well-founded and corresponds accurately to the real world.

Bibliography

Abberley, P. (1991) *Handicapped by Numbers – A Critique of the OPCS Surveys*, Bristol Polytechnic Occasional Papers in Sociology No. 9. Available at http://disability-studies.leeds.ac.uk/files/library/Abberley-occ-paper.pdf (accessed 4 April 2014).

Abel, E. M., Chung-Canine, U. and Broussard, K. (2013) 'A Quasi-Experimental Evaluation of a School-Based Intervention for Children Experiencing Family Disruption', *Journal of Evidence-Based Social Work*, 10(2): 136–44.

Abley, C., Manthorpe, J., Bond, J., Keady, J., Samsi, K., Campbell, S., Watts, S. and Robinson, L. (2013) 'Patients' and Carers' Views on Communication and Information Provision when Undergoing Assessments in Memory Services', *Journal of Health Services Research & Policy*, 18(3): 167–73.

Advisory Council on the Misuse of Drugs (2003) *Hidden Harm. Responding to the Needs of Children of Problem Drug Users* (London: Home Office).

AERC Alcohol Academy (2010) *Clarifying Brief Interventions*, Briefing Paper. Available at http://www.alcoholacademy.net/news/19/65/Clarifying-brief-interventions-Academy-briefing-paper.html (accessed 1 September 2012).

Ainsworth, M. D. S., Blehar, M. C., Waters, E. and Wall, S. (1978) *Patterns of Attachment: A Psychological Study of the Strange Situation* (Hillsdale, NJ: Lawrence Erlbaum Associates).

Alcohol Learning Centre (2012) *Identification and Brief Advice*. Available at http://www.alcohol-learningcentre.org.uk/Topics/Browse/BriefAdvice/ (accessed 1 September 2012).

Aldgate, J. and McIntosh, M. (2006) *Looking After the Family: A Study of Children Looked After in Kinship Care in Scotland* (Edinburgh: Astron).

Allebeck, P. (1989) 'Schizophrenia: A Life Shortening Disease', *Psychiatric Bulletin*, 15: 81–9.

Allen, G. (2011) *Early Intervention: The Next Steps* (London: Her Majesty's Government).

Alzheimer's Society (2011) *Short Changed. Protecting People with Dementia from Financial Abuse* (London: Alzheimer's Society).

Alzheimer's Society (2012) *Dementia 2012: A National Challenge* (London: Alzheimer's Society).

Alzheimer Disease International (2012) *World Alzheimer Report 2012: Overcoming the Stigma of Dementia* (London: Alzheimer Disease International).

Alzheimer's Society (2012) 'Assistive Technology – Devices to Help With Everyday Living'. Available at http://www.alzheimers.org.uk/site/scripts/documents_info.php?document ID=109 (accessed 19 March 2014).

Alzheimer's Society (2013) 'Position Statement: Safer Walking Technology' Available at http://www.alzheimers.org.uk/site/scripts/documents_info.php?documentID=579 (accessed 19 March 2014).

Andrews, D. A. (2011) 'The Impact of Nonprogrammatic Factors on Criminal-Justice Interventions', *Legal and Criminological Psychology*, 16(1): 1–23.

Andrews, D. A., Bonta, J. and Hoge, R. D. (1990) 'Classification for Effective Rehabilitation: Rediscovering Psychology', *Criminal Justice and Behavior*, 17: 19–52.

Andrews, D. A. and Kiessling, J. J. (1980) 'Program Structure and Effective Correctional Practices: A Summary of the CaVIC Research', in Ross, R. and Gendreau, P. (eds), *Effective Correctional Treatment* (Toronto: Butterworths): 441–63.

Australian Association of Social Workers (2013) *Practice Standards* (Canberra: Australian Association of Social Workers).

Aveyard, H. (2011) *Doing a Literature Review in Health and Social Care*, 2nd edn (Maidenhead: McGraw Hill).

Aveyard, H. and Sharp, P. (2009) *A Beginner's Guide to Evidence-Based Practice in Health and Social Care*, 1st edn (Maidenhead: Open University Press).

Aveyard, H. and Sharp, P. (2013) *A Beginner's Guide to Evidence-Based Practice in Health and Social Care*, 2nd edn (Maidenhead: Open University Press).

Axford, N. (2010) 'Conducting Needs Assessments in Children's Services', *British Journal of Social Work*, 40: 4–25.

Babor, T. F., Higgins-Biddle, J. C., Saunders, J. B. and Monteiro, M. G. (2001) *AUDIT: The Alcohol Use Disorders Identification Test* (Geneva: World Health Organization).

Baker, K., Kelly, G. and Wilkinson, B. (2011) *Assessment in Youth Justice* (Bristol: Polity Press).

Banerjee, S., Willis, R., Matthews, D., Contell, F., Chan, J. and Murray, J. (2007) 'Improving the Quality of Care for Mild to Moderate Dementia: An Evaluation of the Croydon Memory Service Model', *International Journal of Geriatric Psychiatry*, 22(8): 782–8.

Barber, J. G. (1995) *Social Work with Addictions* (London: Macmillan).

Barlow, J. (1998) 'Parent Training Programmes and Behaviour Problems: Findings From a Systematic Review', in Buchanan, A. and Hudson, B. (eds), *Parenting, Schooling and Childrens Behaviour: Interdisciplinary Approaches* (Alton: Ashgate Publishers): 221–36.

Barlow, J., Jones, D. and Fisher, J. D. (2012) *Systematic Review of Models of Analysing Significant Harm* (London: Department for Education).

Barnes, C. (1991) *Disabled People in Britain and Discrimination: A Case for Anti-Discrimination Legislation* (London: Hurst & Co.).

Barnes, C. (1996) 'Disability and the Myth of the Independent Researcher', in Barton, L. and Oliver, M. (eds), *Disability Studies: Past Present and Future* (Leeds: Disability Press): 239–43.

Barnes, C. (2014) 'Reflections on Doing Emancipatory Disability Research', in Swain, J., French, S., Barnes, C. and Thomas, C. (eds), *Disabling Barriers – Enabling Environments*, 3rd edn (London: Sage): 37–44.

Barnes, C. and Mercer, G. (1997) 'Breaking the Mould? An Introduction to Doing Disability Research', in Barnes, C. and Mercer, G. (eds), *Doing Disability Research* (Leeds: Disability Press).

Barnes, C. and Mercer, G. (2004) *Disability Policy and Practice: Applying the Social Model* (Leeds: Disability Press).

Barnes, C. and Mercer, G. (2006) *Independent Futures: Creating User Led Services in a Disabling Society* (Bristol: Policy Press).

Barry, M. (2010) 'Youth Transitions: From Offending to Desistance', *Journal of Youth Studies*, 13(1): 113–29.

Bartels, S. J., Blow, F. C., Van Citters, A. D. and Brockmann, L. M. (2006) 'Dual Diagnosis Among Older Adults Co-occurring Substance Abuse and Psychiatric Illness', *Journal of Dual Diagnosis*, 2(3): 9–30.

Barton, L. (1992) 'Introduction', *Disability, Handicap and Society*, 7(2): 99.

Bebbington, A. and Miles, J. (1989) 'The Background of Children Who Enter Local Authority Care', *British Journal of Social Work*, 19(1): 349–68.

Beckett, C. (2010) *Assessment and Intervention in Social Work: Preparing for Practice* (London: Sage).

Beddoes, D., Sheikh, S., Khanna, M. and Francis, R. (2010a) *The Impact Of Drugs on Different Minority Groups: A Review Of The UK Literature. Part 3: Disabled People* (London: UK Drugs Policy Commission).

Beddoes, D., Sheikh, S., M., K. and Prlat, R. (2010b) *The Impact of Drugs on Different Minority Groups: A Review of the UK Literature. Part 1 Ethnic Groups* (London: UK Drugs Policy Commission).

Beech, R., Russell, W., Little, R. and Sherlow-Jones, S. (2004) 'An Evaluation of a Multidisciplinary Team for Intermediate Care at Home', *International Journal of Integrated Care*, 4 (e02).

Beresford, P. (2000) 'Service Users' Knowledge and Social Work Theory: Conflict or Collaboration', *British Journal of Social Work*, 30: 489–503.

Beresford, P. (2001) 'Service Users, Social Policy and The Future of Welfare', *Critical Social Policy*, 21(4): 494–512.

Beresford, P. (2003) *Its Our Lives. A Short History of Knowledge, Distance and Experience* (London: OSP for Citizen Press in association with Shaping Our Lives).

Beresford, P. (2014) 'Personal Budgets: Not What They Seem'. Available at http://disability now.org.uk/article/personal-budgets-not-what-they-seem (accessed 4 April 2014).

Beresford, P. and Boxall, K. (2012) 'Service Users, Social Work Education and Knowledge for Social Work Practice', *Social Work Education*, 31(2): 154–66.

Beresford, P. and Croft, S. (2012) *User Controlled Research. Scoping Review* (London: NIHR School for Social Care Research).

Beresford, P., Fleming, J., Glynn, M., Bewley, C., Croft, S., Branfield, F. and Postle, K. (2011) *Supporting People: Towards a Person-Centred Approach* (Bristol: Policy Press).

Bhui, K., Stansfeld, S., Hull, S., Priebe, S., Mole, F. and Feder, G. (2003) 'Ethnic Variations in Pathways To and Use of Specialist Mental Health Services in the UK: Systematic Review', *British Journal of Psychiatry*, 182(2): 105–16.

Biehal, N. (2006) *Reuniting Looked After Children with Their Families. A Review* (London: National Children's Bureau).

Biestek, F. (1957) *The Casework Relationship* (Chicago: Loyola University Press).

Blakeman, K. (2014) 'Google Search Tips'. Available at http://www.rba.co.uk/search/ (accessed 19 March 2014).

Bookle, M. and Webber, M. (2011) 'Ethnicity and Access to an Inner City Home Treatment Service: A Case-Control Study', *Health and Social Care in the Community*, 19(3): 280–8.

Booth, A., Papaioannou, D. and Sutton, A. (2011) *Systematic Approaches to a Successful Literature Review* (London: Sage).

Booth, C. (1889) *Life and Labour of the People in London* (London: Macmillan).

Booth, S. H., Booth, A. and Falzon, L. J. (2003) 'The Need for Information and Research Skills Training to Support Evidence-Based Social Care: A Literature Review and Survey', *Learning in Health and Social Care*, 2(4): 191–201.

Bowes, A., Dawson, A. and Greasley-Adams, C. (2013) *Literature Review: The Cost Effectiveness of Assistive Technology in Supporting People with Dementia* (Stirling: University of Stirling).

Bowlby, J. (1969) *Attachment and Loss. Vol. 1: Attachment* (New York: Basic Books).

Bowlby, J. (1973) *Attachment and Loss. Vol. 2: Separation: Anxiety and Anger* (London: Hogarth Press).

Brandon, M., Bailey, S., Belderson, P., Gardner, R., Sidebotham, P., Dodsworth, J., Warren, C. and Black, J. (2009) *Understanding Serious Case Reviews and their Impact: A Biennial Analysis of Serious Case Reviews 2005–7* (London: Department for Children Schools and Families).

Brandon, M., Belderson, P., Warren, P. C. R., Howe, A., Sidebotham, P., Dodsworth, J. and Black, J. (2008) *Analysing Child Death and Injury Through Abuse and Neglect: What Can We Learn? A Biennial Analysis of Serious Case Reviews 2003–5* (Norwich: University of East Anglia).

Brayne, H. and Carr, H. (2010) *Law for Social Workers* (Oxford: Oxford University Press).

Brendel, D. H. (2006) *Healing Psychiatry: Bridging the Science/Humanism Divide* (Cambridge, MA: MIT Press).

Brent Borough Council and Brent Health Authority (1985) *Jasmine Beckford: A Child in Trust: Jasmine Beckford. Report of the Panel of Inquiry into the Circumstances Surrounding the Death of Jasmine Beckford* (London: Brent Borough Council and Brent Health Authority).

Brinkborg, H., Michanek, J., Hesser, H. and Berglund, G. (2011) 'Acceptance and Commitment Therapy for the Treatment of Stress Among Social Workers: A Randomized Controlled Trial', *Behaviour Research and Therapy*, 49(6/7): 389–98.

Britton, J. (2007) *Assessing Young People for Substance Use* (London: National Treatment Agency).

Broadhurst, K. (2009) 'Supporting Parents under New Labour. How Does Every Parent Matter?', in Broadhurst, K., Grover, C. and Jamieson, J. (eds), *Critical Perspectives on Safeguarding Children* (Oxford: Wiley-Blackwell): 111–30.

Broadhurst, K., Hall, C., Wastell, D., White, S. and Pithouse, A. (2010a) 'Risk, Instrumentalism and the Humane Project in Social Work: Identifying the Informal Logics of Risk Management in Children's Statutory Services', *British Journal of Social Work*, 40(4): 1046–64.

Broadhurst, K. and Mason, C. (2012) 'Social Work Beyond the VDU: Foregrounding Co-Presence in Situated Practice. Why Face-to-Face Practice Matters', *British Journal of Social Work*, Advance Access, doi:10.1093/bjsw/bcs124

Broadhurst, K. and Pithouse, A. (2009) 'The Common Assessment Framework: Technical Fix or Framework for Change in Meeting the 'Additional' Needs of Children and Young People?', in Broadhurst, K., Grover, C. and Jamieson, J. (eds), *Safeguarding Children: Critical Perspectives* (London: Wiley).

Broadhurst, K., Wastell, D., White, S., Hall, C., Peckover, S., Thompson, K., Pithouse, A. and Davey, D. (2010b) 'Performing "Initial Assessment": Identifying the Latent Conditions for Error at the Front-Door of Local Authority Children's Services', *British Journal of Social Work*, 40(2): 352–70.

Brodie, I., Goldman, R. and Clapton, J. (2011) *Mental Health Service Transitions for Young People. SCIE Research Briefing 37* (London: Social Care Institute for Excellence).

Bronfenbrenner, U. (1979) *The Ecology of Human Development* (Cambridge, MA: Harvard University Press).

Brooks, N. (2002) 'Intermediate Care Rapid Assessment Support Service: An Evaluation', *British Journal of Community Nursing*, 7(12): 623–33.

Buckley, H., Holt, S. and Whelan, S. (2007) 'Listen to Me! Children's Experiences of Domestic Violence', *Child Abuse Review*, 16(5): 296–310.

Burkhart, G., Olszewski, D., Martel, C., Nilson, M. and Wallon, A. (2003) *Drug Use Amongst*

Vulnerable Young People (Lisbon: European Monitoring Centre for Drugs and Drug Addiction).

Burns, T. (2010) 'The Rise and Fall of Assertive Community Treatment?', *International Review of Psychiatry*, 22(2): 130–7.

Burns, T., Catty, J., Dash, M., Roberts, C., Lockwood, A. and Marshall, M. (2007) 'Use of Intensive Case Management to Reduce Time in Hospital in People with Severe Mental Illness: Systematic Review and Meta-Regression', *British Medical Journal*, 335(7615): 336–40.

Burns, T., Creed, F., Fahy, T., Thompson, S., Tyrer, P. and White, I. (1999) 'Intensive Versus Standard Case Management for Severe Psychotic Illness: A Randomised Trial', *The Lancet*, 353(9171): 2185–9.

Burns, T., Knapp, M., Catty, J., Healey, A., Henderson, A. S., Watt, H. and Wright, C. (2001) 'Home Treatment for Mental Health Problems: A Systematic Review', *Health Technology Assessment*, 5(15): 1–139.

Burns, T., Rugkasa, J., Molodynski, A., Dawson, J., Yeeles, K., Vasquez-Montes, M., Voysey, M., Sinclair, J. and Priebe, S. (2013) 'Community Treatment Orders for Patients with Psychosis (OCTET): A Randomised Controlled Trial,' *The Lancet*, 381(9878): 1627–33.

Butler, I. and Drakeford, M. (2005) 'Trusting in Social Work', *British Journal of Social Work*, 35(5): 639–53.

Byrne, M. and Onyett, S. R. (2010) *Teamwork Within Mental Health Services In Ireland – Resource Paper* (Dublin: Mental Health Commission).

Cabinet Office (1999) *Modernising Government* (London: HMSO).

Caldwell, K., Coleman, K., Copp, G., Bell, L. and Ghazi, F. (2007) 'Preparing for Professional Practice: How Well does Professional Training equip Health and Social Care Practitioners to engage in Evidence-based Practice?', *Nurse Education Today*, 27 (6), 518–28.

Callaghan, L. and Towers, A.-M. (2013) 'Feeling in Control: Comparing Older People's Experiences in Different Care Settings', *Ageing & Society*, FirstView, doi:10.1017/S0144686X13000184

Cameron, A. and Lart, R. (2003) 'Factors Promoting and Obstacles Hindering Joint Working: A Systematic Review of the Research Evidence', *Journal of Integrated Care*, 11(2): 9–17.

Cameron, A., Lart, R., Bostock, L. and Coomber, C. (2012) *SCIE Research Briefing 41: Factors That Promote and Hinder Joint and Integrated Working Between Health and Social Care Services* (London: Social Care Institute for Excellence).

Cameron, M. and Keenan, E. K. (2010) 'The Common Factors Model: Implications for Transtheoretical Clinical Social Work Practice', *Social Work*, 55(1): 63–73.

Carers UK (2008) *Choice or Chore? Carers' Experiences of Direct Payments* (London: Carers UK).

Carew, R. (1987) 'The Place of Intuition in Social Work', *Australian Social Work*, 40(3): 5–9.

Carr, S. (2012) *Personalisation: A Rough Guide. SCIE Guide 47* (London: Social Care Institute for Excellence).

Cattan, M., Kime, N. and Bagnall, A.-M. (2010) *Low-Level Support for Socially Isolated Older People: An Evaluation of Telephone Befriending* (London: Help the Aged).

Cattan, M., Kime, N. and Bagnall, A.-M. (2011) 'The Use of Telephone Befriending in Low Level Support for Socially Isolated Older People – An Evaluation', *Health & Social Care in the Community*, 19(2): 198–206.

Centre for Economic Performance's Mental Health Policy Group (2012) *How Mental Illness Loses Out in the NHS* (London: Centre for Economic Performance, London School of Economics).

Children in Scotland (2005) *My Turn To Talk? The Participation Of Looked After And Accommodated Children in Decision-Making Concerning Their Care* (Edinburgh: Scottish Executive).

Chitty, C. (2005) 'The Impact of Corrections on Re-Offending: Conclusions and the Way Forward', in Harper, G. and Chitty, C. (eds), *The Impact of Corrections on Re-Offending: A Review of 'What Works' (Home Office Research Study 291)*. (London: Home Office).

Christie, N. (1997) 'Four Blocks Against Insight: Notes on the Oversocialization of Criminologists', *Theoretical Criminology*, 1(1): 13–23.

Churchill, R. (2007) *International Experiences of Using Community Treatment Orders* (London: Institute of Psychiatry, King's College London).

CILIP Information Literacy Group (2014) 'Information Literacy'. Available at http://www.informationliteracy.org.uk/ (accessed 19 March 2014).

Clapton, J. (2010) *Bibliographic Databases for Social Care Searching. Knowledge and Research Report 34* (London: Social Care Institute for Excellence).

Clarke, K. (2006) 'Childhood, Parenting and Early Intervention: A Critical Examination of the Sure Start National Programme', *Critical Social Policy*, 26(4): 699–721.

Clarke, R. V. G. and Cornish, D. B. (1975) *The Controlled Trial in Institutional Settings (Home Office Research Study 32)* (London: HMSO).

Clarkson, P., Brand, C., Hughes, J. and Challis, D. (2011) 'Integrating Assessments of Older People: Examining Evidence and Impact from a Randomised Controlled Trial', *Age and Ageing*, 40(3): 388–91.

Cleaver, H. (2000) *Fostering Family Contact: Studies in Evaluating the Children Act 1989* (London: HMSO).

Cleaver, H., Nicholson, D., Tarr, S. and Cleaver, D. (2007) *Child Protection, Domestic Violence and Parental Substance Misuse: Family Experiences and Effective Practice* (London: Jessica Kingsley).

Cochrane, A. L. (1972) *Effectiveness and Efficiency. Random Reflections on Health Services* (London: Nuffield Provincial Hospitals Trust).

Cochrane Collaboration (2007) 'How to Develop a Search Strategy for a Cochrane Review'. Available at http://chmg.cochrane.org/sites/chmg.cochrane.org/files/uploads/ How%20to%20develop%20a%20search%20strategy-support-manual.pdf (accessed 27 March 2014).

College of Social Work (2012) *Professional Capabilities Framework* (London: College of Social Work).

Collins, H. (1985) *Changing Order: Replication and Induction in Scientific Practice* (London: Sage).

Collins, H. and Evans, R. (2007) *Rethinking Expertise* (Chicago: Chicago University Press).

Collins, S. (ed.) (1990) *Alcohol, Social Work and Helping* (London: Routledge).

Collins, S. and Keene, J. (2000) *Alcohol, Social Work and Community Care* (Birmingham: Venture Press).

Commission for Healthcare Audit and Inspection (2007) *Count Me In 2007. Results of the 2007 National Census of Inpatients in Mental Health and Learning Disability Services in England and Wales* (London: Commission for Healthcare Audit and Inspection).

Committee of Inquiry into the Care and Supervision Provided in Relation to Maria Colwell (1974) *Report of the Committee of Inquiry Into the Care and Supervision Provided by Local Authorities and Other Agencies in Relation to Maria Colwell and the Co-ordination Between Them* (London: HMSO).

Cooke, J., Bacigalupo, R., Halladay, L. and Norwood, H. (2008) 'Research Use and Support Needs, and Research Activity in Social Care: A Cross-sectional Survey in Two Councils with Social Services Responsibilities in the UK', *Health & Social Care in the Community*, 16(5): 538–47.

Cooper, D. L., Petherick, E. S. and Wright, J. (2013) 'The Association Between Binge Drinking and Birth Outcomes: Results from the Born in Bradford Cohort Study', *Journal of Epidemiology and Community Health*, doi: 10.1136/jech-2012-202303

Cope, R. (1989) 'The Compulsory Detention of Afro-Caribbeans under the Mental Health Act', *New Community*, 15(3): 343–56.

Copello, A., Orford, J., Hodgson, R., Tober, G., Barrett, C. and the UKATT Research Team (2002) 'Social Behaviour and Network Therapy: Basic Principles and Early Experiences', *Addictive Behaviors*, 27(2): 345–66.

Copello, A., Orford, J., Velleman, R., Templeton, L. and Krishnan, M. (2000a) 'Methods for Reducing Alcohol and Drug Related Family Harm in Non-Specialist Settings', *Journal of Mental Health*, 9(3): 329–43.

Copello, A., Templeton, L., Krishnan, M., Orford, J. and Velleman, R. (2000b) 'A Treatment Package to Improve Primary Care Services for Relatives of People with Alcohol and Drug Problems', *Addiction Research & Theory*, 8: 471–81.

Copello, A., Williamson, E., Orford, J. and Day, E. (2006) 'Implementing and Evaluating Social Behaviour and Network Therapy in Drug Treatment Practice in the UK: A Feasibility Study', *Addictive Behaviors*, 31(5): 802–10.

Corby, B. (2006) *Applying Research in Social Work Practice* (Maidenhead: Open University Press).

Coulter, S. (2011) 'Systemic Family Therapy for Families who have Experienced Trauma: A Randomised Controlled Trial', *British Journal of Social Work*, 41(3): 502–19.

Council on Social Work Education (2008) *Educational Policy and Accreditation Standards* (Alexandria, VA: Council on Social Work Education).

Cox, C. (2007) 'Social Work and Dementia', in Cox, C. (ed.), *Dementia and Social Work Practice: Research and Interventions* (New York: Springer): 4–13.

Coyle, D., Macpherson, R., Foy, C., Molodynski, A., Biju, M. and Hayes, J. (2013) 'Compulsion in the Community: Mental Health Professionals' Views and Experiences of CTOs', *Psychiatrist*, 37(10): 315–21.

Cree, V. (2002) 'The Changing Nature of Social Work', in Adams, R., Dominelli, L. and Payne, M. (eds), *Social Work: Themes, Issues and Critical Debates* (Basingstoke: Palgrave Macmillan).

Crombie, I. (1996) *The Pocket Guide to Critical Appraisal* (London: BMJ Publishing Group).

Cullen, F. T. (2012) 'Taking Rehabilitation Seriously: Creativity, Science, and the Challenge of Offender Change', *Punishment and Society*, 14(1): 94–114.

D'Cruz, H. and Jones, M. (2004) *Social Work Research: Ethical and Political Contexts* (London: Sage).

Daniel, B., Wassell, S. and Gilligan, R. (2010) *Child Development for Child Care and Protection Workers* (London: Jessica Kingsley).

Davey, B., Levin, E., Iliffe, S. and Kharicha, K. (2005) 'Integrating Health and Social Care: Implications for Joint Working and Community Care Outcomes for Older People', *Journal of Interprofessional Care*, 19(1): 22–34.

Davies, C., English, I., Lodwick, A., McVeigh, J. and Bellis, M. A. (eds) (2012) *United Kingdom Drug Situation: Annual Report to the European Monitoring Centre for Drugs and Drug Addiction (EMCDDA)* (London: Department of Health).

Davies, C. and Ward, H. (2011) *Safeguarding Children Across Services: Messages from Research on Identifying and Responding to Child Maltreatment* (London: Jessica Kingsley).

Davies, H. and Nutley, S. (2002) *Discussion Paper 2. Evidence-Based Policy and Practice: Moving from Rhetoric to Reality* (St Andrews, Research Unit for Research Utilisation).

de Shazer, S. (1985) *Keys to Solution in Brief Therapy* (New York: W.W. Norton & Co.).

de Shazer, S. (1988) *Clues: Investigating Solutions in Brief Therapy* (New York: W.W. Norton & Co.).

Department for Children Schools and Families (2010) *NI 51 Statistical Release – Effectiveness of Child and Adolescent Mental Health Services (CAMHS)* (London: Department for Children, Schools and Families).

Department for Education (2013a) *The Common Assessment Framework for Children and Young People* (London: Department for Education).

Department for Education (2013b) *Working Together to Safeguard Children* (London: HMSO).

Department of Health (1997) *Developing Partnerships in Mental Health* (London: HMSO).

Department of Health (1999) *National Service Framework for Mental Health. Modern Standards and Service Models* (London: Department of Health).

Department of Health (2000) *Framework for the Assessment of Children in Need and their Families* (London: HMSO).

Department of Health (2004) *Choosing Health: Making Healthy Choices Easier* (London: Department of Health).

Department of Health (2007) *Safe. Sensible. Social. The Next Steps in the National Alcohol Strategy* (London: Department of Health).

Department of Health (2008) *Refocusing the Care Programme Approach* (London: Department of Health).

Department of Health (2009) *The Community Care, Services for Carers and Children's Services (Direct Payments) (England) Regulations 2009* (London: Department of Health).

Department of Health (2009b) *Living Well with Dementia: National Dementia Strategy* (London: Department of Health).

Dimigen, G., Del Priore, C., Butler, S., Evans, S., Ferguson, L. and Swan, M. (1999) 'Psychiatric Disorder Among Children at Time of Entering Local Authority Care', *British Medical Journal*, 319: 675–6.

Dingwall, R., Eekalaar, J. and Murray, T. (1983) *The Protection of Children: State, Intervention and Family Life* (Oxford: Blackwell).

Dixon, J. and Stein, M. (2002) *Still a Bairn: Throughcare and Aftercare Services in Scotland* (Edinburgh: Scottish Executive).

Dixon-Woods, M., Bonas, S., Booth, A., Jones, D. R., Miller, T., Sutton, A. J., Shaw, R. L., Smith, J. A. and Young, B. (2006) 'How Can Systematic Reviews Incorporate Qualitative Research? A Critical Perspective', *Qualitative Research*, 6(1): 27–44.

Dodd, S.-J. and Epstein, I. (2011) *Practice-Based Research in Social Work: A Guide for Reluctant Researchers* (London: Routledge).

Dominelli, L. (2002) *Anti-Oppressive Social Work Theory and Practice* (Basingstoke: Palgrave Macmillan).

Dominelli, L. (2004) *Social Work Theory and Practice for a Changing Profession* (Cambridge: Policy Press).

Dominelli, L. (2009) 'Social Work Research: Contested Knowledge for Practice', in Adams, R., Dominelli, L. and Payne, M. (eds), *Practising Social Work in a Complex World*, 2nd edn (Basingstoke: Palgrave Macmillan), 241–56.

Donnellan, C. (2003) *Parenting Issues* (Cambridge: Independence Publishers).

Dowden, C. and Andrews, D. A. (2004) 'The Importance of Staff Practices in Delivering Effective Correctional Treatment: A Meta-Analysis of Core Correctional Practices', *International Journal of Offender Therapy and Comparative Criminology*, 48: 203–14.

Drake, R. E., McHugo, G. J., Bebout, R. R., Becker, D. R., Harris, M., Bond, G. R. and Quimby, E. (1999) 'A Randomized Clinical Trial of Supported Employment for Inner-City Patients With Severe Mental Disorders', *Archives of General Psychiatry*, 56(7): 627–33.

Duffy, S. (2010) *Personalisation in Mental Health: A Model for the Integration of Health and Social Care* (Sheffield: Centre for Welfare Reform).

Dunn, L. (2001) 'Mental Health Act Assessments: Does a Community Treatment Team Make a Difference?', *International Journal of Social Psychiatry*, 47(2): 1–19.

Dunstan, S. (ed.) (2012) *General Lifestyle Survey Overview. A Report on the General Lifestyle Survey 2010* (London: Office for National Statistics).

Durnescu, I. (2012) 'What Matters Most on Probation Supervision: Staff Characteristics, Staff Skills or Programme?', *Criminology and Criminal Justice*, 12(2): 93–216.

Dutt, K. and Webber, M. (2010) 'Access to Social Capital and Social Support Amongst South East Asian Women with Severe Mental Health Problems: A Cross-Sectional Survey', *International Journal of Social Psychiatry*, 56(6): 593–605.

Dworkin, R. (1978) *Taking Rights Seriously* (London: Duckworth).

Enguídanos, S. M. and Jamison, P. M. (2006) 'Moving from Tacit Knowledge to Evidence-based Practice: The Kaiser Permanente Community Partners Study', *Home Health Care Services Quarterly*, 25(1/2): 13–31.

EPPI-Centre (2010) *EPPI-Centre Methods for Conducting Systematic Reviews* (London: Evidence for Policy and Practice Information and Co-ordinating Centre, Institute of Education, University of London).

Epstein, I. (1987) 'Pedagogy of the Perturbed: Teaching Research to the Reluctants', *Journal of Teaching in Social Work*, 1(1): 71–89.

Epstein, I. (2001) 'Using Available Information in Practice-Based Research: Mining for Silver While Dreaming of Gold', *Social Work in Health Care*, 33(3/4): 15–32.

Epstein, I. (2009) 'Promoting Harmony Where There is Commonly Conflict: Evidence-Informed Practice as an Integrative Strategy', *Social Work in Health Care*, 48(3): 216–31.

Epstein, I. (2010) *Clinical Data-Mining: Integrating Practice and Research* (New York: Oxford University Press).

Epstein, I. (2011) 'Reconciling Evidence-based Practice, Evidence-informed Practice, and Practice-based Research: The Role of Clinical Data-Mining', *Social Work*, 56(3): 284–8.

Epstein, L. (1996) "The Trouble with the Researcher – Practitioner Idea', *Social Work Research*, 20(2): 113–17.

Eriksson, B. G. and Hummelvoll, J. K. (2012) 'To Live as Mentally Disabled in the Risk Society', *Journal of Psychiatric and Mental Health Nursing*, 19(7): 594–602.

Evans, S. and Huxley, P. (2012) 'What Research Findings Tell Social Workers About Their Work in Mental Health', in Davies, M. (ed.), *Social Work with Adults* (Basingstoke: Palgrave Macmillan): 141–63.

Evans, T. (2010) *Professional Discretion in Welfare Services* (Aldershot: Ashgate).

Evans, T. and Hardy, M. (2010) *Evidence and Knowledge for Practice* (Cambridge: Polity).

Evans, T. and Harris, J. (2004) 'Street-Level Bureaucracy, Social Work and the (Exaggerated) Death of Discretion', *British Journal of Social Work*, 34(6): 871–95.

Farmer, E. and Moyers, S. (2008) *Kinship Care: Fostering Effective Family and Friends Placements* (London: Jessica Kingsley).

Farmer, E. and Owen, M. (1995) *Child Protection Practice: Private Risks and Public Remedies* (London: HMSO).

Farmer, E. and Wijedasa, D. (2013) 'The Reunification of Looked After Children with Their Parents: What Contributes to Return Stability?', *British Journal of Social Work*, 43(8): 1611–29.

Ferguson, I. (2007) 'Increasing User Choice or Privatizing Risk? The Antinomies of Personalization', *British Journal of Social Work*, 37(3): 387–403.

Ferguson, I. and Lavalette, M. (eds) (2014) *Adult Social Care* (Bristol: Policy Press).

Fernando, S. (2010) *Mental Health, Race and Culture*, 3rd edn (Basingstoke: Palgrave Macmillan).

Fingeld, D. L. (2003) 'Metasynthesis: The State of the Art – So Far', *Qualitative Health Research*, 13: 893–904.

Finkelstein, V. (2001) 'A Personal Journey into Disability Politics'. Available at http://disability-studies.leeds.ac.uk/files/library/finkelstein-presentn.pdf (accessed 4 April 2014).

Fitzgibbon, W. (2011) *Probation and Social Work on Trial* (Basingstoke: Palgrave Macmillan).

Folkard, M. S., Smith, D. E. and Smith, D. D. (1976) *IMPACT Vol. II: The Results of the Experiment (Home Office Research Study 36)* (London: HMSO).

Fonagy, P., Target, M., Cottrell, D., Phillips, J. and Kurtz, Z. (2002) *What Works for Whom? A Critical Review of Treatments for Children and Adolescents* (New York and London: Guilford).

Fook, J. and Gardner, F. (2007) *Practising Critical Reflection: A Resource Handbook* (Maidenhead: Open University Press).

Forrester, D. (2008) 'Is the Care System Failing Children?', *Political Quarterly*, 79(2): 206–11.

Forrester, D., Copello, A., Waisbein, C. and Pokhrel, S. (2008) 'Evaluation of an Intensive Family Prevention Service for Families Affected by Substance Misuse', *Child Abuse Review*, 17(6): 410–26.

Forrester, D., Glynn, G. and McMann, M. (2012) 'Social Work Research and Substance Misuse', in Davies, M. (ed.), *Social Work with Adults* (Basingstoke: Palgrave Macmillan).

Forrester, D. and Harwin, J. (2011) *Parents who Misuse Drugs and Alcohol. Effective Interventions in Social Work and Child Protection* (London: Wiley-Blackwell).

Fowles, A. J. (1978) *Prison Welfare: An Account of an Experiment in Liverpool (Home Office Research Study 45)* (London: HMSO).

Fraser, M. W. and Wu, S. (2013) *Satisfaction with Social Welfare Services: A Review* (Stockholm: National Board of Health and Welfare).

Fraser, S., Lewis, V., Ding, S., Kellett, M. and Robinson, C. (2004) *Doing Research with Children and Young People* (London: Sage).

Freidson, E. (1994) *Professionalism Reborn: Theory, Prophecy and Policy* (Cambridge: Polity).

Freire, P. (1972) *Pedagogy of the Oppressed* (Harmondsworth: Penguin).

Fryers, T., Melzer, D. and Jenkins, R. (2003) 'Social Inequalities and the Common Mental Disorders: A Systematic Review of the Evidence', *Social Psychiatry and Psychiatric Epidemiology*, 38(5): 229–37.

Furminger, E. and Webber, M. (2009) 'The Effect of Crisis Resolution and Home Treatment on Assessments under the 1983 Mental Health Act: An Increased Workload for Approved Social Workers?', *British Journal of Social Work*, 39(5): 901–17.

Furness, S. and Gilligan, P. (2010) *Religion, Belief and Social Work: Making a Difference* (Bristol: Policy Press).

Gadda, A. (2012) *Looking After Young People? An Exploratory Study of Home Supervision Requirements in Scotland. PhD Summary Report for the Scottish Government* (Edinburgh: University of Edinburgh).

Galvani, S. (2007) 'Refusing to Listen: Are We Failing the Needs of People with Alcohol and Drug Problems?', *Social Work Education*, 26(7): 697–707.

Galvani , S. (2012) *Supporting People with Alcohol and Drug Problems. Making a Difference* (Bristol: Policy Press).

Galvani, S. and Forrester, D. (2011) *Social Work Services and Recovery from Substance Misuse. A Review of the Evidence* (Edinburgh: Scottish Government).

Galvani, S., Hutchinson, A. and Dance, C. (2013) 'Identifying and Assessing Substance Use: Findings From a National Survey of Social Work and Social Care Professionals', *British Journal of Social Work*, Advance Access, doi:10.1093/bjsw/bct033

Galvani, S. and Livingston, W. (2012a) *Mental Health and Substance Use. A BASW Pocket Guide* (Birmingham: British Association of Social Workers).

Galvani, S. and Livingston, W. (2012b) *Young People and Alcohol. A BASW Pocket Guide* (Birmingham: British Association of Social Workers).

Gambrill, E. (1999) 'Evidence Based Practice: An Alternative to Authority-Based Practice', *Families in Society: The Journal of Contemporary Human Services*, 80(4): 341–50.

Gambrill, E. (2011) 'Evidence-Based Practice and the Ethics of Discretion', *Journal of Social Work*, 11(1), 26–48.

Garbarino, J. (1981) 'An Ecological Approach to Child Maltreatment', in Pelton, L. H. (ed.), *The Social Context of Child Abuse and Neglect*. (New York: Human Sciences Press): 228–67.

Gardner, A. (2012) 'Curriculum Guide – Personalisation'. Available at http://www.tcsw.org.uk/uploadedFiles/TheCollege/Media_centre/CG_Personalisation.pdf (accessed 4 April 2014).

Garety, P. A., Craig, T. K. J., Dunn, G., Fornells-Ambrojo, M., Colbert, S., Rahaman, N., Read, J. and Power, P. (2006) 'Specialised Care for Early Psychosis: Symptoms, Social Functioning and Patient Satisfaction: Randomised Controlled Trial', *British Journal of Psychiatry*, 188(1): 37–45.

Garety, P. A., Fowler, D. G., Freeman, D., Bebbington, P., Dunn, G. and Kuipers, E. (2008)

'Cognitive-Behavioural Therapy and Family Intervention for Relapse Prevention and Symptom Reduction in Psychosis: Randomised Controlled Trial', *British Journal of Psychiatry*, 192(6): 412–23.

Garland, D. (1996) 'The Limits of the Sovereign State', *British Journal of Criminology*, 36(4): 445–71.

Geertz, C. (1973) *The Interpretation of Cultures: Selected Essays* (New York: Basic Books).

Ghate, D. and Daniels, A. (1997) *Talking About My Generation* (London: NSPCC).

Gibbs, L. and Gambrill, E. (2002) 'Evidence-Based Practice: Counterarguments to Objections', *Research on Social Work Practice*, 12(3): 452–76.

Gilgun, J. (1994) 'Hand Into Glove. The Grounded Theory Approach and Social Work Practice Research', in Sherman, E. and Reid, W. J. (eds), *Qualitative Research in Social Work* (New York: Columbia University Press): 115–25.

Gilligan, P. and Manby, M. (2008) 'The Common Assessment Framework: Does the Reality Match the Rhetoric?', *Child and Family Social Work*, 13(2): 177–87.

Gilligan, R. (1997) 'Beyond Permanence? The Importance of Resilience in Child Placement Practice and Planning', *Adoption and Fostering*, 21: 12–20.

Gilligan, R. (2000) 'Adversity, Resilience and Young People. The Protective Value of Positive School and Spare Time Experiences', *Children and Society*, 14: 37–47.

Glasby, J. (2011) 'From Evidence Based to Knowledge Based Policy and Practice', in Glasby, J. (ed.), *Evidence, Policy and Practice: Critical Perspectives in Health and Social Care* (Bristol: Policy Press).

Glasby, J. (2014) 'The Controversies of Choice and Control: Why Some People Might Be Hostile to English Social Care Reforms', *British Journal of Social Work*, 44(2): 252–66.

Glasby, J. and Beresford, P. (2006) 'Commentary and Issues : Who Knows Best? Evidence-Based Practice and the Service User Contribution', *Critical Social Policy*, 26: 268–84.

Glendinning, C., Challis, D., Fernández, J.-L., Jacobs, S., Jones, K., Knapp, M., Manthorpe, J., Moran, N., Netten, A., Stevens, M. and Wilberforce, M. (2008) *Evaluation of the Individual Budgets Pilot Programme: Final Report* (York: Social Policy Research Unit, University of York).

Glenndenning, J. (2012) *Children Looked After by Local Authorities in England (Including Adoption and Care Leavers) – Year Ending 31 March 2012* (London: Department for Education).

Goggin, C. and Gendreau, P. (2006) 'The Implementation of Quality Services in Offender Rehabilitation Programmes', in Hollin, C. R. and Palmer, E. J. (eds), *Offender Behaviour Programmes: Development, Application and Controversies* (Chichester: Wiley): 69–111.

Goldblatt, P. and Lewis, C. (1998) *Reducing Offending: An Assessment of Research Evidence on Ways of Dealing with Offending Behaviour (Home Office Research Study 187)* (London: Home Office).

Goldmeier, J. (1994) 'Intervention with Elderly Substance Abusers in the Workplace', *Families in Society*, 75(10): 624–9.

Goodman, A. (2007) *Social Work with Drug and Substance Misusers* (Exeter: Learning Matters).

Goodman, R. (1997) 'The Strengths and Difficulties Questionnaire: A Research Note', *Journal of Child Psychology and Psychiatry*, 38: 581–6.

Gordon, J., Cooper, B. and Dumbleton, S. (2009) *How do Social Workers use Evidence in Practice?* (Milton Keynes: Open University).

Gossop, M. (2006) *Treating Drug Misuse Problems: Evidence of Effectiveness* (London: National Treatment Agency).

Gough, D. (2007) 'Weight of Evidence: A Framework for the Appraisal of the Quality and Relevance of Evidence', *Research Papers in Education*, 22(2): 213–28.

Gould, N. (1989) 'Reflective Learning for Social Work Practice', *Social Work Education*, 8(2): 9–20.

Gould, N. (2006) 'An Inclusive Approach to Knowledge for Mental Health Social Work Practice and Policy', *British Journal of Social Work*, 36(1): 109–25.

Gould, N. (2008) 'Research', in Davies, M. (ed.), *The Blackwell Companion To Social Work* (Oxford: Blackwell).

Gould, N. (2010) *Mental Health Social Work in Context* (London: Routledge).

Gould, N. and Taylor, I. (eds) (1996) *Reflective Learning for Social Work: Theory, Research and Practice* (Aldershot: Arena).

Gray, M., Coates, J. and Yellow Bird, M. (eds) (2010) *Indigenous Social Work Around the World: Towards Culturally Relevant Education and Practice* (Aldershot: Ashgate).

Gray, M., Joy, E., Plath, D. and Webb, S. A. (2013a) 'Implementing Evidence-Based Practice: A Review of the Empirical Research Literature', *Research on Social Work Practice*, 23(2): 157–66.

Gray, M., Joy, E., Plath, D. and Webb, S. A. (2013b) 'What Supports and Impedes Evidence-Based Practice Implementation? A Survey of Australian Social Workers', *British Journal of Social Work*, Advance Access, 10.1093/bjsw/bct123

Grayson, L. and Gomersall, A. (2003) *A Difficult Business: Finding the Evidence for Social Science Reviews. ESRC UK Working Paper 19* (London: ESRC).

Green, H., McGinnity, A., Meltzer, H., Ford, T. and Goodman, R. (2005) *Mental Health of Children and Young People in Great Britain* (London: Ashford Press).

Gridley, K., Brooks, J. and Glendinning, C. (2012) *Good Support for People with Complex Needs: What Does It Look Like and Where Is the Evidence? Research Findings* (London: National Institute for Health Research School for Social Care Research).

Gross, D., Fogg, L. and Tucker, S. (1995) 'The Efficacy of Parent Training for Promoting Positive Parent–Toddler Relationships', *Research in Nursing and Health*, 18: 489–99.

Grover, C. and Mason, C. (2013) 'The Allen Report: Class, Gender and Disadvantage', *Families, Relationships & Societies*, doi: 10.1332/204674313X669829

Hahn, H. (1985) 'Toward a Politics of Disability: Definitions, Disciplines, and Policies', *Social Science Journal*, 22(4): 87–105.

Hammersley, M. (2013) *The Myth of Research Based Policy and Practice* (London: Sage).

Hardy, M. (2012) 'Overstating the Case? The Trials and Tribulations of Social Work with Offenders', *Qualitative Social Work*, 11(6): 677–90.

Haringey Local Safeguarding Children Board (2009) *Serious Case Review: Baby Peter. Executive Summary* (London: Haringey Local Safeguarding Children Board).

Harris, J. (2003) *The Social Work Business* (London: Routledge).

Harris, N. (2002) 'Neuroleptic Drugs and Their Management', in Harris, N., Williams, S. and Bradshaw, T. (eds), *Psychosocial Interventions for People with Schizophrenia A Practical Guide for Mental Health Workers* (Basingstoke: Palgrave Macmillan): 68–83.

Harrison, L. (1992) 'Substance Misuse and Social Work Qualifying Training in the British Isles: A Survey of CQSW Courses', *British Journal of Addiction*, 87(4): 635–42.

Harrison, L. (1996) *Alcohol Problems in the Community* (London: Routledge).

Hasler, F. (1993) 'Developments in the Disabled People's Movement', in Swain, J., Finkelstein, V., French, S. and Oliver, M. (eds), *Disabling Barriers – Enabling Environments*. (London: Sage): 278–84.

Hatton, C. and Waters, J. (2011) *The National Personal Budget Survey* (Lancaster: In Control/Lancaster University).

Hatton, C. and Waters, J. (2013) *The Second POET Survey of Personal Budget Holders and Carers* (Lancaster, In Control/Lancaster University).

Health Advisory Service (2001) *The Substance of Young Needs: Review 2001* (Brighton: Pavilion Publishing).

Health and Care Professions Council (2011) *Standards of Proficiency – Social Workers in England* (London: Health and Care Professions Council).

Health and Care Professions Council (2012) *Standards of Proficiency – Social Workers in England* (London: Health and Care Professions Council).

Her Majesty's Government (2008) *Drugs: Protecting Families and Communities. The 2008 Drug Strategy* (London: Home Office).

Her Majesty's Government (2010) *Drugs Strategy 2010. Reducing Demand, Restricting Supply, Building Recovery: Supporting People to Live a Drug Free Life* (London: Home Office).

Her Majesty's Treasury (2011) *Magenta Book: Guidance for Evaluation* (London: HM Treasury).

Hewitt-Taylor, J. (2011) *Using Research in Practice* (Basingstoke: Palgrave Macmillan).

Heyman, B., Shaw, M., Alaszewski, A. and Titterton, M. (2010) *Risk, Safety and Clinical Practice: Healthcare Through the Lens of Risk* (Oxford: Oxford University Press).

Hoare, J. and Moon, D. (eds) (2010) *Drug Misuse Declared: Findings from the 2009/10 British Crime Survey England and Wales* (London: HMSO).

Holland, S. (2011) *Child and Family Assessment in Social Work Practice*, 2nd edn (London: Sage).

Holland, S., Faulkner, A. and Perez-del-Aguila, R. (2005) 'Promoting Stability and Continuity of Care for Looked After Children: A Survey and Critical Review', *Child and Family Social Work*, 10: 29–41.

Hollis, F. (1964) *Casework: A Psychosocial Therapy* (New York: Random House).

Hollomotz, A. (2012) 'Are We Valuing People's Choices Now? Restrictions to Mundane Choices Made by Adults with Learning Difficulties', *British Journal of Social Work*, 44(2): 234–51.

Home Office (2012) *Drug Misuse Declared: Findings from the 2011/12 Crime Survey for England and Wales*, 2nd edn (London: Home Office).

Horwarth, J. (2013) *Child Neglect: Planning and Intervention* (Basingstoke: Palgrave Macmillan).

Howard, P., Francis, B., Soothill, K. and Humphreys, L. (2009) *OGRS 3: The Revised Offender*

Group Reconviction Scale (Ministry of Justice Research Summary 7/09) (London: Ministry of Justice).

Howe, D. (1995) *Attachment Theory for Social Work Practice* (Basingstoke: Palgrave Macmillan).

Howe, D. (2005) *Child Abuse and Neglect: Attachment, Development and Intervention* (Basingstoke: Palgrave).

Howe, D., Brandon, M., Hinings, D. and Schofield, G. (1999) *Attachment Theory, Child Maltreatment and Family Support: A Practice and Assessment Model* (Basingstoke: Macmillan).

Hudson, C. G. (2009) 'Decision Making in Evidence Based Practice: Science and Art', *Smith College Studies in Social Work*, 79: 155–74.

Humphreys, K. (2004) *Circles of Recovery: Self-Help Organisations for Addiction* (Cambridge: Cambridge University Press).

Humphreys, K. and Moos, R. H. (2007) 'Encouraging Posttreatment Self-Help Group Involvement to Reduce the Demand for Continuing Care Services: Two Year Clinical and Utilisation Outcomes', *Alcoholism: Clinical and Experimental Research*, 31(1): 64–8.

Humphries, B. (2008) *Social Work Research and Social Justice* (Basingstoke: Palgrave Macmillan).

Hunt, J., Waterhouse, S. and Lutman, E. (2008) *Keeping Them in the Family: Outcomes for Children Placed in Kinship Care Through Proceedings* (London: British Association for Adoption and Fostering).

Hunt, P. (1981) 'Settling Accounts with the Parasite People: A Critique of "A Life Apart" by E.J Miller and G.V.Gwynne', *Disability Challenge*, 1: 37–50.

Hurcombe, R., Bayley, M. and Goodman, A. (2010) *Ethnicity and Alcohol: A Review of the Literature* (York: Joseph Rowntree Foundation).

Hutchings, J., Nash, S., Smith, M. and Parry, G. (1998) *Long-Term Outcome for Pre-School Children Referred to CAMH Team for Behaviour Management Problems* (Bangor: School of Psychology, University of Wales).

Hutchinson, A., Galvani, S. and Dance, C. (2013) 'Working with Substance Use: Levels and Predictors of Positive Therapeutic Attitudes Across Social Care Practitioners in England', *Drugs: Education, Prevention and Policy*, 20(4): 312–21.

Huxley, A., Copello, A. and Day, E. (2005) 'Substance Misuse and the Need for Integrated Services', *Learning Disability Practice*, 8(6): 14–17.

Huxley, P., Baker, C., White, J., Madge, S., Onyett, S. and Gould, N. (2012) 'The Social Care Component of Multidisciplinary Mental Health Teams: A Review and National Survey', *Journal of Health Services Research & Policy*, 17 (Supplement 2): 23–9.

Huxley, P., Mohamad, H., Korer, J., Jacob, C., Raval, H. and Anthony, P. (1989a) 'Psychiatric Morbidity in Clients of Social Workers: Social Outcome', *Social Psychiatry & Psychiatric Epidemiology*, 24(5): 258–65.

Huxley, P., Raval, H., Korer, J. and Jacob, C. (1989b) 'Psychiatric Morbidity in the Clients of Social Workers: Clinical Outcome', *Psychological Medicine*, 19(1): 189–97.

Huxley, P. and Thornicroft, G. (2003) 'Social Inclusion, Social Quality and Mental Illness', *British Journal of Psychiatry*, 182(4): 289–90.

Iganski, P., Smith, D., Dixon, L., Kielinger, V., Mason, G., McDevitt, J., Perry, B., Stelman, A., Bargen, J., Lagou, S. and Pfeffer, R. (2011) *Rehabilitation of Hate Crime Offenders* (Glasgow: Equality and Human Rights Commission).

International Federation of Social Workers (2013) 'Gobal Definition of Social Work: Update'. Available at http://ifsw.org/get-involved/global-definition-of-social-work/ (accessed 3 December 2013).

Jolley, D. (2005) 'Why Do People with Dementia Become Disabled', in Marshall, M. (ed.), *Perspectives on Rehabilitation and Dementia.* (London: Jessica Kingsley): 20–9.

Kaambwa, B., Bryan, S., Barton, P., Parker, H., Martin, G., Hewitt, G., Parker, S. and Wilson, A. (2008) "Costs and Health Outcomes of Intermediate Care: Results From Five UK Case Sites', *Health & Social Care in the Community*, 16(6): 573–81.

Kazi, M. (2003) *Realist Evaluation in Practice* (London: Sage).

Keene, J. (2010) *Understanding Drug Misuse. Models of Care and Control* (Basingstoke: Palgrave Macmillan).

Kelleher, I., Keeley, H., Corcoran, P., Lynch, F., Fitzpatrick, C., Devlin, N., Molloy, C., Roddy, S., Clarke, M. C., Harley, M., Arseneault, L., Wasserman, C., Carli, V., Sarchiapone, M., Hoven, C., Wasserman, D. and Cannon, M. (2012) 'Clinicopathological Significance of Psychotic Experiences in Non-Psychotic Young People: Evidence From Four Population-Based Studies', *British Journal of Psychiatry*, 201(1): 26–32.

Kemshall, H. (1998) 'Defensible Decisions for Risk: Or "It's the Doers Wot Get the Blame"', *Probation Journal*, 45(6): 67–72.

Kendrick, A. (2008) 'Introduction: Residential Child Care', in Kendrick, A. (ed.), *Residential Child Care: Prospects and Challenges* (London: Jessica Kingsley), 7–15.

Kerson, T. (2004) 'Boundary Spanning: An Ecological Reinterpretation of Social Work Practice in Health and Mental Health Systems', *Social Work in Mental Health*, 2(2): 39–57.

Khoo, E. and Skoog, V. (2014) 'The Road to Placement Breakdown: Foster Parents' Experiences of the Events Surrounding the Unexpected Ending of a Child's Placement in Their Care', *Qualitative Social Work*, 13(2): 255–69.

Killaspy, H., Bebbington, P., Blizard, R., Johnson, S., Nolan, F., Pilling, S. and King, M. (2006) 'The REACT Study: Randomised Evaluation of Assertive Community Treatment in North London', *British Medical Journal*, 332: 815–19.

Kingsford, R. and Webber, M. (2010) 'Social Deprivation and the Outcomes of Crisis Resolution and Home Treatment for People With Mental Health Problems: A Historical Cohort Study', *Health & Social Care in the Community*, 18(5): 456–64.

Kirk, S. A. and Reid, W. J. (2002) *Science and Social Work: A Critical Appraisal* (New York: Columbia University Press).

Knapp, M. and Prince, M. (2007) *Dementia UK* (London: Alzheimer's Society).

Kosonen, M. (1996) 'Maintaining Sibling Relationships: Neglected Dimension in Child Care Practice', *British Journal of Social Work*, 26: 809–22.

Kroll, B. and Taylor, A. (2003) *Parental Substance Use and Child Welfare* (London: Jessica Kingsley).

Kuhn, T. (1970) *The Structure of Scientific Revolutions* (Chicago: University of Chicago Press).

Kurtz, E. (1991) *Not-God: A History of Alcoholic Anonymous* (Minnesota: Hazelden Pittman Archive Press).

Kurtz, Z., Thornes, R. and Wolind, S. (1995) *Services for the Mental Health of Children and Young People in England: Assessment of Needs and Unmet Need* (London: HMSO).

Lambert, H. (2006) 'Accounting for EBM: Notions of Evidence in Medicine', *Social Science & Medicine*, 62: 2633–45.

Langan, J. and Lindow, V. (2004) *Living with Risk. Mental Health Service User Involvement in Risk Assessment and Management* (Bristol: Policy Press/Joseph Rowntree Foundation).

Lavalette, M. (ed.) (2011) *Radical Social Work Today: Social Work at the Crossroads* (Bristol: Polity Press).

Lavoie, D. (2010) 'Alcohol Identification and Brief Advice in England: A Major Plank in Alcohol Harm Reduction Policy', *Drug and Alcohol Review*, 29(6): 608–11.

Le Mesurier, N. and Cumella, S. (2001) 'The Rough Road and the Smooth Road: Comparing Access to Social Care for Older People via Area Teams and GP Surgeries', *Managing Community Care*, 9(1): 7–13.

Leff, J. P., Kuipers, L., Berkowitz, R., Eberlein-Fries, R. and Sturgeon, D. (1982) 'A Controlled Trial of Social Intervention in Schizophrenia Families', *British Journal of Psychiatry*, 141: 121–34.

Leonard, P. (1997) *Postmodern Welfare: Reconstructing an Emancipatory Project* (London: Sage).

Lewis, J. (2001) 'What Works in Community Care?', *Managing Community Care*, 9(1), 3–6.

Lightfoot, P. and Orford, J. (1986) 'Helping Agents Attitudes Towards Alcohol Related Problems: Situations Vacant? A Test of an Elaboration of a Model', *British Journal of Addiction*, 81: 749–56.

Lipsey, M., Landenberger, N. A. and Wilson, S.J. (2007) 'Effects of Cognitive-Behavioral Programs for Criminal Offenders', *Campbell Systematic Reviews*, 6.

Lishman, J. (ed.) (2007) *Handbook for Practice Learning in Social Work and Social Care. Knowledge and Theory*, 2nd edn (London: Jessica Kingsley).

Livingston, W., Baker, M., Atkins, B. and Jobber, S. (2011) 'A Tale of the Spontaneous Emergence of a Recovery Group and the Characteristics That Are Making It Thrive: Exploring the Politics and Knowledge of Recovery', *Journal of Groups in Addiction and Recovery*, 6(1): 176–96.

Livingston, W. and Galvani, S. (2012) *Older People and Alcohol. A BASW Pocket Guide* (Birmingham: British Association of Social Workers).

Lloyd, E. (ed.) (1999) *Parenting Matters: What Works in Parenting Education?* (London: Barnardos).

Long, A., Grayson, L. and Boaz, A. (2006) 'Assessing the Quality of Knowledge in Social Care: Exploring the Potential of a Set of Generic Standards', *British Journal of Social Work*, 36: 207–26.

Lord Laming (2003) *The Victoria Climbié inquiry. Report of an Inquiry by Lord Laming. Cm 5730* (London: HMSO).

Lord Laming (2009) *The Protection of Children in England: A Progress Report* (London: HMSO).

Lundahl, B. W., Kunz, C., Brownell, C., Tollefson, D. and Burke, B. L. (2010) 'A Meta-Analysis of Motivational Interviewing: Twenty-Five Years of Empirical Studies', *Research on Social Work Practice*, 20(2): 137–60.

Lutman, E. and Farmer, E. (2013) 'What Contributes to Outcomes for Neglected Children Who Are Reunified with Their Parents? Findings from a Five-Year Follow-Up Study', *British Journal of Social Work*, 43(3): 559–78.

Macdonald, G. (2001) *Effective Interventions for Child Abuse and Neglect: An Evidence-Based Approach to Planning and Executing Interventions* (Chichester: Wiley).

Macdonald, G. (2003) *Using Systematic Reviews to Improve Social Care* (London: Social Care Institute for Excellence).

Macdonald, G. and Sheldon, B. (1998) 'Changing One's Mind: The Final Frontier?', *Issues in Social Work Education*, 18(1): 3–25.

MacIntyre, G. and Paul, S. (2012) 'Teaching Research in Social Work: Capacity and Challenge', *British Journal of Social Work*, doi: 10.1093/bjsw/bcs010

Magill, M. (2006) 'The Future of Evidence in Evidence-Based Practice: Who Will Answer the Call for Clinical Relevance?', *Journal of Social Work*, 6: 101.

Magill, M. and Ray, L. A. (2009) 'Cognitive Behavioral Treatment with Adult Alcohol and Illicit Drug Users: A Meta-Analysis of Randomized Controlled Trials', *Journal of Studies on Alcohol and Drugs*, 70(4): 516–27.

Maguire, M. (2004) 'The Crime Reduction Programme in England and Wales: Reflections on the Vision and the Reality', *Criminology and Criminal Justice*, 4(3): 213–37.

Mair, G. (ed.) (2004) *What Matters in Probation.* (Cullompton: Willan).

Mair, G., Cross, N. and Taylor, S. (2008) *The Community Order and the Suspended Sentence Order: The Views and Attitudes of Sentencers* (London: Centre for Crime and Justice Studies).

Maluccio, A. N., Fein, E. and Olmstead, K. A. (1986) *Permanency Planning for Children: Concepts and Methods* (New York: Tavistock Publications).

Manning, V., Best, D., Faulkner, N. and Titherington, E. (2009) 'New Estimates of the Number of Children Living with Substance Misusing Parents: Results from UK National Household Surveys', *BMC Public Health*, 9(1): 377.

Manning, V. C., Strathdee, G., Best, D., Keaney, F. and McGillivray, L. (2002) 'Dual Diagnosis Screening: Preliminary Findings on the Comparison of 50 Clients Attending Community Mental Health Services and 50 Clients Attending Community Substance Misuse Services', *Journal of Substance Use*, 7(4): 221–8.

Manthorpe, J. and Samsi, K. (2013) '"Inherently Risky?": Personal Budgets for People with Dementia and the Risks of Financial Abuse: Findings from an Interview-Based Study with Adult Safeguarding Coordinators', *British Journal of Social Work*, 43(5): 889–903.

Mari, J. and Streiner, D. (1999) *Family Intervention for Schizophrenia (Cochrane Review), Cochrane Library, Issue 1* (Oxford: Update Software).

Marmot, M. (2010) *Fair Society, Healthy Lives. The Marmot Review. Strategic Review of Health Inequalities in England Post-2010* (London: Institute of Health Equity, University College London).

Marsh, P. and Fisher, M. (2005) *Developing the Evidence Base for Social Work and Social Care Practice* (London: Social Care Institute for Excellence).

Marshall, L. E. and Marshall, W. L. (2012) 'The Risk/Needs/Responsivity Model: The Crucial Features of General Responsivity', in Bowen, E. and Brown, S. (eds), *Perspectives on Evaluating Criminal Justice and Corrections* (Bingley: Emerald): 29–45.

Marshall, M. and Lockwood, A. (1998) 'Assertive Community Treatment for People with Severe Mental Disorders', *Cochrane Library, Issue 2* (Oxford: Update Software).

Martinez-Brawley, E. E. and Zorita, P. M. B. (1998) 'At the Edge of the Frame: Beyond Science and Art in Social Work', *British Journal of Social Work*, 28(2): 197–212.

Martinez-Brawley, E. E. and Zorita, P. M. B. (2007) 'Tacit and Codified Knowledge in Social Work: A Critique of Standardization in Education and Practice', *Families in Society*, 88(4): 534–42.

Martinson, R. (1974) 'What Works? Questions and Answers About Prison Reform', *Public Interest*, 35: 22–54.

Maruna, S. (2001) *Making Good: How Ex-convicts Reform and Rebuild Their Lives* (Washington, DC: American Psychological Association).

Mayer, J. E. and Timms, N. (1970) *The Client Speaks: Working Class Impressions of Casework* (New York: Atherton).

Maynard-Campbell, S., Maynard, A. and Winchombe, M. (2007) *Mapping the Capacity and Potential for User-Led Organisations in England: A Summary of the Main Findings from a*

National Research Study Commissioned by the Department of Health (London: Department of Health).

McCarthy, T. and Galvani, S. (2012) *Children and Families and Alcohol use. A BASW Pocket Guide* (Birmingham: British Association of Social Workers).

McClung, M. and Gayle, V. (2010) 'Exploring the Care Effects of Multiple Factors on the Educational Achievement of Children Looked After at Home and Away From Home: An Investigation of Two Scottish Local Authorities', *Child and Family Social Work*, 15(4): 409–31.

McCracken, D. (1988) *The Long Interview* (Newbury Park, CA: Sage).

McCracken, S. G. and Marsh, J. C. (2008) 'Practitioner Expertise in Evidence-Based Practice Decision Making', *Research on Social Work Practice*, 18(4): 301–10.

McCrae, N., Murray, J., Huxley, P. and Evans, S. (2005) 'The Research Potential of Mental Health Social Workers: A Qualitative Study of the Views of Senior Mental Health Service Managers', *British Journal of Social Work*, 35(1): 55–71.

McCrory, E. S., De Brito, A. and E., V. (2012) 'The Link Between Child Abuse and Psychopathology: A Review of the Neurobiological and Genetic Research', *Journal of the Royal Society of Medicine*, 105: 151–6.

McGorry, P. D., Edwards, J., Mihalopoulos, C., Harrigan, S. M. and Jackson, H. J. (1996) 'EPPIC: An Evolving System of Early Detection and Optimal Management', *Schizophrenia Bulletin*, 22(2): 305–26.

McGuire, J. (1995) What Works: Reducing Re-offending. Guidelines from Research and Practice (Chichester: Wiley).

McIvor, G. (1990) *Sanctions for Serious and Persistent Offenders* (Stirling: Social Work Research Centre).

McLaughlin, H. (2007) *Understanding Social Work Research* (London: Sage).

McLaughlin, H. (2010) 'Keeping Service User Involvement in Research Honest', *British Journal of Social Work*, 40(5): 1591–608.

McLaughlin, H. (2012) *Understanding Social Work Research*, 2nd edn (London: Sage).

McNeill, F. (2006) 'A Desistance Paradigm for Offender Management', *Criminology and Criminal Justice*, 6(1): 39–62.

McNeill, F. (2009) *Towards Effective Practice in Offender Supervision* (Glasgow: Scottish Centre for Crime and Justice Research).

McNeill, F., Raynor, P. and Trotter, C. (eds) (2010) *Offender Supervision: New Directions in Theory, Research and Practice* (Cullompton: Willan).

McNeill, F. and Weaver, B. (2010) *Changing Lives? Desistance Research and Offender Management* (Glasgow: Scottish Centre for Crime and Justice Research).

McNicoll, A. (2013) 'Councils Split on Integration of Mental Health Social Workers in the NHS'. Available at http://www.communitycare.co.uk/blogs/mental-health/2013/09/councils-split-on-full-integration-of-mental-health-social-workers-in-nhs/ (accessed 7 April 2014).

Meacher, M. (1972) *Taken for a Ride: Special Residential Homes for Confused Old People: A Study of Separatism in Social Policy* (London: Longman).

Meltzer, H., Gatward, R., Goodman, R. and T. F. (2003) *The Mental Health of Young People Looked After by Local Authorities in England* (London: HMSO).

Meltzer, H., Singleton, N., Lee, A., Bebbington, P., Brugha, T. and Jenkins, R. (2002) *The Social and Economic Circumstances of Adults with Mental Disorders* (London: HMSO).

Mental Health Foundation (1999) *The Big Picture: A National Survey of Child Mental Health in Britain* (London: Mental Health Foundation).

Mental Health Foundation (2011) *Personal Budgets for People with Dementia* (London: Mental Health Foundation).

Mental Health Foundation (2014) *Research on MCA* (London: Mental Health Foundation).

Mikulincer, M. and Shaver, P. R. (2007) *Attachment in Adulthood: Structure, Dynamics and Change* (New York: Guilford Press).

Miller, E. J. and Gwynne, G. V. (1972) *A Life Apart: A Pilot Study of Residential Institutions for the Physically Handicapped and Young Chronically Sick* (London: Tavistock Publications).

Miller, G. and Prinz, R. (1990) 'Enhancement of Social Learning Family Interventions for Childhood Conduct Disorders', *Psychological Bulletin*, 108: 291–307.

Miller, W. and Rollnick, S. (2002) *Motivational Interviewing: Preparing People for Change*, 2nd edn (New York: Guilford Press).

Milner, J. and O'Byrne, P. (2009) *Assessment in Social Work*, 3rd edn (Basingstoke: Palgrave Macmillan).

Ministry of Justice (2011) *National Standards for the Management of Offenders in England and Wales* (London: Ministry of Justice).

Moore, N. (2002) 'A Model of Social Information Need', *Journal of Information Science*, 28(2): 297–303.

Morgan, H. (2012) 'The Social Model of Disability as a Threshold Concept: Troublesome Knowledge and Liminal Spaces in Social Work Education', *Social Work Education*, 31(2): 215–26.

Morgan, H. (2014) 'User-Led Organisations: Facilitating Independent Living?', in Swain, J., French, S., Barnes, C. and Thomas, C. (eds), *Disabling Barriers – Enabling Environments*, 3rd edn (London: Sage): 206–13.

Morgan, H. and Roulstone, A. (2012) 'Special Issue: Disability Studies and Social Work Education', *Social Work Education*, 31(2).

Moriarty, J. (2012) 'Carers and the Role of the Family', in Sinclair, A. J., Morley, J. E. and Vellas, B. (eds), *Pathy's Principles and Practice of Geriatric Medicine*, 5th edn (Chichester: Wiley): 2838–55.

Moriarty, J. and Manthorpe, J. (2012) *Diversity in Older People and Access to Services: An Evidence Review* (London: Age UK).

Morrow, V. (1998) *Understanding Families: Children's Perspectives* (London: National Children's Bureau).

Moselhy, H. F. (2009) 'Co-morbid Post-Traumatic Stress Disorder and Opioid Dependence Syndrome', *Journal of Dual Diagnosis*, 5(1): 30–40.

Moyer, A., Finney, J., Swearingen, C. and Vergun, P. (2002) 'Brief Interventions for Alcohol Problems: A Meta-Analytic Review of Controlled Investigations in Treatment-Seeking and Non-Treatment Seeking Populations', *Addiction*, 97(3): 279–92.

Mullen, E. J. and Bacon, W. (2004) 'Implementation of Practice Guidelines and Evidence Based Treatment: A Survey of Psychiatrists, Psychologists and Social Workers', in Roberts, A. R. and Yeager, K. (eds), *Evidence Based Practice Manual: Research and Outcome Measures in Health and Human Services* (New York: Oxford University Press): 210–18.

Mullen, E. J., Bledsoe, S. E. and Bellamy, J. L. (2008) 'Implementing Evidence-Based Social Work Practice', *Research on Social Work Practice*, 18(4): 325–38.

Munro, E. (1999) 'Common Errors of Reasoning in Child Protection Work', *Child Abuse and Neglect*, 23(8): 745–58.

Munro, E. (2003) *Formal Risk Assessment Instruments or Intuitive Knowledge?* (Houten, Netherlands: Bohn Stafleu Van Loghum).

Munro, E. (2005) 'Improving Practice: Child Protection as a Systems Problem', *Children and Youth Services Review*, 27(4): 375–91.

Munro, E. (2008) *Effective Child Protection*, 2nd edn (Los Angeles, CA: Sage).

Munro, E. (2010) 'Learning to Reduce Risk in Child Protection', *British Journal of Social Work*, 40(4): 1135–51.

Munro, E. (2011) *The Munro Review of Child Protection: Final Report. A Child-Centred System* (London: Department for Education).

Murphy, M. (2004) *Developing Collaborative Relationships in Interagency Child Protection Work* (Lyme Regis: Russell House Publishing).

Murray, G. K. and Jones, P. B. (2012) 'Psychotic Symptoms in Young People Without Psychotic Illness: Mechanisms and Meaning', *British Journal of Psychiatry*, 201(1): 4–6.

Nathan, J. and Webber, M. (2010) 'Mental Health Social Work and the Bureau-Medicalisation of Mental Health Care: Identity in a Changing World', *Journal of Social Work Practice*, 24(1): 15–28.

National Centre for Independent Living (2008) *Review of Peer Support Activity in the Context of Self-Directed Support and the Personalisation of Adult Social Care* (London: National Centre for Independent Living).

National Collaborating Centre for Mental Health (2010) *Schizophrenia. The NICE Guideline on Core Interventions in the Treatment and Management of Schizophrenia in Primary and Secondary Care. Updated edn* (London: National Institute for Health and Clinical Excellence).

National Collaborating Centre for Mental Health (2012) *Service User Experience in Adult Mental Health* (London: British Psychological Society and Gaskell).

National Evaluation of Sure Start (2005) *Implementing Sure Start Local Programmes: An In-Depth Study. Part Two: A Close Up On Services* (London: Department for Education and Skills).

National Institute for Health and Care Excellence (2014) *Psychosis and Schizophrenia in Adults: Treatment and Management. NICE Clinical Guideline 178* (London: National Institute for Health and Care Excellence).

National Institute for Health and Clinical Excellence (2009) *Depression in Adults. The Treatment and Management of Depression in Adults. NICE Clinical Guideline 90* (London: National Institute for Health and Clinical Excellence).

Needham, M. (2007) *Changing Habits. North West Dual Diagnosis Intelligence Report. Informing the Commissioning, Management and Provision of Integrated Service Provision for Dual Diagnosis Treatment Populations. Emerging Findings – Access to Mental Health Treatment for Adults with Substance and/or Alcohol Misuse Problems Part of the CSIP National Dual Diagnosis Programme* (Hyde, Cheshire: North West CSIP).

Neil, E., Cossar, J., Lorgelly, P. and Young, J. (2010) *Helping Birth Families: Services, Costs and Outcomes* (London: British Association for Adoption and Fostering).

Neil, E. and Howe, D. (eds) (2004) *Contact in Adoption and Permanent Foster Care.* (London: British Association for Adoption and Fostering).

Netten, A., Jones, K., Knapp, M., Fernandez, J. L., Challis, D., Glendinning, C., Jacobs, S., Manthorpe, J., Moran, N., Stevens, M. and Wilberforce, M. (2012) 'Personalisation Through Individual Budgets: Does it Work and for Whom?', *British Journal of Social Work*, 42(8): 1556–73.

Nevo, I. and Slonim-Nevo, V. (2011) 'The Myth of Evidence-Based Practice: Towards Evidence-Informed Practice', *British Journal of Social Work*, 41(6): 1176–97.

Newman, T., Moseley, A., Tierney, S. and Ellis, A. (2005) *Evidence-based Social Work: A Guide for the Perplexed* (Lyme Regis: Russell House).

NSPCC (2013) 'Statistics on Looked After Children'. Available at http://www.nspcc.org.uk/Inform/resourcesforprofessionals/lookedafterchildren/statistics_wda88009.html (accessed 22 August 2013).

Nutley, S., Powell, A. and Davies, H. (2013) 'What Counts as Good Evidence?'. Available at http://www.alliance4usefulevidence.org/assets/What-Counts-as-Good-Evidence-WEB.pdf (accessed 23 August 2013).

Nutley, S. M., Davies, H. T. O. and Smith, P. C. (2000) *What Works? Evidence-based Policy and Practice in Public Services* (Bristol: Policy Press).

Nuttall, C. (2003) 'The Home Office and Random Allocation Experiments', *Evalaution Review*, 27(3): 267–89.

Nybell, L. M., Snook, J. J. and Finn, J. L. (2009) *Childhood, Youth and Social Work in Transformation: Implications for Policy and Practice* (New York: Columbia University Press).

O'Hare, T. (2003) 'Evidence-Based Social Work Practice with Mentally Ill Persons Who Abuse Alcohol and Other Drugs', *Social Work in Mental Health*, 1(1): 43–62.

Oakley, A., Strange, V., Toroyan, T., Wiggins, M., Roberts, I. and Stephenson, J. (2003) 'Using Random Allocation to Evaluate Social Interventions: Three Recent U.K. Examples', *ANNALS of the American Academy of Political and Social Science*, 589(1): 170–89.

Office for National Statistics (2007) *Child and Adolescent Mental Health Statistics* (London: HMSO).

Office for Public Management (2007) *The Implications of Individual Budgets for Service Providers: Report from a Workshop held on 19th July 2007* (London: Department of Health and Office for Public Management).

Office for Standards in Education Children's Services and Skills (2009) *Keeping in Touch. A Report of Children's Experience by the Children's Rights Director for England* (London: OFSTED).

Office of the Deputy Prime Minister (2004) *Mental Health and Social Exclusion: Social Exclusion Unit Report* (London: Office of the Deputy Prime Minister).

Office of the Public Guardian (2007) *Mental Capacity Act 2005 Code of Practice* (London: Department of Constitutional Affairs).

Oliver, M. (1983) *Social Work with Disabled People* (Basingstoke: Macmillan).

Oliver, M. (1990) *The Politics of Disablement* (Basingstoke: Macmillan).

Oliver, M. (1992) 'Changing the Social Relations of Research Production?', *Disability, Handicap & Society*, 7(2): 101–14.

Oliver, M. (2004) 'The Social Model in Action: If I Had a Hammer', in Barnes, C. and Mercer, G. (eds), *Implementing the Social Model of Disability: Theory and Research.* (Leeds: Disability Press): 18–31.

Orford, J. (2008) 'Asking the Right Questions in the Right Way: The Need for a Shift in Research on Psychological Treatments for Addiction', *Addiction*, 103(6): 875–85.

Orford, J., Templeton, L., Patel, A., Copello, A. and Velleman, R. (2007) 'The 5-Step Family Intervention in Primary Care: I. Strengths and Limitations According to Family Members', *Drugs: Education, Prevention and Policy*, 14(1): 29–47.

Orme, J. and Powell, J. (2008) 'Building Research Capacity in Social Work: Process and Issues', *British Journal of Social Work*, 38(5): 988–1008.

Palmer, J. and Smith, D. (2010) 'Promoting Human Dignity: An Evaluation of a Programme for Racially Motivated Offenders', *Probation Journal*, 57(4): 368–82.

Pardeck, T. (1988) 'Social treatment through an ecological approach', *Journal of Clinical Social Work*, 16(1): 92–104.

Parker, J. and Bradley, G. (2010) *Social Work Practice: Assessment, Planning, Intervention and Review* (Exeter: Learning Matters).

Parker, J. and van Teijlingen, E. (2012) 'The Research Excellence Framework (REF): Assessing the Impact of Social Work Research on Society', *Practice*, 24(1): 41–52.

Parkinson, G. (1970) 'I Give Them Money', *New Society*, February, 220–1.

Parrott, L., Jacobs, G. and Roberts, D. (2008) *Stress and Resilience Factors in Parents with Mental Health Problems and their Children. SCIE Research Briefing 23* (London: Social Care Institute for Excellence).

Parton, N. (2008) 'Changes in the Form of Knowledge in Social Work: From the "Social" to the "Informational"', *British Journal of Social Work*, 38(2): 253–69.

Parton, N. and O'Byrne, P. (2000) *Constructive Social Work: Towards a New Practice* (London: Macmillan).

Pawson, R. (2006) *Evidence-Based Policy: A Realist Perspective* (London: Sage).

Pawson, R., Boaz, A., Grayson, L., Long, A. and Barnes, C. (2003) *Types and Quality of Knowledge in Social Care. Knowledge Review 3* (London and Bristol: Social Care Institute for Excellence/Policy Press).

Pawson, R., Greenhalgh, T., Harvey, G. and Walshe, K. (2004) *Realist Synthesis: An Introduction. ESRC Research Methods Programme Methods Paper 2* (Manchester: University of Manchester).

Pawson, R. and Tilley, N. (1997) *Realistic Evaluation* (London: Sage).

Paylor, I., Measham, F. and Asher, H. (2012) *Social Work and Drug Use* (Maidenhead: Open University Press).

Payne, M. (2002) 'The Politics of Systems Theory within Social Work', *Journal of Social Work*, 2(3): 269–92.

Payne, M. (2014) *Modern Social Work Theory*, 4th edn (Basingstoke: Palgrave Macmillan).

Penn, H. and Gough, D. (2002) 'The Price of a Loaf of Bread: Some Conceptions of Family Support', *Children and Society*, 16(1): 17–32.

Petr, C. (ed.) (2009) *Multi-Dimensional Evidence-Based Practice: Synthesizing Knowledge, Research and Values* (New York: Routledge).

Philips, C. and Shaw, I. (2011) 'Innovation and the Practice of Social Work Research (Editorial for Special Edn)', *British Journal of Social Work*, 41(4): 609–24.

Pierson, J. (2011) *Understanding Social Work: History and Context* (Berkshire: Open University Press/McGraw Hill).

Pilling, S., Bebbington, P., Kuipers, E., Garety, P., Geddes, J., Orbach, G. and Morgan, C. (2002) 'Psychological Treatments in Schizophrenia: I. Meta-Analysis of Family Intervention and Cognitive Behaviour Therapy', *Psychological Medicine*, 32(5): 763–82.

Pincus, A. and Minahan, A. (1973) *Social Work Practice: Model and Method* (Illinois: F.E. Peacock).

Pithouse, A. (2006) 'A Common Assessment for Children in Need? Mixed Messages from a Pilot Study in Wales', *Child Care in Practice*, 12(3): 199–217.

Pithouse, A., Batchelor, C., Crowley, A., Webb, A. and Ward, H. (2004) *Developing a Multi-Agency Pre-Referral Common Assessment Approach to the Identification of Children in Need in the Community* (Cardiff: School of Social Sciences, Cardiff University).

Pithouse, A., Broadhurst, K., Hall, C., Peckover, S., Wastell, D. and White, S. (2012) 'Trust, Risk and the (Mis)management of Contingency and Discretion Through New Information Technologies in Children's Services', *Journal of Social Work*, 12(2): 158–78.

Pithouse, A., Hall, C., Peckover, S. and White, S. (2009) 'A Tale of Two CAFs: The Impact of the Electronic Common Assessment Framework', *British Journal of Social Work*, 39(4): 599–612.

Plath, D. (2013) 'Organizational Processes Supporting Evidence-Based Practice', *Administration in Social Work*, 37(2): 171–88.

Polanyi, M. (1958) *Personal Knowledge: Toward a Post-Critical Philosphy* (London: Routledge).

Polkinghorne, D. E. (2004) *Practice and the Human Sciences: The Case for a Judgment-Based Practice of Care* (Albany: State University of New York Press).

Pope, N. D., Rollins, L., Chaumba, J. and Risler, E. (2011) 'Evidence-Based Practice Knowledge and Utilization Among Social Workers', *Journal of Evidence-Based Social Work*, 8(4): 349–68.

Popper, K. (1944) 'The Poverty of Historicism, II. A Criticism of Historicist Methods', *Economica, New Series*, 11(43): 119–37.

Popper, K. (2002) *The Logic of Scientific Discovery* (London: Routledge Classics Press).

Porporino, F. J. (2010) 'Bringing Sense and Sensitivity to Corrections: From Programmes to "Fix" Offenders to Services to Support Desistance', in Brayford, J., Cowe, F. and Deering, J. (eds), *What Else Works? Creative Work with Offenders* (Cullompton: Willan): 61–85.

Powell, J. and Lovelock, R. (1992) *Changing Patterns of Mental Health Care* (London: Avebury).

Quinton, D. (2004) *Supporting Parents: Messages from Research* (London: Jessica Kingsley).

Quinton, D. and Rutter, M. (1988) *Parenting Breakdown: The Making and Breaking of Intergenerational Links* (Aldershot: Avebury).

Quirk, A., Lelliott, P. and Seale, C. (2006) 'The Permeable Institution: An Ethnographic Study of Three Acute Psychiatric Wards in London', *Social Science & Medicine*, 63(8): 2105–17.

Raistrick, D., Heather, N. and Godfrey, C. (2006) *Review of the Effectiveness of Treatment for Alcohol Problems* (London: National Treatment Agency for Substance Misuse).

Rapp, C. (1998) *The Strengths Model: Case Management with People Suffering from Severe and Persistent Mental Illness* (New York: Oxford University Press).

Ray, L., Smith, D. and Wastell, L. (2003) 'Understanding Racist Violence', in Stanko, E. A. (ed.), *The Meanings of Violence* (London and New York: Routledge): 112–29.

Ray, L., Smith, D. and Wastell, L. (2004) 'Shame, Rage and Racist Violence', *British Journal of Criminology*, 44(3): 350–68.

Raynor, P. (1988) *Probation as an Alternative to Custody* (Aldershot: Avebury).

Raynor, P. (2004) 'The Probation Service "Pathfinders": Finding the Path and Losing the Way?', *Criminology and Criminal Justice*, 4(3): 309–25.

Raynor, P., Ugwudike, P. and Vanstone, M. (2010) 'Skills and Strategies in Probation Supervision: The Jersey Study', in Mcneill, F., Raynor, P. and Trotter, C. (eds), *Offender Supervision: New Directions in Theory, Research and Practice*. (Cullompton: Willan): 113–29.

Redmond, B. (2005) 'Homelessness and Mental Health', in Quin, S. and Redmond, B. (eds), *Mental Health and Social Policy in Ireland* (Dublin: University College Dublin): 158–75.

Rees, R. (2001) *Poverty and Public Health 1815–1949* (Oxford: Heinemann).

Research in Practice for Adults (2013) 'Critical Appraisal Skills: Why Should we Critically Appraise?'. Available at http://www.ripfa.org.uk/onetoone/projectoutputs/doc_details/323-06-ld-health-facilitation-and-learning-disability?tmpl=component (accessed 15 August 2013).

Rethink (2008) *Briefing – Physical Health and Mental Health* (London: Rethink).

Richards, S., Sullivan, M. P., Tanner, D., Beech, C., Milne, A., Ray, M., Phillips, J. and Lloyd, L. (2013) 'On the Edge of a New Frontier: Is Gerontological Social Work in the UK Ready to Meet Twenty-First-Century Challenges?', *British Journal of Social Work*, Advance Access, doi:10.1093/bjsw/bct082

Richmond, M. E. (1917) *Social Diagnosis* (New York: Russell Sage Foundation).

Robbins, D. (1998) 'The Refocusing Children's Initiative: An Overview of Practice', in Bayley, R. (ed.), *Transforming Children's Lives: The Importance of Early Intervention*. (London: Family Policy Studies Centre): 86–90.

Roberts, C. (1989) *Hereford and Worcester Probation Service Young Offender Project: First Evaluation Report* (Oxford: Department of Social and Administrative Studies, University of Oxford).

Robinson, L. (2013) 'Racism and Mental Health', in Walker, S. (ed.), *Modern Mental Health Critical Perspectives on Psychiatric Practice* (St. Albans: Critical Publishing).

Robinson, S. and Harris, H. (2011) *Smoking and Drinking Among Adults, 2009. A Report on the 2009 General Lifestyle Survey* (London: Office for National Statistics).

Rose, N. (2005) 'In Search of Certainty: Risk Management in a Biological Age', *Journal of Public Health*, 4(3): 14–22.

Rosenhan, D. L. (1973) 'On Being Sane in Insane Places', *Science*, 179: 250–8.

Roulstone, A. (2012) '"Stuck In The Middle With You": Towards Enabling Social Work with Disabled People', *Social Work Education*, 31(2): 142–54.

Roulstone, A. and Morgan, H. (2009) 'Neo-Liberal Individualism or Self-Directed Support: Are We All Speaking the Same Language on Modernising Adult Social Care?', *Social Policy and Society*, 8: 333–45.

Rowntree, B. S. (1901) *Poverty. A Study of Town Life* (London: Macmillan).

Ruch, G. (2012) 'Where Have All the Feelings Gone? Developing Reflective and Relationship-Based Management in Child-Care Social Work', *British Journal of Social Work*, 42(7): 1315–32.

Ruch, G., Turney, D. and Ward, A. (2010) *Relationship-Based Social Work: Getting to the Heart of Practice* (London: Jessica Kingsley).

Rushton, A. and Dance, C. (2003) 'Preferentially Rejected Children and their Development in Permanent Family Placements', *Child & Family Social Work*, 8(4): 257–67.

Rushton, A., Dance, C., Quinton, D. and Mayes, D. (2001) *Siblings in Late Permanent Placements* (London: British Association for Adoption and Fostering).

Rushton, A. and Minnis, H. (2008) 'Residential and Foster Family Care', in Rutter, M., Bishop, A., Pine, D., Scott, D., Stevenson, J., Taylor, E. and Thapar, A. (eds), *Child and Adolescent Psychiatry* 5th edn (Oxford: Blackwell): 487–501.

Rutter, D. and Fisher, M. (2013) *Knowledge Transfer in Social Care and Social Work: Where is the Problem? PSSRU Discussion Paper 2866* (London, Personal Social Services Research Unit/Social Care Institute for Excellence).

Rutter, D., Francis, J., Coren, E. and Fisher, M. (2010) *SCIE Systematic Research Reviews: Guidelines*, 2nd edn (London: Social Care Institute for Excellence).

Rutter, M. (1981) *Maternal Deprivation Reassessed*, 2nd edn (Harmondsworth: Penguin).

Rutter, M. (1995) *Psychosocial Disturbances in Young People: Challenges for Prevention* (Cambridge: Cambridge University Press).

Rutter, M. (2007) 'Sure Start Local Programmes: An Outsider's Perspective', in Belsky, J., Barnes, J. and Melhuish, E. (eds), *The National Evaluation of Sure Start Does Area-Based Early Intervention Work?* (Bristol: Policy Press): 197–210.

Rutter, M. and Smith, D. (1995) *Psychosocial Disorders in Young People* (London: Wiley).

Ryan, T. (2000) 'Exploring the Risk Management Strategies of Mental Health Service Users', *Health, Risk & Society*, 2(3): 267–82.

Sackett, D. L., Rosenberg, W. M. C., Gray, J. A. M., Haynes, R. B. and Richardson, W. S. (1996) 'Evidence Based Medicine: What It Ss and What It Isn't', *British Medical Journal*, 312(7023): 71–2.

Sadlier, G. (2010) *Evaluation of the Impact of the HM Prison Service Enhanced Thinking Skills Programme on Reoffending Outomces of the Surveying Prisoner Crime Reduction (SPCR) Sample (Ministry of Justice Research Series 19/10)* (London: Ministry of Justice).

Saini, M. and Shlonsky, A. (2012) *Systematic Synthesis of Qualitative Research* (New York: Oxford University Press).

Sainsbury Centre for Mental Health (2002) *Breaking the Circles of Fear* (London: Sainsbury Centre for Mental Health).

Sainsbury Centre for Mental Health (2009) *Commissioning What Works: The Economic and Financial Case for Supported Employment* (London: Sainsbury Centre for Mental Health).

Saleeby, D. (2005) *The Strengths Perspective in Social Work Practice* (Boston: Allyn & Bacon).

Samsi, K., Abley, C., Campbell, S., Keady, J., Manthorpe, J., Robinson, L., Watts, S. and Bond, J. (2014) 'Negotiating a Labyrinth: Experiences of Assessment and Diagnostic Journey in Cognitive Impairment and Dementia', *International Journal of Geriatric Psychiatry*, 29(1): 58–67.

Sapey, B. (2004) 'Practice for What? The Use of Evidence in Social Work with Disabled People', in Smith, D. (ed.), *Evidence-Based Practice and Social Work* (London: Jessica Kingsley).

Sapey, B. J. and Pearson, J. (2004) 'Do Disabled People Need Social Workers?', *Social Work and Social Sciences Review*, 11(3): 52–70.

Schaffer, H. and Rudolph, R. (1990) *Making Decisions About Children. Psychological Questions and Answers* (Oxford: Blackwell).

Schofield, G. and Beek, M. (2005) 'Providing a Secure Base: Parenting Children in Long-Term Foster Family Care', *Attachment & Human Development*, 7(1): 3–25.

Schon, D. (1987) *Educating the Reflective Practitioner* (San Francisco: Jossey-Bass).

Scottish Social Services Council (2009) *Scottish Social Services Council Codes of Practice for Social Service Workers and Employers* (Dundee: Scottish Social Services Council).

Scourfield, J. (2003) *Gender and Child Protection* (Basingstoke: Palgrave Macmillan).

Scourfield, J., Tolman, R., Maxwell, N., Holland, S., Bullock, A. and Sloan, L. (2012) 'Results of a Training Course for Social Workers on Engaging Fathers in Child Protection', *Children and Youth Services Review*, 34(8): 1425–32.

Selwyn, J. (2010) 'The Challenges in Planning for Permanency', *Adoption and Fostering*, 34(3): 32–7.

Selwyn, J., Sturgess, W., Quinton, D. and Baxter, C. (2006) *Cost and Outcomes of Non-infant Adoptions* (London: British Association for Adoption and Fostering).

Sen, R. and Broadhurst, K. (2011) 'Contact Between Children in Out-of-Home Placements and Their Family and Friends Networks: A Research Review', *Child and Family Social Work*, 16: 298–309.

Shakespeare, T. (1996) 'Rules of Engagement: Doing Disability Research', *Disability & Society*, 11(1): 115–21.

Shaw, I. (1999) *Qualitative Evaluation* (London: Sage).

Shaw, I. (2011) *Evaluating in Practice*, 2nd edn (Aldershot: Ashgate).

Shaw, I. (2012a) 'The Positive Contributions of Quantitative Methodology to Social Work Research: A View From the Sidelines', *Research on Social Work Practice*, 22(2): 129–34.

Shaw, I. (2012b) *Practice and Research* (Farnham: Ashgate).

Shaw, I., Briar-Lawson, K., Orme, J. and Ruckdeschel, R. (2010a) 'Editorial Essay. Mapping Social Work Research: Pasts, Presents and Futures', in Shaw, I., Briar-Lawson, K., Orme, J. and Ruckdeschel, R. (eds), *The Sage Handbook of Social Work Research*. (London: Sage): 1–20.

Shaw, I., Briar-Lawson, K., Orme, J. and Ruckdeschel, R. (eds) (2010b) *The SAGE Handbook of Social Work Research* (London: Sage).

Shaw, I. and Gould, N. (2001) *Qualitative Social Work Research* (London: Sage Publications).

Shaw, M. (1974) *Social Work in Prison (Home Office Research Study 22)* (London, HMSO).

Sheldon, B. (2001) 'The Validity of Evidence-Based Practice in Social Work: A Reply to Stephen Webb', *British Journal of Social Work*, 31(5): 801–9.

Sheldon, B. and Chilvers, R. (2000) *Evidence-Based Social Care. A Study of Prospects and Problems* (Lyme Regis: Russell House Publishing).

Sheldon, B. and Chilvers, R. (2002) 'An Empirical Study of the Obstacles to Evidence-Based Practice', *Social Work and Social Sciences Review*, 10(1): 6–26.

Sheldon, B. and Macdonald, G. (1999) *Research and Practice in Social Care: Mind the Gap* (Exeter University: Centre for Evidence-Based Social Services).

Sheldon, B. and Macdonald, G. (2008) *A Textbook of Social Work* (London: Routledge).

Sheppard, M. (1995) 'Social Work, Social Science and Practice Wisdom', *British Journal of Social Work*, 25: 265–93.

Sheppard, M. (2006) *Social Work and Social Exclusion* (Aldershot: Ashgate).

Sheppard, M. (2007) 'Assessment: From Reflexivity to Process Knowledge', in Lishman, J. (ed.), *Handbook for Practice Learning in Social Work and Social Care*, 2nd edn (London: Jessica Kingsley Publishers).

Sheridan, M. (2000) 'Chart Illustrating the Developmental Progress of Infants and Young Children', in Department of Health (ed.), *Assessing Children in Need and Their Families: Practice Guidance*. (London: HMSO): 23–8.

Shlonsky, A. (2010) 'A Fine Balancing Act: Kinship Care, Subsidized Guardianship and Outcomes', in Kerman, B., Freundlich, M. and Maluccio, A. (eds), *Achieving Permanence for Older Children and Youth in Foster Care* (New York: Columbia University Press): 176–86.

Shlonsky, A., Webster, D. and Needell, B. (2003) 'The Ties That Bind: A Cross-Sectional Analysis of Siblings in Foster Care', *Journal of Social Service Research*, 29: 27–52.

Sidebotham, P., Brandon, M., Powell, C., Solebo, C., Koistenen, J. and Ellis, C. (2010) *Learning from Serious Case Reviews: Report of a Research Study on the Methods of Learning Lessons Nationally from Serious Case Reviews* (London: Department for Education).

Sinclair, I. (2005) *Fostering Now. Messages from Research* (London: Jessica Kingsley).

Sinclair, I., Baker, C., Lee, J. and Gibbs, I. (2007) *The Pursuit of Permanence. A Study of the English Care System* (London: Jessica Kingsley).

Sinclair, I., Baker, C., Wilson, K. and Gibbs, I. (2005a) *Foster Children: Where They Go and How They Get On* (London: Jessica Kingsley).

Sinclair, I., Wilson, K. and Gibbs, I. (2005b) *Foster Placements: Why They Succeed and Why They Fail* (London: Jessica Kingsley).

Sirey, J. A., Hannon, C. P., D'Angelo, D. and Knies, K. (2012) 'A Community Treatment Intervention Advancing Active Treatment in the Elderly (ACTIVATE): A Pilot Study', *Journal of Gerontological Social Work*, 55(5): 382–91.

Slack, K. and Webber, M. (2008) 'Do We Care? Adult Mental Health Professionals' Attitudes Towards Supporting Service Users' Children', *Child and Family Social Work*, 13: 72–9.

Smart, C. and Williams, B. (1973) *Utilitarianism For and Against* (Cambridge: Cambridge University Press).

Smith, C. and White, S. (1997) 'Parton, Howe and Postmodernity: A Critical Commentary on Mistaken Identity', *British Journal of Social Work*, 27(2): 275–95.

Smith, D. (2012) 'Arguments about Methods in Criminal Justice Evaluation', in Bowen, E. and Brown, S. (eds), *Perspectives on Evaluating Criminal Justice and Corrections*. (Bingley: Emerald): 49–69.

Social Care Institute for Excellence (2005) *Therapies and Approaches for Helping Children and Adolescents who Deliberately Self-Harm (DSH). SCIE Research Briefing 17* (London: Social Care Institute for Excellence).

Social Work Reform Board (2010) *Building a Safe and Confident Future: One Year On. Detailed Proposals from the Social Work Reform Board* (London: Department for Education).

Soydan, H. (1999) *The History of Ideas in Social Work* (Birmingham: Venture Press).

Spector, A., Thorgrimsen, L., Woods, B., Royan, L., Davies, S., Butterworth, M. and Orrell, M. (2003) 'Efficacy of an Evidence-Based Cognitive Stimulation Therapy Programme for People with Dementia: Randomised Controlled Trial', *British Journal of Psychiatry*, 183: 248–54.

Spencer, L., Ritchie, J., Lewis, J. and Dillon, L. (2003) *Quality in Qualitative Evaluation: A Framework for Assessing Research Evidence. A Quality Framework* (London: Cabinet Office).

Srivastava, O. P., Foundation, R., Ayre, P. and Stewart, J. (2003) 'The Graded Carer Profile: A Measure of Care', in Calder, M. C. and Hackett, S. (eds), *Assessment in Child Care Using and Developing Frameworks For Practice* (Lyme Regis: Russell House Publishing): 227–46.

Staller, K. (2013) 'Epistemological Boot Camp: The Politics of Science and What Every Qualitative Researcher Needs to Know to Survive in the Academy', *Qualitative Social Work: Research and Practice*, 12(4): 395–413.

Stanford, S. (2008) 'Taking a Stand or Playing it Safe: Revisiting the Moral Conservatism of Risk in Social Work Practice', *European Journal of Social Work*, 3: 209–20.

Stanley, N., Miller, P. and Richardson Foster, H. (2012) 'Engaging with Children's and Parents' Perspectives on Domestic Violence', *Child and Family Social Work*, 17(2): 192–201.

Stein, L. I. and Test, M. A. (1980) 'Alternative to Mental Hospital Treatment. I. Conceptual Model, Treatment Program, and Clinical Evaluation', *Archives of General Psychiatry*, 37: 392–7.

Stein, M. (2012) *Young People Leaving Care: Supporting Pathways to Adulthood* (London: Jessica Kingsley).

Stoesz, D. (2010) 'Second-Rate Research for Second Class Citizens', *Research on Social Work Practice*, 20: 329–32.

Stokes, J. and Schmidt, G. (2012) 'Child Protection Decision Making: A Factorial Analysis Using Case Vignettes', *Social Work*, 57(1): 83–90.

Straus, S. E. and McAlister, D. C. (2000) 'Evidence-based Medicine: A Commentary on Common Criticisms', *Canadian Medical Journal*, 163(7): 837–41.

Sullivan, J. (2010) 'Helping People Who Hear Voices and Have False Beliefs', in Grant, A. (ed.), *Cognitive Behavioural Interventions for Mental Health Practitioners* (Exeter: Learning Matters).

Swain, J., French, S., Barnes, C. and Thomas, C. (eds) (2014) *Disabling Barriers – Enabling Environments*, 3rd edn (London: Sage).

Swinkels, A., Albarran, J. W., Means, R. I., Mitchell, T. and Stewart, M. C. (2002) 'Evidence-Based Practice in Health and Social Care: Where Are We Now?', *Journal of Interprofessional Care*, 16(4): 335–47.

Taylor, B. (2013) *Professional Decision Making and Risk in Social Work* (London: Sage).

Tearse, M. (2010) 'Love Fostering – Need Pay. A UK-Wide Survey of Foster Carers about Fees'. Available at http://www.fostering.net/sites/www.fostering. net/files/public/resources/reports/love_fostering_need_pay_0310.pdf (accessed 22 August 2013).

Templeton, L., Zohhadi, S., Galvani, S. and Velleman, R. (2006) *'Looking Beyond Risk'. Parental Substance Misuse: Scoping Study* (Edinburgh: Scottish Executive).

Tew, J., Gould, N., Abankwa, D., Barnes, H., Beresford, P., Carr, S., Copperman, J., Ramon, S., Rose, D., Sweeney, A. and Louise, W. (2006) *Values and Methodologies for Social Research in Mental Health* (Bristol: Policy Press).

Tew, J., Ramon, S., Slade, M., Bird, V., Melton, J. and Le Boutillier, C. (2012) 'Social Factors and Recovery From Mental Health Difficulties: A Review of the Evidence', *British Journal of Social Work*, 42(3): 443–60.

Thomas, C. L., Man, M.-S., O'Cathain, A., Hollinghurst, S., Large, S., Edwards, L., Nicholl, J., Montgomery, A. A. and Salisbury, C. (2014) 'Effectiveness and Cost-Effectiveness of a Telehealth Intervention to Support the Management of Long-Term Conditions: Study Protocol for Two Linked Randomized Controlled Trials', *Trials*, 15(1): 36.

Thomas, N. (2009) 'Listening to Children and Young People', in Schofield, G. and Simmonds, J. (eds), *The Child Placement Handbook Research, Policy and Practice.* (London: British Association for Adoption and Fostering): 63–80.

Thyer, B. A. (ed.) (2010) *The Handbook of Social Work Research Methods*, 2nd edn (Thousand Oaks, CA: Sage).

Thyer, B. A. (2012) 'The Scientific Value of Qualitative Research for Social Work', *Qualitative Social Work*, 11(2): 115–25.

Thyer, B. A. and Pignotti, M. (2011) 'Evidence-Based *Practices* Do Not Exist', *Clinical Social Work Journal*, 39(4): 328–33.

TOPPS UK Partnership (2002) *The National Occupational Standards for Social Work* (Leeds: TOPPS).

Toseland, R. W. and Hacker, L. (1982) 'Self-Help Groups and Professional Involvement', *Social Work*, 27(4): 341–7.

Trappes-Lomax, T., Ellis, A., Fox, M., Taylor, R., Power, M., Stead, J. and Bainbridge, I. (2006) 'Buying Time I: A Prospective, Controlled Trial of a Joint Health/Social Care Residential

Rehabilitation Unit for Older People on Discharge from Hospital', *Health & Social Care in the Community*, 14(1): 49–62.

Travis, J. and Petersilia, J. (2001) 'Reentry Reconsidered: A New Look at an Old Question', *Crime and Delinquency*, 47(3): 291–313.

Triseliotis, J. (1983) 'Identity and Security in Adoption and Long-Term Fostering', *Adoption and Fostering*, 7: 22–31.

Tunnard, J. (2004) *Parental Mental Health Problems: Messages from Research, Policy and Practice* (Dartington: Research in Practice).

Turner, R. J., Lloyd, D. A. and Taylor, J. (2006) 'Physical Disability and Mental Health: An Epidemiology of Psychiatric and Substance Disorders', *Rehabilitation Psychology*, 51(3): 214–23.

UK Drugs Policy Commission (2010) *The Impact of Drugs on Different Minority Groups: Ethnicity and Drug Treatment* (London: UK Drugs Policy Commission).

UPIAS (1976) 'Fundamental Principles of Disability'. Available at http://disability-studies.leeds.ac.uk/files/library/UPIAS-fundamental-principles.pdf (accessed 4 April 2014).

Utting, D. (1995) *Family and Parenthood: Supporting Families, Preventing Breakdown* (York: Joseph Rowntree Foundation).

Van Ijzendoorn, M. H. and Juffer, F. (2006) 'The Emmanuel Miller Memorial Lecture 2006. Adoption as Intervention. Meta-Analytic Evidence for Massive Catch-up and Plasticity in Physical, Socio-Emotional, and Cognitive Development', *Journal of Child Psychology and Psychiatry*, 47: 1228–45.

Wadd, S., Lapworth, K., Sullivan, M., Forrester, D. and Galvani, S. (2011) *Working with Older Drinkers* (Luton: University of Bedfordshire).

Wade, J., Biehal, N., Farrelly, N. and Sinclair, I. (2011) *Caring for Abused and Neglected Children: Making the Right Decisions for Reunification or Long-term Care* (London: Jessica Kingsley).

Walker, S. (2001) 'Family Support and Social Work Practice: Opportunities for Child Mental Health Work', *Social Work and Social Sciences Review*, 9(2): 25–40.

Walker, S. (2003) *Social Work and Child and Adolescent Mental Health* (Lyme Regis: Russell House Publishers).

Walker, S. (2011) *The Social Workers Guide to Child and Adolescent Mental Health* (London: Jessica Kingsley).

Walker, S. (2012) 'Family Support Services', in Gray, M., Midgeley, J. and Webb, S. (eds), *The Sage Handbook of Social Work* (London: Sage): 613–26.

Ward, H., Brown, R. and Westlake, D. (2012) *Safeguarding Babies and Very Young Children* (London: Jessica Kingsley).

Ward, H. and Peel, M. (2003) *Evaluation of the Introduction of Inter-Agency Referral Documentation (Children in Need and Need of Protection Assessment and Consent Form)* (Loughborough: Children's Research Centre, Loughborough University).

Wardle, I. (2009) *Recovery and the UK Drug Treatment System: Key Dimensions of Change* (Manchester: Lifeline Project Limited).

Warner, J. and Sharland, E. (2010) 'Editorial for Special Issue on Risk and Social Work', *British Journal of Social Work*, 40(4): 1035–45.

Warner, R. (2010) *Recovery from Schizophrenia: Psychiatry and Political Economy* (Hove: Routledge).

Warr, P. and Jackson, P. (1985) 'Factors Influencing the Psychological Impact of Prolonged Unemployment and of Re-employment', *Psychological Medicine*, 15(4): 795–807.

Webb, S. A. (2001) 'Some Considerations on the Validity of Evidence-Based Practice in Social Work', *British Journal of Social Work*, 31(1): 57–79.

Webb, S. A. (2006) *Social Work in a Risk Society* (Basingstoke: Palgrave Macmillan).

Webber, M. (2011) *Evidence-Based Policy and Practice in Mental Health Social Work*, 2nd edn (Exeter: Learning Matters).

Webber, M. (2012) 'Developing Advanced Practitioners in Mental Health Social Work: Pedagogical Considerations', *Social Work Education*, 32(7): 944–55.

Webber, M. (2014) 'From Ethnography to Randomized Controlled Trial: An Innovative Approach to Developing Complex Social Interventions', *Journal of Evidence-Based Social Work*, 11 (1/2): 173–82.

Webber, M., Currin, L., Groves, N., Hay, D. and Fernando, N. (2009) 'Social Workers Can e-Learn: Evaluation of a Pilot Post-Qualifying e-Learning Course in Research Methods and Critical Appraisal Skills for Social Workers', *Social Work Education*, 29(1): 48–66.

Webber, M. and Currin Salter, L. (2011) 'Gearing Practitioners up for Research: Evaluation of a Pilot Online Research Training Course for Social Workers', *Research, Policy and Planning*, 28(3): 185–97.

Webber, M., Morris, D., Newlin, M., Howarth, S., Treacy, S. and McCrone, P. (under review) 'Effect of the Connecting People Intervention on Access to Social Capital: A Pilot Study', *Research on Social Work Practice*.

Webber, M. and Nathan, J. (eds) (2010) *Reflective Practice in Mental Health: Advanced Psychosocial Practice with Children, Adolescents and Adults* (London: Jessica Kingsley).

Webber, M., Reidy, H., Ansari, D., Stevens, M. and Morris, D. (under review) 'Developing and Modelling Complex Social Interventions: Introducing the Connecting People Intervention', *Research on Social Work Practice*.

Webber, M., Reidy, H., Ansari, D., Stevens, M. and Morris, D. (in press) 'Enhancing Social Networks: A Qualitative Study of Health and Social Care Practice in UK Mental Health Services', *Health & Social Care in the Community*.

Weinberg, M. (2010) 'The Social Construction of Social Work Ethics: Politicizing and Broadening the Lens', *Journal of Progressive Human Services*, 21(1): 32–44.

Wells, P. (2007) 'New Labour and Evidence Based Policy Making: 1997–2007', *People, Place and Policy Online*, 1(1): 22–9.

Welsh Assembly Government (2008) *Consultation on Stronger Families Through a New Approach to Integrated Family Support* (Cardiff: Welsh Assembly Government).

White, S., Hall, C. and Peckover, S. (2009) 'The Descriptive Tyranny of the Common Assessment Framework: Technologies of Categorization and Professional Practice in Child Welfare', *British Journal of Social Work*, 39(7): 1197–217.

White, W. L. (2009) 'The Mobilization of Community Resources to Support Long-Term Addiction Recovery', *Journal of Substance Abuse Treatment*, 36(2): 146–58.

Williams, V., Porter, S. and Marriott, A. (2013) 'Your Life, Your Choice: Support Planning Led by Disabled People's Organisations', *British Journal of Social Work*, doi:10.1093/bjsw/bct005

Williams, B. (1993) *Ethics and the Limits of Philosophy* (London: Fontana).

Wilson, K., Ruch, G., Lymbery, M. and Cooper, A. (2008) *Social Work: An Introduction to Contemporary Practice* (Harlow: Pearson).

Wilson, K., Sinclair, I., Taylor, C., A., P. and Sellick, C. (2004) *Fostering Success. An Exploration of the Research Literature in Foster Care. Knowledge Review 5* (London: Social Care Institute for Excellence).

Winnicott, D. (1965) *The Maturational Process and the Facilitating Environment* (London: Hogarth).

Winokur, M., Holtan, A. and Batchelder, K. (2014) 'Kinship Care for the Safety, Permanency, and Well-Being of Children Removed from the Home for Maltreatment: A Systematic Review', *Campbell Systematic Reviews*, 10(2).

Wolpert, M., Fuggle, P., Cottrell, D., Fonagy, P., Phillips, J., Pilling, S., Stein, S. and Target, M. (2006) *Drawing on the Evidence. Advice for Mental Health Professionals Working with Children and Adolescents,*, 2nd edn (London: CAMHS Evidence Based Practice Unit).

Wong, Y. and Vinsky, J. (2009) 'Speaking From the Margins: A Critical Reflection on the "Spiritual but not Religious" Discourse in Social Work', *British Journal of Social Work*, 39(7): 1343–59.

World Health Organization (2010) *Mental Health* (Geneva: WHO).

Young, A. F. and Ashton, E.T (1956) *British Social Work in the Nineteenth Century* (London: Routledge & Kegan Paul).

Young Minds (2010) *Briefing on Section 131A of the Mental Health Act 1983* (London: Young Minds).

Zarb, G. and Nadash, P. (1994) *Cashing in on Independence: Comparing the Costs and Benefits of Cash and Services* (London: BCODP).

Index